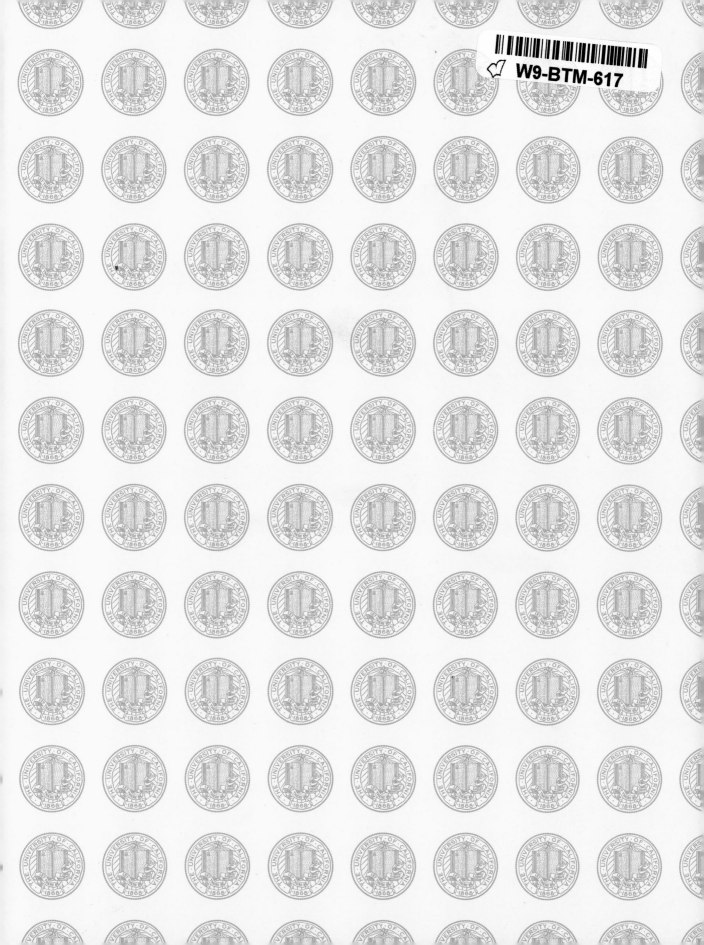

the wellness
kitchen

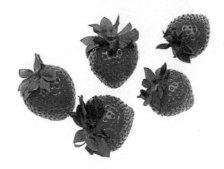

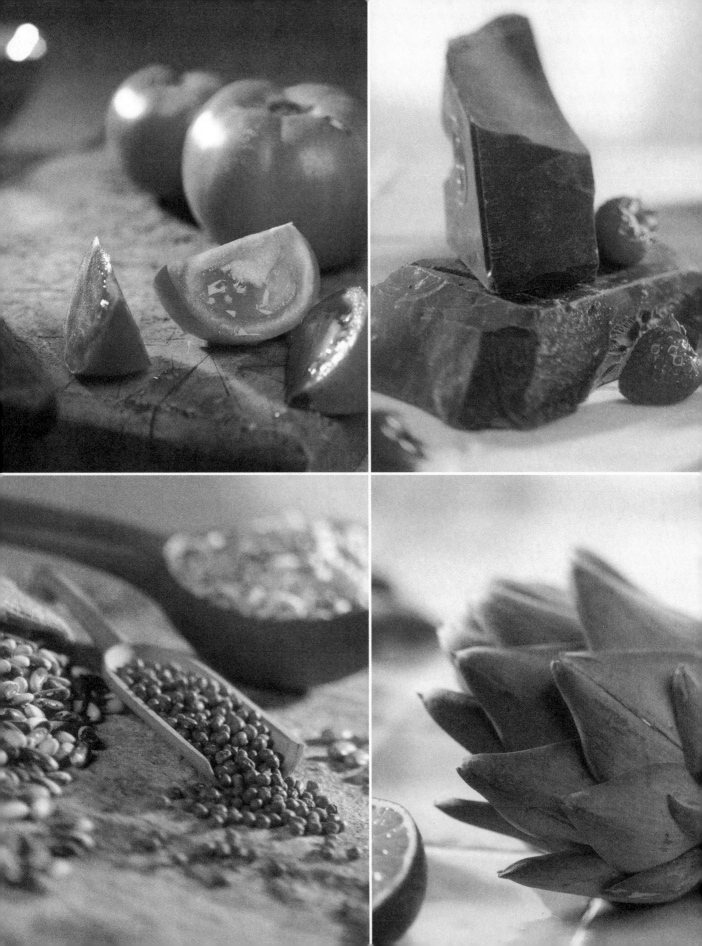

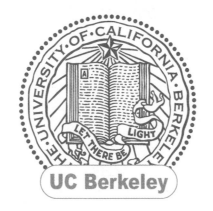

UC Berkeley

the wellness kitchen

Bringing the latest nutrition information
to your table

by the staff of The Wellness Kitchen *and the editors of the*
UC Berkeley Wellness Letter

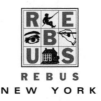

REBUS
NEW YORK

THE UNIVERSITY OF CALIFORNIA, BERKELEY WELLNESS LETTER

www.WellnessLetter.com

The Wellness Letter is a monthly eight-page newsletter that draws on the expertise of the world-famous School of Public Health at the University of California, Berkeley to cover health, nutrition, and exercise topics in language that is clear, engaging, and nontechnical. It's a unique resource that tells you about fundamental ways to prevent illness. *The Wellness Letter* has been rated #1 among all health newsletters by *U.S. News & World Report*.

To view sample articles from the current issue and see information on our other publications, visit us online at **www.WellnessLetter.com**.

You can also order a trial subscription of this award-winning newsletter by calling 386-447-6328 or by writing to Wellness Letter, P.O. Box 420148, Palm Coast, FL 32142.

This book was created and produced by Rebus, Inc.
New York, NY 10012

COVER PHOTOGRAPH: **Alan Richardson**
INTERIOR PHOTOGRAPHS: **Lisa Koenig**

For information about permission to reproduce selections from this book, write to Permissions, Health Letter Associates, 632 Broadway, New York, NY 10012

Library of Congress Cataloging-in-Publication Data

The wellness kitchen : bringing the latest nutrition information to your table / by the staff of the Wellness Kitchen and the editors of the UC Berkeley Wellness Letter.
    p. cm.
Includes index.
ISBN 0-929661-80-X
  1. Nutrition—Popular works. 2. Health—Popular works. 3. Cookery—Popular works. I. University of California, Berkeley, wellness letter.

RA784.W447 2003
614.5'63—dc21   20030041415

Printed in the United States of America
10 9 8 7 6 5 4 3 2 1

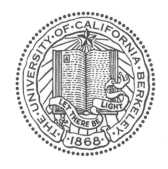

contents

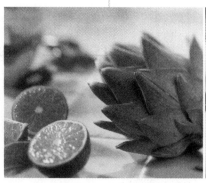 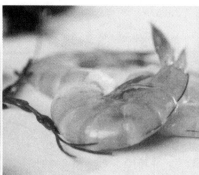 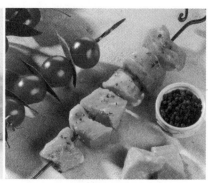

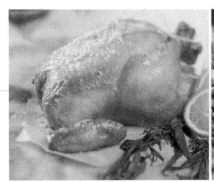

**poultry
102**

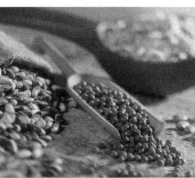

**meatless main
dishes 138**

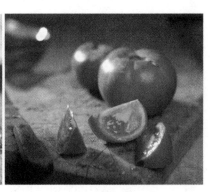

**side dishes
162**

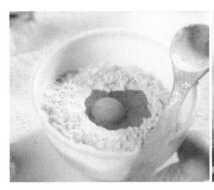

**breads &
muffins 208**

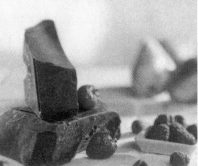

**desserts
224**

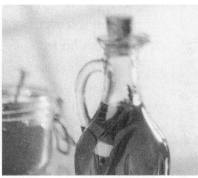

**the pantry
250**

how to use this

In recent years, Americans have become more and more familiar with the role that nutrition plays in disease prevention—about dietary fat and dietary fiber; carbohydrates and protein; about vitamins and minerals; and about certain plant compounds called phytochemicals. Unfortunately, there has been a tendency to concentrate on these nutrients in their supplement form, instead of in foods themselves. Singling out an individual nutrient ignores the likelihood that any health benefit is the result of all the nutrients in a food working in concert. So, eating a variety of whole foods—and learning how to cook with them—is an important step toward health and well-being.

the recipes

In *The Wellness Kitchen* we have created recipes using a variety of whole foods, with an emphasis on fruits, vegetables, grains, and fish (although meat, poultry, and dairy are here, too, as they bring important nutrients to the diet). We hope to teach, by creative example, basic cooking methods as well as tricks for maximizing the nutrition in recipes. We have limited the cooking methods used to those that we consider the most healthful. For example, we have included no information on deep-frying (for obvious reasons); and with just a couple of exceptions we provide no information on boiling vegetables, since we think that there are other more healthful methods.

The book is divided into chapters that follow a typical cookbook format. The opening chapter, Starters & Nibbles, deals with dishes that either begin a multi-course meal (such as appetizers and soups) or that can be eaten as a snack any time of day. The next four chapters—Fish & Shellfish, Meat, Poultry, and Meatless—are all for entrees, followed by a chapter of Side Dishes (including grains, vegetables, and salads). Next up are Breads & Muffins, and finally Desserts. There is also a special chapter called The Pantry, with recipes for sauces, salsas, chutneys, and more.

the nutritional analyses

Each recipe in the book is accompanied by a nutritional analysis, including values for calories, total fat (including grams of saturated fat), cholesterol, dietary fiber, carbohydrates, protein, and sodium. If you are trying to keep track of specific nutrients in your diet, the most important thing to understand is that you should be evaluating your intake not for an individual dish in a meal, and not even for the meal itself, but for a day's intake—and, ideally, for a week's intake.

good source of

Following the main nutritional analysis for each recipe is a section called "good source of," which includes an alphabetical listing of vitamins, minerals, and other healthful compounds. To qualify as a "good source of" a nutrient, the recipe must provide a certain percent-

book

age of the recommended daily intake for that nutrient. (For nutrients that have different values for different age groups, the calculation uses the highest value—see the chart on page 308.) In the case of a main-course dish, it must provide at least 25% of the recommended intake. First courses, side dishes, breads, and desserts must provide at least 10%. If the dish also happens to be on the high side for calories (for example, over 250 calories for a dessert), then we expect it to pull its weight and provide at least 20% of the recommended intake for a nutrient.

"recipe creators"

Sprinkled throughout the recipe chapters you will find our "Recipe Creators." These are charts that allow you to choose your own combination of flavors and ingredients in a dish. For example, for Sweet Smoothies (*"Recipe Creator," page 19*), you are asked to choose 1 fruit + 1 liquid + 1 flavoring + 1 spice. Your smoothie might be Banana-Maple, or Strawberry-Soy, or Ginger-Cantaloupe. If you tried every single possibility presented in this chart, you could have 225 unique smoothie recipes.

foods A to Z

In this A-to-Z compendium, you will find nutrition profiles of foods from acorn squash to zucchini. The nutrients that are highlighted as important for

each food are those that provide 10% or more of the recommended daily intake in a single portion. The portion sizes used are amounts that an average person would consume at one sitting. For meat, poultry, and fish, the portion size has been standardized at 3 ounces cooked. For vegetables, it tends to be 1 cup cooked or 2 cups uncooked (salad greens, for example). Fruit portions are generally either 1 cup of cut-up fruit or individual whole fruits. Portions of high-fat foods, such as nuts and cheese, are 1 ounce.

Following each nutrition profile are some tips for maximizing the nutrients in the food. For example, to enhance the bioavailability of the beta carotene in carrots, you should cook them with a small amount of healthful oil.

recommended daily intakes

The baseline values that help us determine when a food or a recipe conains nutrients in significant quantity are derived from the Recommended Dietary Allowances (RDAs) for adults. Where the RDA has not been established for a nutrient, a value called Adequate Intake (AI) is used. The RDAs and AIs were reviewed and updated between 1997 and 2002, and the values in this book reflect those updates. A chart of the current RDAs and AIs can be found on page 308.

the right choices for the wellness kitchen

Whoever said that nothing is simple must have been thinking about dietary advice. Turn on the television, read the newspaper, or go to a dinner party, and you're likely to encounter one debate or another about some aspect of healthy eating. In recent years, the debate at center stage has involved carbohydrates and fats—macronutrients that, along with protein, provide energy and help to maintain and repair the body. One side of this debate says that "carbs"—which come mainly from plant-based foods—are what you're supposed to fill up on when you cut down on fat. Another side claims that carbohydrates are what have made Americans so overweight, and that they should be replaced largely by high-protein foods.

Likewise, we've been told often enough that "low-fat" is the key to a healthy diet—meaning that fat should provide less than 30 percent of your total calories. But how can you make such a calculation? Unless you have a dietician in residence, it's impossible to figure out what your total calorie intake is, let alone what percentage of those calories comes from fat. And you've undoubtedly heard some experts say that oils such as olive and canola are heart-protective, since they are rich in monounsaturated fats. In fact, the American Heart Association (AHA), the most influential backer of low-fat eating, has fine-tuned its advice on fats to allow for more monounsaturated fat—at least under some circumstances—because of its potential health ben-

efits. Does this mean you should eat more of these oils?

Clearly, even nutrition experts don't agree about the benefits of the standard low-fat, high-carbohydrate diet. There is some evidence that, in some people, this kind of diet over the long term promotes high blood sugar levels and high triglycerides (fats in the blood) and lowers HDL ("good") cholesterol. Thus, some nutritionists recommend eating more monounsaturated oils, not more carbohydrates. They cite the example of Italy, where the typical diet is rich in monounsaturated fats (mostly from olive oil) and heart disease rates are low. Yet other researchers insist that consuming too much of any fat is bad, since fats are high in calories and thus promote obesity. Some actually recommend a very-low-fat diet, with less than 15 percent of calories derived from fat.

the good-carb, good-fat diet

Developing healthy eating habits isn't as confusing or restrictive as many people imagine. The first principle of a healthy diet is simply to eat a wide variety of foods—and that is also the first principle behind the recipes in *The Wellness Kitchen*. The second principle is that, for most people, it's best to stick to a diet that is relatively low in fat and rich in carbohydrates—but with certain qualifications. Actually, it doesn't help to

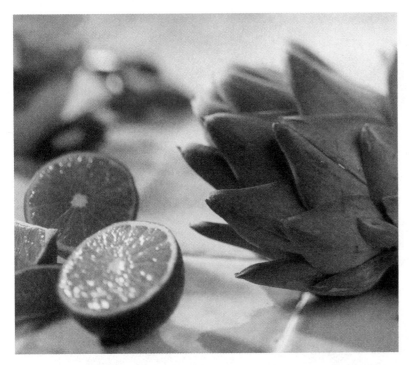

by fruits, whole grains, legumes, and vegetables (so-called "complex" carbohydrates), not by sugary, highly processed foods.

Whole grains (such as oats, whole wheat, brown rice) are more nutritious than refined grains, since they retain the bran and the germ, which are rich in vitamins, minerals, fiber, and beneficial phytochemicals. Whole grains are digested more slowly, and thus have a more modest effect on blood sugar than refined carbs or sugars. The same is true of vegetables and beans. The fiber in these foods has many health benefits. In particular, soluble fiber (found in oats, barley, and beans) may help lower LDL ("bad") cholesterol, triglycerides, and blood pressure. People whose diet is rich in whole grains and other high-fiber foods tend to have a lower risk of heart disease, diabetes, high blood pressure, and some cancers.

talk about "fats" and "carbohydrates"—the terms are confusing. There are good fats and bad fats, and not-so-good carbohydrates. Moreover, nearly all foods are combinations of various fats, carbohydrates, and protein.

Here is what these distinctions mean for you, in terms of the specific components of a healthy diet.

Make fruits, vegetables, and whole grains the basis of your diet. The bulk of your calories should come from carbohydrates—but mainly the carbohydrates provided

Limit your intake of sugary foods and refined-grain products. Many foods high in sugar (especially sucrose and other added sugars, notably fructose) supply "empty calories"—that

---

carbohydrates & obesity

Carbohydrates (especially, but not only, sugars) have come under attack for being the leading cause of obesity. The fact of the matter is that weight gain is caused by eating more calories than you burn—it's that simple. It doesn't matter where those calories come from, as far as weight is concerned. (Many overweight people get into trouble by satisfying their "sweet tooth" with foods—such as candy, ice cream, and cakes—that also contain excessive amounts of fat.)

Furthermore, there is no evidence that eating carbohydrates stimulates appetite or leads to more or easier fat storage and weight gain, as some carbohydrate-bashers claim. (Exercise also plays an important role in weight control, and a combination of exercise and diet is the best strategy for permanent weight loss.)

The recipes in *The Wellness Kitchen* tend to be carbohydrate-rich dishes that are also relatively low in fat—*and* low in calories.

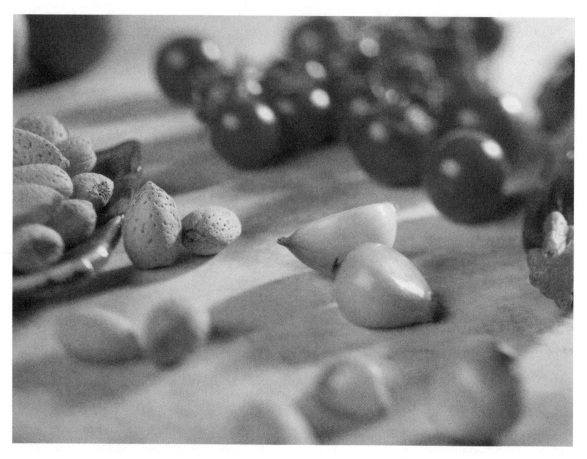

is, they have few nutrients but lots of calories. Many sugary foods are also high in fat. Refined grains such as plain pasta and bread, by themselves, are not high in calories, but what's typically put on top of them (meat or cream sauces, butter, cheese) can double or triple the calories.

By contrast, the calories in foods rich in complex carbs usually bring many nutritional extras with them. It depends on the food, though. Dairy products and fruit, for example, contain sugars, but are important parts of a healthy diet because of the other nutrients they contain.

Be careful not only about how much fat you eat, but also the *kind* of fat. Your consumption of calories derived from fat should be at or below 30 percent of your daily calories. You can reduce your intake by choosing to eat small servings of skinless chicken and turkey breast and/or lean meat, and fat-free or low-fat dairy products. You needn't give up high-fat foods such as cheese, but eat them only occasionally and in small amounts.

The American Heart Association (AHA) has long recommended that less than one-third of fat calories should come from saturated fatty acids, less than one-third polyunsaturated, and the rest monounsaturated (*see box, opposite page, for more about these kinds of fats*). Recently, the AHA has emphasized reducing saturated fats even more and replacing them with monounsaturated fats.

Exact calculations are impossible in real life, but you can move in the right direction, for instance, by replacing butter with a highly monounsaturated oil such as canola or olive oil (or peanut, walnut, or almond oil). All it takes is a small change: replacing just two tablespoons of butter with the same amount of olive or canola oil may be enough to shift your daily fat balance to meet the new AHA recommendation. Small amounts of peanuts, almonds, or peanut butter are also healthful choices.

Eat more fish and nuts. Fish contains heart-protective omega-3 fatty acids, which are polyunsaturated. Omega-3s make platelets in the blood less likely to stick together, or clot, and so help lower the risk of a fatal heart attack. They may also make the heart less susceptible to dangerous, sometimes fatal, rhythm abnormalities. One study published in *The New England Journal of Medicine* found that healthy men with high blood levels of omega-3s had a significantly lower risk of sudden cardiac death. Many experts recommend eating fish at least twice a week. Fatty fish, such as mackerel, salmon, herring, and tuna contain the highest amounts of omega-3s.

Nuts, too, contain healthy unsaturated fats that help lower cholesterol, especially when substituted for foods high in saturated fat. Moreover, certain phytochemicals in nuts, such as sterols, may inhibit the formation of cholesterol. Remember, though, that nuts are calorie-dense and should be consumed in moderation.

Limit your intake of foods containing hydrogenated oils. These are found in many packaged foods, including stick margarine, puddings, crackers, cookies, and potato chips. Hydrogenation makes some of the unsaturated fats more saturated, and also results in "trans fats," which act like saturated fat, boosting blood cholesterol and increasing the risk of heart disease. Manufacturers hydrogenate—that is, add hydrogen to—polyunsaturated vegetable oils in order to give them (and the processed foods made with them) a more solid consistency and a longer shelf life. It's nearly impossible to tell exactly how much trans fat you're eating, since it isn't listed on food labels. This will change, now that the FDA plans to require food makers to list the amount of trans fats on labels.

---

which fats are which?

All fats are combinations of saturated and unsaturated fatty acids, which is why fats are described with terms such as "highly saturated" or "highly polyunsaturated." For instance, only about half the fatty acids in beef are saturated, but that's a high proportion. Fatty acids vary in length and in degree of saturation (that is, how many carbon and hydrogen atoms they carry), both of which help determine whether a fat is solid or liquid (oil) at room temperature.

▶ **Saturated fatty acids** carry all the hydrogen atoms that the carbon atoms can hold. Highly saturated fats come chiefly from animal sources and include butter, milk fat, and the fat in meats. Two vegetable oils—coconut and palm kernel oils—are also highly saturated. These fats are generally solid at room temperature.

▶ **Unsaturated fatty acids** do not carry all the hydrogen atoms that the carbon atoms are capable of holding. If one pair of hydrogen atoms is missing, the fatty acids are called *monounsaturated* (olive, peanut, and canola oils are largely monounsaturated). If two pairs or more of hydrogen atoms are missing, the fatty acids are called *polyunsaturated* (corn, safflower, and sesame oils are primarily polyunsaturated). These fats generally are liquid at room temperature. Plants and fish are important sources of unsaturated fats.

daily guidelines

The USDA's recommendations are a good, practical place to start when choosing your high-carb, low-fat foods. It shows 6 to 11 daily servings of grains, 2 to 4 servings of fruit, 3 to 5 servings of vegetables, and 2 to 3 servings of dairy products (along with small amounts of meat, poultry, or fish). The more calories you consume each day, the more servings you should consume in each category.

Servings are small: just one slice of bread or a medium piece of fruit; half a cup of cooked rice, pasta, beans, or vegetables; a cup of raw leafy vegetables; or ¾ cup of juice. A large apple or banana, a cup of broccoli, or a medium-size salad each counts as two servings.

Such a semi-vegetarian diet will derive more than half its calories from carbohydrates. Include as many whole grains as you can (at least 3 servings a day), according to the government's new dietary guidelines. Limit your intake of highly refined, low-fiber grain products such as white bread. It's much better to get simple carbs (sugars) from fruit, milk, and juice than from cake, cookies (even if low-fat), or soda. There's nothing wrong with small amounts of foods and beverages high in added sugar, but many Americans eat too much of them, adding lots of calories, leaving little room for more nutritious foods, and increasing the risk of chronic disease.

adding more disease protection

The previous points form the basics of a healthy diet. But you can enhance your diet, and thereby increase its potential health benefits, with the following food choices, all of which are well-represented in the recipes throughout the book.

Consume enough calcium. Calcium builds strong bones and helps maintain bone density and strength through a lifetime. This is especially important for women, whose bone density declines at menopause, increasing the risk of osteoporosis. The habit of eating calcium-rich foods should begin in childhood, when bone density is on the increase. The more bone you build early in life, the better you can withstand bone loss later. Low-fat and fat-free dairy products are good sources of calcium. So are foods as varied as canned sardines (with bones), orange juice and cereals fortified with calcium, canned white beans, turnip greens, and tofu (when processed with calcium). To reach the government's recommended daily intake of 1,200 milligrams for adults over age 50, you may have to supplement your diet with calcium pills. However, the pills should be taken in addition to calcium-rich foods, not in place of them.

Increase your intake of green, orange, red, and yellow fruits and vegetables. Foods such as broccoli, carrots, tomatoes, cantaloupe, and citrus fruits are high in antioxidant nutrients such as vitamin C and carotenoids. Acting at the molecular level, these antioxidants inactivate a class of particles known as free radicals, highly reactive molecules in the body that can cause damage to cells. A high intake of antioxidants may be protective against heart disease, cancer, and other disorders. Researchers are only beginning to understand their importance.

Consume some foods rich in alpha-linolenic acid. This compound is an omega-3 fatty acid related to those in fish, and studies suggest that it, too, helps protect the heart. Not many foods are rich in alpha-linolenic acid (ALA)—only canola and soybean oils, ground flaxseeds and flaxseed oil, and walnuts and walnut oil are good sources. In a recent study, women who consumed the equivalent of a daily tablespoon of canola oil, half an ounce of wal-

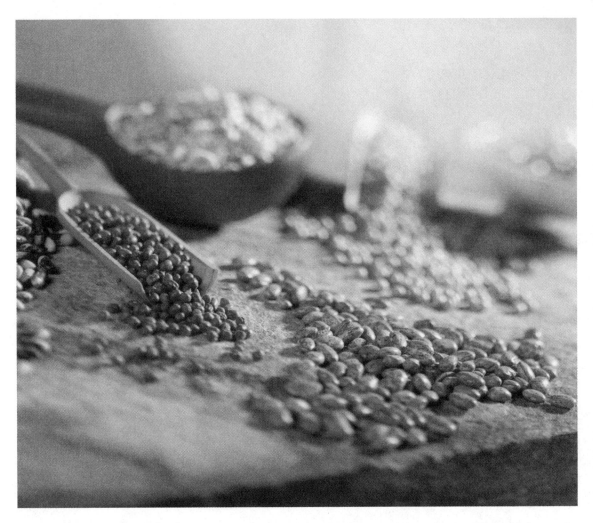

nuts, or a little ground flaxseed had a one-third to one-half lower risk of a fatal heart attack than those consuming little ALA.

Take advantage of beans. Lima, kidney, black, and other beans are all excellent low-fat sources of protein. In addition, beans are some of the best sources of cholesterol-lowering soluble fiber. Studies have shown that eating 4 ounces of beans a day can significantly reduce both total and LDL ("bad") cholesterol.

Add some soy to your diet. Soy foods may reduce the risk of heart disease. Other possible health benefits—not so well established—include protection against prostate cancer and osteoporosis. Just remember that even soyfoods

with a heart-healthy label may be high in salt, sugar, and calories, so be sure to read labels.

a wellness bounty

The recipes in *The Wellness Kitchen* were created to help make healthy eating a life-long habit. They are made with everyday ingredients and contain simple step-by-step instructions. In addition, you will find complete nutrition information for every dish; delicious ways to obtain more nutrients in every meal; and menu suggestions that take the guesswork out of serving balanced meals. Throughout, you will also find many additional facts and tips based on the latest nutrition research.

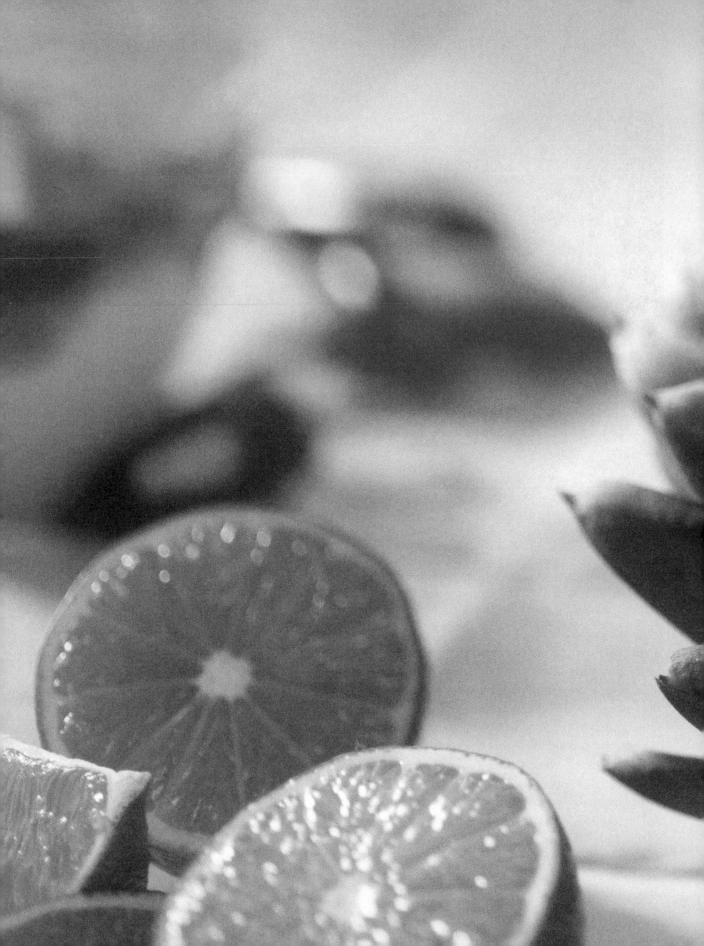

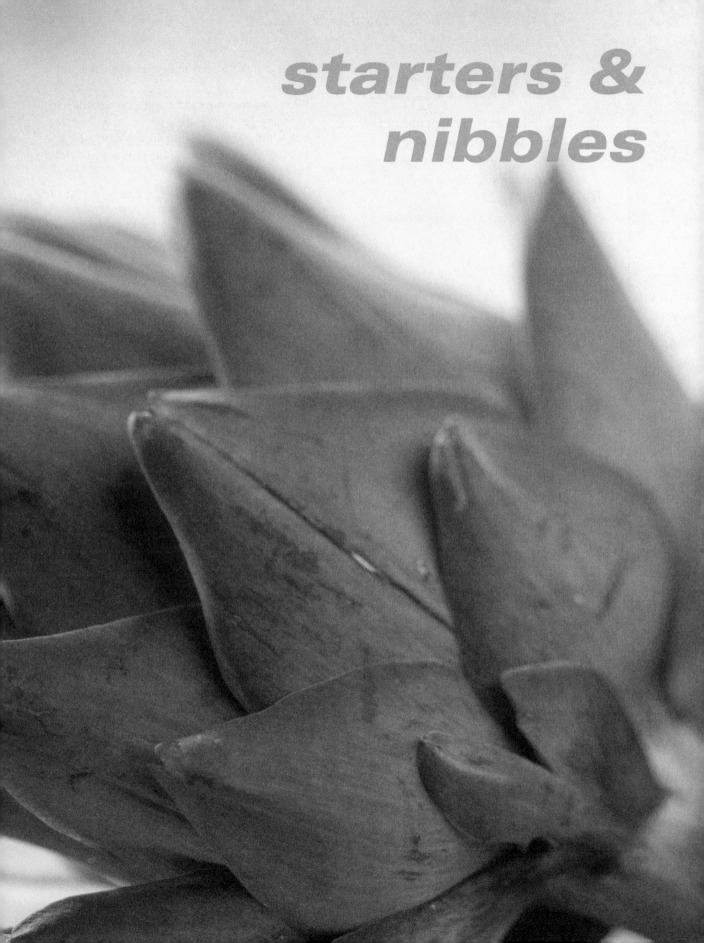

starters &
nibbles

beverages

Thirst is only one of the reasons to buy, make, or drink a beverage. Drinks can also be:

▶ Refreshing (*try homemade Gingerale, page 20*)

▶ Comforting (*how about a mug of Powerhouse Hot Chocolate?, page 20*)

▶ Nourishing (*invent your own smoothie with the "Recipe Creator," opposite page*).

Cranberry-Lime Spritzer

To remove the lime zest (the thin colored portion of the peel), use a vegetable peeler to take it off in strips. Try to get just the zest portion, because that's where all of the flavor is.

> 2 bags (12 ounces each) fresh or frozen cranberries
>
> 4 cups apple juice
>
> 3 tablespoons honey
>
> Zest of 1 lime
>
> ⅔ cup fresh lime juice (about 5 limes)

1 In a large saucepan, combine the cranberries, apple juice, honey, and lime zest. Bring to a boil. Reduce to a simmer and cook until the berries have all popped, about 15 minutes.

2 Strain the mixture through a fine-mesh sieve,

---

different spins

▶ **Cranberry-Grape Spritzer** Follow the directions for *Cranberry-Lime Spritzer*, but use white grape juice instead of apple juice. Use lemon zest and juice instead of lime, and reduce the lemon juice to ½ cup.

▶ **Gingery Lime-Lemonade** Follow the directions for *Minted Lime-Lemonade*, but omit the cinnamon, and use 2 teaspoons ground ginger and ¼ teaspoon white pepper.

---

pushing on the berries to extract as much liquid as possible.

3 Let cool to room temperature, then transfer the cranberry-lime juice to a jar or juice container with a tight-fitting lid. Stir in the lime juice and shake to combine. Store in the refrigerator. *Makes 5 cups juice*

per ¼ cup juice: 51 calories, 0.1g total fat (0g saturated), 0mg cholesterol, 2g dietary fiber, 13g carbohydrate, 0g protein, 4mg sodium. **good source of:** anthocyanins.

For one spritzer Spoon ¼ cup of cranberry-lime juice into a tall glass and add ½ cup chilled seltzer. Add ice if desired.

Minted Lime-Lemonade

A fruit ade is sweetened with a "simple syrup," which is made by dissolving sugar in boiling water. The syrup is important because granulated sugar would not dissolve in the cold juice. In this recipe, the sugar syrup is also the vehicle for the cool flavor of mint.

> 8 limes
>
> 2 lemons
>
> 1½ cups sugar
>
> 1 cup water
>
> 1 cup fresh mint leaves, lightly bruised
>
> 1 cinnamon stick

1 With a vegetable peeler, remove strips of zest from 2 of the limes and both the lemons. Squeeze all of the limes to get a total of 1 cup of juice. Squeeze the lemons to get a total of ½ cup of juice. Set the juices aside.

2 In a small saucepan, combine the lime zest, lemon zest, sugar, water, mint, and cinnamon stick. Bring to a boil over medium heat and boil for 5 minutes to dissolve the sugar. Let the syrup cool to room temperature. Strain and discard the solids.

3 Transfer the sugar syrup to a jar or juice container with a tight-fitting lid. Add the lime and

recipe creator
sweet smoothies

Pick ingredients from each of the four categories and follow these basic instructions: In a blender, combine **1 FRUIT, 1 LIQUID, 1 SWEETENER, and 1 SPICE.** Add 6 ice cubes and blend until smooth and frothy. *Makes 1 serving*

FRUITS	LIQUIDS	SWEETENERS	SPICES
▶ Mango, 1 cup sliced	▶ Yogurt, plain low-fat, 1 cup	▶ Honey, 1 Tbsp	▶ Cinnamon, ½ tsp
▶ Banana, 1 cup sliced	▶ Buttermilk, 1 cup	▶ Brown sugar, 2 tsp	▶ Nutmeg, ¼ tsp
▶ Strawberries, 1 cup halved	▶ Milk, low-fat (1%) or fat-free, 1 cup	▶ Maple syrup, 1 Tbsp	▶ Ground ginger, ½ tsp
▶ Cantaloupe, 1 cup cubed	▶ Soymilk, unflavored, 1 cup		
▶ Pineapple, 1 cup cubed	▶ Tofu, soft silken, ½ cup		

savory smoothies

Pick ingredients from each of the four categories and follow these basic instructions: In a blender, combine **1 VEGETABLE, 1 LIQUID, 1 FLAVORING, and 1 HERB.** Add 6 ice cubes and blend until smooth and frothy. *Makes 1 serving*

VEGETABLES	LIQUIDS	FLAVORINGS	HERBS
▶ Cucumber, 1 cup peeled, seeded, and sliced	▶ Yogurt, plain low-fat, 1 cup	▶ Red onion, ¼ cup chopped	▶ Tarragon, ½ tsp
▶ Zucchini, 1 cup sliced	▶ Buttermilk, 1 cup	▶ Scallions, ¼ cup sliced	▶ Cayenne, ⅛ tsp
▶ Green beans, 1 cup cooked	▶ Milk, low-fat (1%) or fat-free, 1 cup + ¼ tsp salt	▶ Tomato, ½ cup chopped	▶ Fresh dill, 2 Tbsp chopped
▶ Avocado, ¼ cup cubes	▶ Soymilk, unflavored, 1 cup + ¼ tsp salt	▶ Chives, 2 Tbsp chopped	▶ Cumin, ½ tsp
			▶ Fresh basil, 1 Tbsp chopped

lemon juices, and shake to combine. Store in the refrigerator. *Makes 3 cups syrup*

per ¼ cup syrup: 107 calories, 0g total fat (0g saturated), 0mg cholesterol, 0g dietary fiber, 28g carbohydrate, 0g protein, 1mg sodium. good source of: vitamin C.

For one serving Spoon ¼ cup of the lime-lemon mixture into an 8-ounce glass. Add ⅓ cup of water or chilled seltzer and stir to combine. Add ice cubes if you like.

Gingerale

Hot and sweet at the same time, this is a very refreshing summer drink. If you like, stir the ginger syrup into water and freeze in ice cube trays, then use the ginger ice cubes to flavor other cold drinks such as cranberry juice or fruit nectars.

2 cups water

¾ cup thinly sliced unpeeled fresh ginger

¼ teaspoon coarsely cracked pepper

1 cup sugar

5 strips (2 x ½-inch) lemon zest

1 vanilla bean, split lengthwise, or
*   1 teaspoon vanilla extract*

1 In a medium saucepan, bring the water, ginger, and pepper to a boil over medium heat. Reduce the heat to low, cover, and simmer for 25 minutes. Strain through a fine-mesh sieve and discard the solids.

2 Return the ginger liquid to the pan. Stir in the sugar, lemon zest, and vanilla bean (if using vanilla extract, do not add it yet). Bring to a boil over medium heat and cook until the sugar has dissolved, about 2 minutes.

3 Remove from the heat, cover, and let stand until cooled to room temperature (if using vanilla extract, add it at this point). Strain the ginger syrup and discard the lemon zest and vanilla bean. Transfer the ginger syrup to a jar and store in the refrigerator. *Makes 2 cups syrup*

per ¼ cup syrup: 104 calories, 0.1g total fat (0g saturated), 0mg cholesterol, 0g dietary fiber, 27g carbohydrate, 0g protein, 2mg sodium.

For one serving Pour ¼ cup of the syrup into a tall glass. Add ¾ cup of chilled seltzer and ice if you like.

different *spins*

▶ **Powerhouse Mocha** Follow the directions for *Powerhouse Hot Chocolate Mix*, and add 8 teaspoons of instant espresso powder along with the other mix ingredients.

did you know?

The antioxidant effect of tea has gotten lots of publicity, but coffee and hot cocoa may have similar, possibly even greater, effects, according to a Swiss laboratory study. The researchers found that coffee and cocoa protected LDL ("bad") cholesterol from oxidation longer than black or herbal teas did (oxidation of LDL increases the risk of coronary artery damage). Of course, what happens in a test tube may not happen in the body, but it has long been known that, like many plant-based foods, coffee, cocoa, and tea contain antioxidant compounds called polyphenols.

Powerhouse Hot Chocolate Mix

Instead of just your garden-variety cocoa, this comforting drink mix is boosted with calcium (from the nonfat milk powder) and high-quality protein from the soy protein powder (which you can buy at health-food stores and many supermarkets. The amount of fat and calories in the hot cocoa will depend on what type of milk you use, ranging from 167 calories and 1.1 grams of fat for fat-free (skim) milk, to 215 calories and 6.7 grams of fat for whole milk.

¾ cup nonfat dry milk powder

½ cup unflavored soy protein powder

½ cup unsweetened cocoa powder

⅓ cup sugar

In a large bowl or in a jar with a tight-fitting lid, combine the milk powder, soy protein powder, cocoa powder, and sugar, and stir or shake well to combine. Store in the refrigerator. *Makes 2 cups mix*

per ¼ cup mix: 103 calories, 0.7g total fat (0.4g saturated), 0mg cholesterol, 2g dietary fiber, 17g carbohydrate, 12g protein, 114mg sodium. good source of: calcium, magnesium, potassium, riboflavin, vitamin B_{12}, vitamin E.

For one serving Spoon ¼ cup of the cocoa mix into a large mug. Add ¾ cup of hot milk and stir until well combined.

appetizers

On one end of the appetizer spectrum is baked Brie, in which an already high-fat cheese is gilded with an extremely high-fat puff-pastry crust. At the other end of the spectrum are carrot and celery sticks. Luckily, there are plenty of healthful, nutrient-dense options in between.

Guacamole

A bowl of guacamole with a basket of chips can add up to quite a few calories and a hefty dose of fat. But substitute pureed frozen peas for some of the avocado, and you can serve a big bowl of this favorite Mexican dip with a clear conscience. The peas add a subtle sweetness and also contribute folate and soluble fiber. **Serving suggestion:** Serve the guacamole with storebought baked tortilla chips, or one of the homemade chips from the "Recipe Creator" on page 23.

> 1½ cups frozen peas, thawed
>
> ½ Hass avocado, peeled
>
> ¼ cup finely chopped red onion
>
> ¼ cup chopped cilantro
>
> 1 tablespoon fresh lime juice
>
> 1½ teaspoons finely chopped jarred or canned jalapeño pepper
>
> ½ teaspoon salt

1 In a food processor, process the peas until finely chopped. Set aside.

2 In a serving bowl, with a potato masher or fork, mash the avocado until not quite smooth (leave it just a little lumpy).

3 Stir in the peas, onion, cilantro, lime juice, jalapeño, and salt. If not serving right away, place a sheet of plastic wrap on the surface and refrigerate. *Makes 6 servings*

per serving: 57 calories, 2.7g total fat (0.4g saturated), 0mg cholesterol, 3g dietary fiber, 7g carbohydrate, 2g protein, 148mg sodium. good source of: lutein, vitamin C.

Roasted Eggplant-Walnut Dip

Although this recipe calls for discarding the eggplant skin, if you don't mind small purple flecks in your dip, just go ahead and puree the whole eggplant (though you should discard the tough parts at the stem end). The compounds that are responsible for the color of fruits and vegetables are being investigated for their health potential, so why not go ahead and eat the deeply colored eggplant skin? **Serving suggestion:** Serve this silky dip with vegetable crudités or wedges of pita bread. Or make your own pita "chips" using the Homemade Chips "Recipe Creator" on page 23.

> 2 eggplants (about 1 pound each), halved lengthwise
>
> 4 slices firm-textured whole-wheat sandwich bread, toasted and torn into pieces
>
> 3 cloves garlic, peeled
>
> 2 tablespoons coarsely chopped walnuts
>
> 2 tablespoons fresh lemon juice
>
> 2 teaspoons dark sesame oil
>
> ¾ teaspoon salt
>
> ¾ teaspoon ground coriander
>
> ¼ cup chopped cilantro

1 Preheat the oven to 400°F. Place the eggplant halves, cut-sides down, on a baking sheet and bake for 25 minutes, or until tender. When cool enough to handle, scoop out the flesh with a spoon.

2 Transfer the eggplant to a food processor. Add the toast pieces, garlic, walnuts, lemon juice, sesame oil, salt, and ground coriander, and process to a smooth puree.

3 Spoon the dip into a serving bowl and stir in the cilantro. *Makes 4 cups*

per ½ cup: 91 calories, 3g total fat (0.3g saturated), 0mg cholesterol, 4g dietary fiber, 14g carbohydrate, 3g protein, 289mg sodium. good source of: fiber, omega-3 fatty acids, thiamin.

Yogurt Cheese

Although cream cheese comes in a range of fat levels, from fat-free to full-fat, it does not come with much calcium. Yogurt, on the other hand, is a leading source of this important mineral. So, to make a spread to use for breakfast or for appetizers, a good bone-health choice is to make your own yogurt cheese. Though it's called cheese, it's really just yogurt that's been thickened to a fresh cheese consistency by draining off some of the whey. The nutrition analysis below is for the yogurt cheese alone; the actual calorie counts will vary depending on what mix-in you use. **Timing alert:** You should start the yogurt in the morning (or the night before), because it needs to drain for at least 8 hours.

> *1 quart plain fat-free yogurt*
> *Mix-ins (recipes follow)*

1 Set a paper coffee filter or a fine-mesh sieve lined with dampened cheesecloth over a bowl. Spoon the yogurt into the filter or sieve and place in the refrigerator overnight to drain.

2 Transfer the yogurt cheese to a bowl and discard the whey. Stir in one of the mix-ins listed below. *Makes 1½ cups*

per 2 tablespoons: 23 calories, 0.1g total fat (0.1g saturated), 1mg cholesterol, 0g dietary fiber, 3g carbohydrate, 2g protein, 31mg sodium.

Strawberry Yogurt Cheese With a potato masher, mash 1 cup of strawberries with 1 teaspoon of sugar. Stir into the yogurt cheese.

Dried Plum (Prune) Yogurt Cheese Stir in ½ cup of prune butter and 1 teaspoon of grated lemon zest.

Herbed Yogurt Cheese Stir in 1 teaspoon of grated lemon zest and ⅓ cup of mixed chopped fresh herbs such as dill, basil, mint, cilantro, parsley, tarragon, or chives.

Roasted Garlic Yogurt Cheese Wrap 1 large bulb of garlic in a sheet of foil and roast at 400°F for 30 minutes, or until soft. Squeeze out the garlic, mash until smooth, and stir into the yogurt cheese.

Pesto Yogurt Cheese Stir in 3 tablespoons of pesto, homemade (*page 256*) or storebought.

Spiced Yogurt Cheese Stir in 2 teaspoons each of ground cumin and ground coriander, 1 teaspoon of chili powder, and ¼ teaspoon of pepper.

Sweet & Spicy Red Lentil Dip

Red lentils (which are small, hulled lentils) cook much more quickly than brown or green lentils and lose their shape more readily. That makes red lentils perfect for this dip—once cooked they're already halfway to being a puree. Carrot juice and an apple lend a slightly sweet note, enhancing the flavors of the curry powder. If you don't have carrot juice, you could use tomato juice, tomato-vegetable juice, or broth.

> *2 cups water*
> *1 cup red lentils*
> *1 tablespoon olive oil*
> *1 Granny Smith apple, unpeeled and thinly sliced*
> *1 small onion, halved and sliced*
> *2 cloves garlic, minced*
> *1 tablespoon curry powder*
> *⅓ cup carrot juice*
> *¾ teaspoon salt*

1 In a medium saucepan, bring the water to a boil over high heat. Add the lentils, reduce the heat to medium, and cook until the lentils are very tender, about 10 minutes. Drain any liquid remaining in the pan. Transfer the lentils to a food processor.

2 Meanwhile, in a large nonstick skillet, heat the oil over medium heat. Add the apple, onion, garlic, and curry powder, and cook, stirring occasionally, until the onion is tender, about 10 minutes.

3 Add the sautéed apple-onion mixture to the lentils in the food processor. Add the carrot juice and salt, and process to a smooth puree. Serve at room temperature or chilled. *Makes 3 cups*

per ⅓ cup: 104 calories, 2.1g total fat (0.3g saturated), 0mg cholesterol, 3g dietary fiber, 17g carbohydrate, 6g protein, 199mg sodium. good source of: folate, thiamin.

recipe creator
homemade chips

Homemade chips are really easy to make and give you a wide range of interesting flavors with a minimum of fat and sodium. Pick ingredients from each of the four categories and follow these basic instructions: Preheat the oven to 400°F. Spray 2 large baking sheets with nonstick cooking spray. In a small bowl, whisk together **1** LIQUID, **1** OIL, **1** SEASONING, and ½ teaspoon salt. Before cutting the "BREAD," brush it evenly with the liquid mixture. Then cut as directed. Place the wedges on the baking sheets and bake 8 to 10 minutes, or until lightly browned, turning them over halfway through the baking time. Transfer the chips to a wire rack to cool. *Makes 48 chips*

LIQUIDS	OILS	SEASONINGS	"BREAD"
▶ Lime juice, ⅓ cup	▶ Olive oil, 2 tsp	▶ Chili powder, 1½ tsp	▶ 8 flour tortillas (6"–7"), cut into 6 wedges
▶ Lemon juice, ⅓ cup	▶ Dark sesame oil, 2 tsp	▶ Garlic powder, 1 tsp	▶ 8 corn tortillas (6"–7"), cut into 6 wedges
▶ Malt vinegar, ⅓ cup	▶ Pumpkin seed oil, 2 tsp	▶ Onion powder, 1 tsp	▶ 4 pita breads (6"–7"), split horizontally, each piece cut into 6 wedges
▶ Tomato-vegetable juice, ⅓ cup		▶ Cumin, 1 tsp	
▶ Carrot juice, ⅓ cup		▶ Coriander, ½ tsp	▶ 3 soft lavash (8 x 10"), each cut into 16 rectangles
		▶ Curry powder, 1 tsp	

Hummus

This Middle Eastern dip is traditionally made with tahini, a paste made of ground sesame seeds. To get the same flavor with significantly less fat, we've used a combination of dark sesame oil and fat-free yogurt—one for deep sesame flavor and the other for a creamy texture.

4 cloves garlic, peeled

3½ cups cooked chick-peas (page 180) or canned (rinsed and drained)

¾ cup plain fat-free yogurt

1 teaspoon grated lemon zest

2 tablespoons fresh lemon juice

4 teaspoons dark sesame oil

½ teaspoon salt

½ teaspoon coriander

¼ teaspoon cayenne pepper

⅛ teaspoon allspice

1 In a small saucepan of boiling water, cook the garlic for 2 minutes to blanch. Drain. Transfer the garlic to a food processor.

2 Add the chick-peas, yogurt, lemon zest, lemon juice, sesame oil, salt, coriander, cayenne, and allspice to the food processor, and pulse until almost smooth but with a little texture. *Makes 4 cups*

per ⅓ cup: 107 calories, 2.9g total fat (0.4g saturated), 0mg cholesterol, 4g dietary fiber, 16g carbohydrate, 6g protein, 209mg sodium. good source of: fiber, folate.

Salmon Mousse

Popular in the '50s and '60s, this traditional appetizer has been updated by the use of fresh salmon instead of canned, and yogurt and reduced-fat sour cream instead of mayonnaise and heavy cream. If you'd prefer, you can substitute one 14¾-ounce can of sockeye salmon for the fresh (and omit the ¼ teaspoon of salt from step 1). If you do, don't bother to drain or remove the skin or bones (which contain calcium) before transferring to the food processor. **Timing alert:** The mousse needs to chill for at least 4 hours before serving.

> 1 pound skinless salmon fillets
>
> 1 teaspoon salt
>
> 1 envelope unflavored gelatin
>
> ½ cup cold water
>
> ¾ cup plain fat-free yogurt
>
> ⅔ cup reduced-fat sour cream
>
> ¼ cup drained white horseradish
>
> 2 tablespoons grated onion
>
> 2 teaspoons grated lemon zest
>
> 3 tablespoons fresh lemon juice

1 Preheat the oven to 450°F. Place the salmon on a baking sheet and sprinkle with ¼ teaspoon of the salt. Roast for about 10 minutes, or until the salmon just barely flakes when tested with a fork (it should still be moist in the center). Let cool to room temperature.

2 Meanwhile, in a small heatproof bowl, sprinkle the gelatin over the water and let stand until softened, about 2 minutes. Set the bowl in a pan of simmering water and heat until the gelatin dissolves, about 3 minutes. Set aside to cool to room temperature.

3 Transfer the gelatin mixture to a food processor along with the salmon, the remaining ¾ teaspoon salt, the yogurt, sour cream, horseradish, onion, lemon zest, and lemon juice. Pulse until the mixture is smooth.

4 Transfer the mousse mixture to a decorative bowl, cover, and refrigerate at least 4 hours for the mousse to set. *Makes 12 servings*

per serving: 82 calories, 3.3g total fat (1.4g saturated), 21mg cholesterol, 0g dietary fiber, 3g carbohydrate, 10g protein, 243mg sodium. good source of: niacin, omega-3 fatty acids, selenium, vitamin B_{12}, vitamin B_6.

did you know?

So, are blue corn chips better for you than other corn chips? Well, blue corn has more protein than white or yellow corn, as well as more zinc and more lysine (an amino acid, which is a building block of protein). It also has a blue pigment that may be healthful, though no one knows how much survives in chips—or how much you would need to eat to get any benefit. Overall, however, any type of corn chip is low in nutrients. And most are also high in calories and fat. You're better off making your choice based on fat and sodium levels than on color.

Bruschetta

From the Italian verb *bruscare*, meaning "to roast over coals," a bruschetta is toasted bread rubbed with garlic and topped with a variety of things, most commonly a chopped tomato and basil concoction. But the variations are infinite. Just use your imagination (think of your favorite pizza toppings) or check out the toppings that follow. The nutrition analysis is for the plain bruschetta; the actual calorie counts will vary depending on what topping you use.

> 8 slices (1 inch thick) whole-wheat Italian bread (4 ounces)
>
> 1 clove garlic, peeled and halved
>
> Toppings (recipes follow)

1 In a toaster or toaster oven, or under the broiler, toast the bread on both sides. Rub both sides of the toast with the cut sides of the garlic halves.

2 Arrange the toast on a large plate or a platter. Spoon any of the following toppings on the toast. *Makes 4 servings*

per serving: 73 calories, 1.2g total fat (0.3g saturated), 0mg cholesterol, 2g dietary fiber, 14g carbohydrate, 3g protein, 150mg sodium. good source of: selenium.

recipe creator
bean dips

Pick ingredients from each of the five categories and follow these basic instructions: Soak 1 cup of DRIED BEANS in water to cover (by 2 inches) for 8 hours. Drain and place in a saucepan with fresh water to cover by 2 inches. Add any 3 AROMATICS and simmer, uncovered, until the beans are tender, about 1 hour. Drain the beans, reserving about 1 cup of the bean cooking water. Transfer the beans to a food processor (along with the aromatics). Add 1 LIQUID, 1 SEASONING, and ¾ teaspoon salt. Puree, adding some of the reserved bean cooking water if the mixture seems too dry. Stir in any or all of the GARNISHES. (For a quick bean dip, skip the first two columns and use 3 cups rinsed and drained canned beans. If the pureed beans seem too dry, add a little bit of water.) *Makes 2½ to 3 cups*

DRIED BEANS	AROMATICS	LIQUIDS	SEASONINGS	GARNISHES
▶ Pinto beans	▶ Lemon, orange, or lime zest, 4 strips	▶ Yogurt, plain low-fat, 3 Tbsp	▶ Cumin, 2 tsp	▶ Scallions or red onion, ⅓ cup chopped
▶ Great Northern beans	▶ Scallions, 3 sliced	▶ Sour cream, reduced-fat, 3 Tbsp	▶ Coriander, 1 tsp	▶ Cilantro, ⅓ cup chopped
▶ Black beans	▶ Garlic, 4 cloves peeled	▶ Tomato paste, ¼ cup	▶ Chili powder, 2½ tsp	▶ Fresh jalapeño peppers, 2 minced
▶ Kidney beans	▶ Canned or bottled jalapeño pepper, 1 whole	▶ Lemon or lime juice, 2 Tbsp	▶ Curry powder, 2 tsp	
▶ Black-eyed peas	▶ Cilantro stems, ½ cup	▶ Dark sesame oil, 2 tsp	▶ Rosemary, ½ tsp minced	
▶ Chick-peas	▶ 1 bay leaf (discard after using)	▶ Walnut oil, 2 tsp		
▶ Chili beans		▶ Pumpkin seed oil, 2 tsp		

Basil-Tomato Bruschetta Combine 2 large diced tomatoes, ¼ cup chopped fresh basil, 2 cloves minced garlic, 2 teaspoons extra-virgin olive oil, and ½ teaspoon salt.

White Bean & Sage Bruschetta Sauté 2 cloves minced garlic in 2 teaspoons olive oil until soft. Stir in ½ teaspoon rubbed sage. Remove from the heat. Add to ½ cup cooked white beans and mash.

Stir in 1 teaspoon grated lemon zest, 1 tablespoon fresh lemon juice, and ¼ teaspoon salt.

Pepper, Onion & Olive Bruschetta Sauté 1 chopped red bell pepper, 1 small chopped onion, and 2 cloves minced garlic in 1 tablespoon olive oil until soft. Stir in 2 tablespoons chopped olives and ¼ teaspoon salt.

recipe creator
appetizer wraps

Flexible soft breads, such as flour tortillas and lahvash (sometimes called shepherd's bread), are the perfect vehicles for any number of filling ingredients. Pick ingredients from each of the four categories and follow these basic instructions: In a small bowl, beat **1** SPREAD with **1** SEASONING. Spread on either 2 burrito-style tortillas (9- or 10-inch) or 2 soft rectangular lahvash sheets (8 x 10). Top with **1** MAIN FILLING and **1** or **2** GARNISHES. Roll up tightly, wrap in foil, and refrigerate for 1 hour. Cut crosswise into ½-inch-thick slices. *Makes about 40 pieces*

SPREADS	SEASONINGS	MAIN FILLINGS	GARNISHES
▶Reduced-fat cream cheese (Neufchâtel), 8 oz	▶Mango chutney, ¼ cup chopped	▶Roast turkey breast, 4 oz thinly sliced	▶Roasted red peppers, ½ cup slivered
▶Low-fat cottage cheese, ¾ cup	▶Fresh basil, ½ cup chopped	▶Albacore tuna, 6-oz can, flaked	▶Red onion, ½ cup very thinly sliced
▶Part-skim ricotta, ¾ cup	▶Cilantro, ½ cup chopped	▶Reduced-sodium, baked ham, 4 oz thinly sliced	▶Shredded lettuce, 1 cup
▶White beans, 1½ cups mashed	▶Taco sauce or thick salsa, ¼ cup	▶Roast chicken breast, 4 oz thinly sliced	
▶Avocado, ⅓ cup diced, mashed with ⅓ cup plain fat-free yogurt	▶Pickle relish, 2 Tbsp	▶Smoked salmon, 4 oz thinly sliced	

Split Pea Salsa

Most people think of salsa as a spicy chopped tomato condiment, but salsa merely means sauce. So, by extension, you can make a salsa out of all sorts of things. Here we use folate- and fiber-rich split peas to make a salsa with Mexican spices. And just so tomato fans won't be disappointed, the salsa also has chopped grape tomatoes.

> 3 cups water
> 1½ cups split peas
> 3 cloves garlic, minced
> ¾ teaspoon salt
> ½ teaspoon oregano
> 1 tablespoon olive oil
> 1½ teaspoons chili powder
> ¾ teaspoon ground coriander
> ⅓ cup fresh lime juice
> ½ cup chopped cilantro
> ¼ cup chopped grape or cherry tomatoes

1 In a medium saucepan, bring the water to a boil over medium heat. Add the split peas, garlic, ¼ teaspoon of the salt, and the oregano, and reduce to a simmer. Cover and cook, stirring occasionally, until the split peas are tender, about 30 minutes. Drain.

2 Meanwhile, in a small skillet, heat the oil over low heat. Add the chili powder and coriander, and cook until fragrant, about 30 seconds.

3 Scrape the spiced oil into a large bowl and whisk in the lime juice and the remaining ½ teaspoon salt. Stir in the hot split peas, the cilantro, and tomatoes. Serve warm, at room temperature, or chilled. *Makes 4 cups*

per ⅓ cup: 100 calories, 1.5g total fat (0.2g saturated), 0mg cholesterol, 7g dietary fiber, 16g carbohydrate, 6g protein, 154mg sodium. good source of: fiber, folate, thiamin.

Roasted Shiitake & Cheese Quesadillas

Spanish Manchego cheese, nutty and buttery tasting, is the perfect foil for earthy mushrooms and corn. If you can't find flavored tortillas, substitute regular flour tortillas.

> ¾ pound fresh shiitake mushrooms,
> stems discarded and caps quartered
>
> 1 large onion, halved and thickly sliced
>
> ¾ cup frozen corn kernels
>
> 1 tablespoon olive oil
>
> ½ teaspoon oregano
>
> ½ teaspoon salt
>
> ½ teaspoon pepper
>
> ½ teaspoon sugar
>
> 4 burrito-size flour tortillas (9 inches),
> preferably tomato and/or spinach
>
> ¼ pound Manchego cheese, shredded

1 Preheat the oven to 400°F. On a jelly-roll pan, stir together the mushrooms, onion, corn, oil, oregano, salt, pepper, and sugar. Bake for 30 minutes, stirring the mixture occasionally, until the onions are tender. Leave the oven on.

2 Place 2 tortillas on a large baking sheet. Top each with the mushroom mixture. Sprinkle with the cheese. Top with the remaining tortillas. Bake for 10 minutes, or until the cheese has melted, the filling is piping hot, and the tortillas are crisp.

3 To serve, cut each quesadilla into 6 wedges. *Makes 12 wedges*

per wedge: 145 calories, 5.6g total fat (2.3g saturated), 6mg cholesterol, 1g dietary fiber, 19g carbohydrate, 6g protein, 394mg sodium. good source of: calcium, selenium, vitamin D.

Egg Roulade with Dill & Mozzarella

Fat-free mozzarella can be difficult to work with, because it can turn rubbery when overheated. However, when it's protected from direct heat (in this recipe, residual heat is used to melt it), it can make a significant contribution to the satisfying mouth-feel of a dish. This appetizer also makes a nice brunch buffet dish.

> 3 large eggs
>
> 2 tablespoons flour
>
> 6 large egg whites
>
> ¼ cup chopped dill
>
> 2 tablespoons grated Parmesan cheese
>
> ¼ teaspoon salt
>
> ¾ cup shredded fat-free mozzarella
> (3 ounces)
>
> ½ cup finely diced red bell pepper

1 Preheat the oven to 400°F. Generously spray a 10 x 15-inch jelly-roll pan with nonstick cooking spray.

2 In a medium bowl, whisk the whole eggs, one at a time, into the flour until smooth. Whisk in the egg whites, dill, Parmesan cheese, and salt until well combined.

3 Pour the mixture into the jelly-roll pan and bake for 8 to 9 minutes, or until just set.

4 Remove from the oven and sprinkle the mozzarella and bell pepper over the top. Let sit for 3 minutes.

5 Run a metal spatula around the edges of the pan to loosen. Beginning at one short side, roll up the mixture, jelly-roll style. To serve, cut the egg roulade crosswise into 12 slices. *Makes 6 servings*

per serving: 106 calories, 3.2g total fat (1.2g saturated), 112mg cholesterol, 0g dietary fiber, 4g carbohydrate, 14g protein, 385mg sodium. good source of: calcium, riboflavin, selenium, vitamin B_{12}, vitamin C.

Artichokes with Creamy Lemon-Garlic Sauce

You can steam the artichokes ahead of time and refrigerate them, but they will have more flavor if you bring them back to room temperature before serving. You can also make the lemon–garlic sauce ahead, but it may stiffen up as it sits in the refrigerator. So save some of the potato cooking water and stir a couple of teaspoons of it into the sauce to loosen it back up before serving.

> 1 baking potato (6 ounces), peeled and thinly sliced
>
> 6 cloves garlic, peeled
>
> ¼ cup fresh lemon juice
>
> ¼ cup light mayonnaise
>
> 2 tablespoons plain fat-free yogurt
>
> ½ teaspoon salt
>
> ⅛ teaspoon cayenne pepper
>
> 4 large artichokes (10 to 12 ounces each), steamed (see below)
>
> 1 teaspoon rosemary, minced

1 In a small pot of boiling water, cook the potato until tender, about 10 minutes. Add the garlic during the last 2 minutes of cooking. Drain, reserving 2 tablespoons of the cooking liquid.

2 Transfer the potato, the reserved cooking liquid, and the garlic to a large bowl and mash until smooth. Add 2 tablespoons of the lemon juice, the mayonnaise, yogurt, salt, and cayenne.

3 Meanwhile, trim off the tough leaves from the artichoke. Trim off the tough end of the stem, then peel the remaining stem.

4 Steam the artichokes, adding the remaining 2 tablespoons lemon juice and rosemary to the steaming water. Serve the artichokes warm or at room temperature with the lemon–garlic sauce. *Makes 4 servings*

per serving: 153 calories, 5.3g total fat (0.6g saturated), 5mg cholesterol, 7g dietary fiber, 25g carbohydrate, 6g protein, 518mg sodium. **good source of:** fiber, folate, magnesium, potassium, vitamin B_6, vitamin C.

how to steam an artichoke

With a sharp, heavy knife, cut off the top one-third of the artichoke, which consists of inedible leaf tips. Pull off any short, coarse leaves from the bottom, and cut off about 1 inch of the tough stem. With a paring knife, peel the remaining stem. Don't cut an artichoke with a carbon-steel knife; it will turn the cut parts black. Rub the cut parts with lemon juice to keep them from darkening.

In a large pot or steamer bottom, bring 2 or 3 inches of water to a boil. You can add herbs or other seasonings to the steaming water to impart a subtle flavor to the artichokes as they cook. Some good choices are rosemary, lemon juice, white wine, garlic, bay leaves, fennel seeds, or tarragon vinegar.

Place the artichokes, stem-sides up, in the steamer and set over the boiling water. Cover and cook until tender, 30 to 45 minutes. To test for doneness, stick a small, sharp knife into the stem where it joins the base of the artichoke.

Remove the artichokes and let them cool slightly, upside down. Serve them warm, at room temperature, or chilled. Try dipping them in the Creamy Lemon-Garlic Sauce (*above*), or one of these sauces: Tofu-Lemon Pepper Dipping Sauce (*page 256*), Dill-Caper Dressing (*page 253*), Orange-Balsamic Dressing (*page 254*), Fresh Ginger & Lime Dressing (*page 254*), or Creamy Carrot Dressing (*page 255*).

Deviled Caribbean Chicken Strips

The Caribbean influence in this spicy chicken appetizer is in the form of dark rum, underscored by the dark brown sugar. The "deviled" aspect comes from the Dijon mustard, whose spiciness is emphasized by cayenne and fresh ginger juice. You can easily make fresh ginger juice, as we do here, but if you can find bottled ginger juice in the supermarket, use 1 tablespoon of it instead. **Serving suggestion:** Serve as part of a buffet with a variety of salsas or dipping sauces.

> 3 tablespoons grated fresh ginger
>
> ¼ cup dark rum
>
> ¼ cup fresh lime juice
>
> 2 cloves garlic, minced
>
> 1 tablespoon Dijon mustard
>
> 1 tablespoon dark brown sugar
>
> ½ teaspoon salt
>
> ¼ teaspoon cayenne pepper
>
> 1 pound skinless, boneless chicken breasts, cut across the grain into ½-inch-wide strips

1 Place the grated ginger in a small fine-mesh sieve set over a large bowl. Press the ginger to extract the juice. Discard the ginger solids.

2 Stir the rum, lime juice, garlic, mustard, brown sugar, salt, and cayenne into the ginger juice. Add the chicken to the marinade, tossing until well coated. Cover and marinate at room temperature for 20 minutes or in the refrigerator for 1 hour.

3 Preheat the broiler. Reserving the marinade, thread the chicken onto eight 6–inch skewers.

4 Broil 4 to 6 inches from the heat, turning the skewers occasionally and brushing with the reserved marinade, for 6 minutes, or until golden brown and cooked through. Don't brush with the marinade during the final minute of cooking (discard any remaining marinade). *Makes 8 servings*

per serving: 92 calories, 1.5g total fat (0.4g saturated), 31mg cholesterol, 0g dietary fiber, 3g carbohydrate, 12g protein, 222mg sodium. good source of: niacin, selenium, vitamin B_6.

Grilled Shrimp Cocktail

These can just as easily be broiled: Spray a broiler pan with nonstick cooking spray. Preheat the broiler. Broil the shrimp 4 to 6 inches from the heat until opaque throughout, about 1 minute per side. **Serving suggestion:** Instead of serving the shrimp as an appetizer, skip the cocktail sauce and serve the shrimp on a salad for a light lunch or dinner dish. Try it on Caesar Salad (*page 201*), Fresh Fennel Salad (*page 203*), Sushi Rice Salad (*page 207*), or a mixed green salad.

> Hot & Spicy Cocktail Sauce (page 256) or 1¼ cups storebought cocktail sauce
>
> 1 teaspoon grated orange zest
>
> ¼ cup orange juice
>
> 1 tablespoon olive oil
>
> ½ teaspoon salt
>
> ½ teaspoon paprika
>
> ¼ teaspoon cayenne pepper
>
> 1 pound jumbo shrimp (about 12), shelled and deveined

1 Make the Hot & Spicy Cocktail Sauce (if using). Refrigerate until serving time.

2 Spray a grill rack with nonstick cooking spray. Preheat the grill to medium.

3 In a large bowl, whisk together the orange zest, orange juice, oil, salt, paprika, and cayenne. Add the shrimp, tossing to coat.

4 Grill the shrimp until opaque throughout, about 1 minute per side. Serve with the cocktail sauce. *Makes 4 servings*

per serving: 120 calories, 4.4g total fat (0.7g saturated), 161mg cholesterol, 0g dietary fiber, 2g carbohydrate, 17g protein, 476mg sodium. good source of: niacin, omega-3 fatty acids, selenium, vitamin B_{12}, vitamin D, zinc.

soups

Time was when the meal called supper was a light meal, taken at night—as opposed to dinner, which was a midday meal and generally a heavy, meat-and-potatoes affair. Supper was often a bowl of soup (a word that shares its origins with "supper"), possibly constructed of leftovers from dinner. Although supper has evolved into the big meal of the day, soups are not often included in the menu, and they should be. Their virtues are many: They can be made ahead of time and frozen, making preparation quick and efficient. They are a perfect medium for using lots and lots of vegetables, and a modest but satisfying amount of meat or poultry. You can round out the meal with whole-grain breads and salads. And best of all, soup recipes tend to be very forgiving, allowing you to substitute ingredients with confidence.

French Onion Soup

Cooking the onions very slowly allows the natural sugars to caramelize, giving the soup a deep, rich flavor. You can make the soup through step 2 ahead of time. Cover and refrigerate the soup, then bring it back to room temperature over low heat before proceeding. **Serving suggestion:** For a light meal, serve the soup with Strawberry, Mango & Lentil Salad (*page 153*) and Toasted Oatmeal Cookies with Cranberries (*page 248*) for dessert.

  2 teaspoons olive oil
  2½ pounds red onions, halved and thinly sliced
  ¼ cup brandy
  2 tablespoons flour
  3 cups chicken broth, homemade (page 252) or canned
  1½ cups water
  1 teaspoon thyme
  ½ teaspoon salt
  ½ teaspoon pepper
  8 thin slices whole-wheat French or Italian bread (about 2 ounces total)
  2 ounces thinly sliced Gruyère or Jarlsberg cheese

1 In a nonstick Dutch oven or large saucepan, heat the oil over medium heat. Add the onions and cook, stirring frequently, until they are very tender and richly browned, about 45 minutes.

2 Stir in the brandy and cook for 1 minute. Sprinkle the flour over the onions, stirring to coat. Stir in the broth, water, thyme, salt, and pepper, and bring to a boil. Reduce to a simmer, cover, and cook until the flavors have developed, about 15 minutes.

3 Meanwhile, preheat the broiler. Place the bread on the broiler rack and broil 4 to 6 inches from the heat for 30 seconds, or until lightly toasted. Turn the bread over and arrange the cheese on top. Return to the broiler and broil for about 30 seconds, or until the cheese has melted.

4 Ladle the soup into bowls and place the cheese toasts on top. *Makes 4 servings*

per serving: 283 calories, 7.1g total fat (3g saturated), 13mg cholesterol, 6g dietary fiber, 36g carbohydrate, 11g protein, 906mg sodium. good source of: calcium, fiber, folate, potassium, quercetin, selenium, thiamin, vitamin B$_6$, vitamin C.

different *spins*

▶**Chili-Spiced Gazpacho with Shrimp**
Follow the directions for *Spicy Gazpacho (opposite page)*, but substitute 4 sliced scallions for the onion. In step 2, add 1 tablespoon chili powder and 1 teaspoon each of cumin and coriander. Replace the vinegar with fresh lime juice. At serving time, stir in ½ cup thawed frozen corn kernels, ¼ cup chopped cilantro, and 1 cup cooked shrimp, halved horizontally.

how (and why) to seed a cucumber

The reason for seeding a cucumber is to remove the excess water that comes with the seeds. It can make salads soggy and soups watery (as in the gazpacho below). But it's easy and quick to seed a cucumber. Just halve it lengthwise, then take a small spoon and use the tip to scrape out the channel of seeds that runs down the center of the cucumber. This will leave you with a cucumber half that looks like a "U" in cross-section. There are some varieties of cucumber—such as hothouse and kirby—that naturally have very few seeds and no liquidy seed core.

Spicy Gazpacho

Carrot juice is the surprise ingredient in this gazpacho. It lends a bright color, a slightly sweet note, and a good amount of beta carotene. **Serving suggestion:** To go with this soup, make one of the flavored tortilla chips from the Homemade Chips "Recipe Creator" on page 23. **Timing alert:** You could actually have this soup at room temperature, but it's especially refreshing chilled, which involves a couple of hours in the refrigerator.

> 1 large cucumber, peeled and seeded
> 3 large tomatoes, quartered
> 2 green bell peppers, cut into large pieces
> 1 medium onion, cut into chunks
> 1 jarred or canned jalapeño pepper
> 2 cloves garlic, peeled
> 1¼ cups carrot juice
> 3 tablespoons red wine vinegar
> ¾ teaspoon salt

1 Cut the cucumber into large chunks.

2 In a food processor, combine the cucumber, tomatoes, bell peppers, onion, jalapeño, garlic, carrot juice, vinegar, and salt, and pulse until chunky but well combined, about 30 seconds.

3 Transfer the gazpacho to a large bowl. Cover and refrigerate for at least 2 hours or until well chilled. *Makes 4 servings*

per serving: 80 calories, 0.7g total fat (0.1g saturated), 0mg cholesterol, 3g dietary fiber, 18g carbohydrate, 3g protein, 488mg sodium. good source of: beta carotene, fiber, potassium, thiamin, vitamin B_6, vitamin C.

Golden Vegetable Soup

This beautiful orange-gold soup gets its wealth of beta carotene (one serving has over 140% of the recommended daily intake) from the carrots and butternut squash. The orange juice intensifies the color, and also adds the B vitamin folate.

> 2½ teaspoons olive oil
> ¾ pound carrots, thinly sliced
> ¾ pound butternut squash, peeled, seeded, and thinly sliced
> ⅔ cup water
> ¼ cup frozen orange juice concentrate
> 1½ cups fat-free milk
> ½ teaspoon salt
> ¼ teaspoon cayenne pepper
> 2 tablespoons reduced-fat sour cream

1 In a large nonstick saucepan, heat the oil over medium heat. Add the carrots and squash, and cook, stirring frequently, until the vegetables begin to color, about 5 minutes.

2 Add the water, cover, and cook until the vegetables are tender, about 15 minutes.

3 Transfer the vegetables and any liquid remaining in the pan to a food processor. Add the orange juice concentrate and process to a smooth puree.

4 Return the puree to the saucepan. Add the milk, salt, and cayenne, and simmer over low heat until heated through. Serve topped with a dollop of sour cream. *Makes 4 servings*

per serving: 172 calories, 4.2g total fat (1.2g saturated), 6mg cholesterol, 6g dietary fiber, 30g carbohydrate, 6g protein, 377mg sodium. good source of: beta carotene, calcium, fiber, folate, potassium, riboflavin, thiamin, vitamin B_6, vitamin C.

Neoclassic Corn Chowder

A classic corn chowder would have heavy cream and lots of bacon; so a neoclassic version is one that has had a health makeover: instead of cream, flour–thickened low-fat milk; instead of pork bacon, turkey bacon. Although turkey bacon is sometimes colored to resemble pork bacon, with its white streaks of fat, it's actually nothing but lean. So to cook it, you need to use a nonstick pan and sometimes a little oil. Here we "stretch" the oil by using some water to keep the bacon from sticking.

> 1 teaspoon olive oil
>
> 2 cups water
>
> 1 medium onion, finely chopped
>
> 3 slices (1 ounce total) turkey bacon, coarsely chopped
>
> 1 red bell pepper, diced
>
> ½ pound red potatoes, cut into ½-inch chunks
>
> ¾ teaspoon salt
>
> ¼ teaspoon black pepper
>
> 1 cup low-fat (1%) or fat-free milk
>
> 2 tablespoons flour
>
> 1 package (10 ounces) frozen corn kernels
>
> 1 teaspoon dark sesame oil

1 In a nonstick Dutch oven or large saucepan, heat the oil and ½ cup of the water over medium heat. Add the onion and bacon, and cook, stirring frequently, until the onion is soft and the water has evaporated, about 7 minutes.

2 Add the bell pepper and cook, stirring frequently, until the pepper is soft, about 5 minutes.

3 Stir in the remaining 1½ cups water, the potatoes, salt, and black pepper, and bring to a boil. Reduce to a simmer, cover, and cook until the potatoes are tender, about 10 minutes.

4 In a small bowl, blend the milk into the flour. Add to the soup, bring to a simmer, and cook, stirring, until slightly thickened, about 3 minutes.

5 Stir in the corn and cook until heated through, about 3 minutes. Stir in the sesame oil and serve. *Makes 4 servings*

per serving: 214 calories, 5.4g total fat (1.4g saturated), 10mg cholesterol, 4g dietary fiber, 37g carbohydrate, 8g protein, 581mg sodium. good source of: lutein, niacin, potassium, riboflavin, thiamin, vitamin B_6, vitamin C.

Herbed Cream of Tomato Soup

To help give the soup a creamy texture, the recipe starts out with a roux, which is a combination of fat and flour (traditionally it would be butter, but we use olive oil instead). When the roux is heated, the starch granules in the flour swell to thicken the soup.

> 1 teaspoon olive oil
>
> 2 tablespoons flour
>
> 1½ cups tomato-vegetable juice
>
> 1 cup evaporated low-fat (2%) milk
>
> ½ cup chopped fresh basil
>
> ¾ teaspoon tarragon
>
> ½ teaspoon salt
>
> ¼ teaspoon pepper
>
> 1 can (15 ounces) crushed tomatoes
>
> ¼ cup tomato paste
>
> 2 teaspoons light brown sugar
>
> 4 teaspoons reduced-fat sour cream

1 In a large nonstick saucepan, heat the oil over medium heat. Add the flour and stir well to coat. Gradually stir in the tomato–vegetable juice and evaporated milk and cook, stirring constantly, until the mixture is smooth and slightly thickened, about 5 minutes.

2 Stir in the basil, tarragon, salt, and pepper. Reduce the heat to low and stir in the crushed tomatoes, tomato paste, and brown sugar. Cover and simmer for 10 minutes, stirring occasionally, to develop the flavors and thicken the soup.

3 Serve the soup topped with a dollop of the sour cream. *Makes 4 servings*

per serving: 167 calories, 3.4g total fat (1.4g saturated), 8mg cholesterol, 3g dietary fiber, 28g carbohydrate, 8g protein, 869mg sodium. good source of: calcium, lycopene, potassium, riboflavin, vitamin B_6, vitamin C.

recipe creator
quick soups

Frozen vegetables are the perfect beginning for a quick "cream of vegetable" soup. Pick ingredients from each of the five categories and follow these basic instructions: In a large nonstick saucepan, sauté 1 small chopped onion and 2 cloves of minced garlic in 2 teaspoons of olive oil until soft. Add **1 VEGETABLE, 1 LIQUID, 1 SEASONING,** and ½ teaspoon salt. Cover and simmer until the vegetables are tender. Transfer the mixture to a food processor or blender and add **1 THICKENER** (do not use a thickener if you are using one of the starchy vegetables, which are marked below with an asterisk). Process to a smooth puree. Reheat gently if necessary. Serve topped with **1** or **2 GARNISHES.** *Makes 4 servings*

FROZEN VEGETABLES	LIQUIDS	SEASONINGS	THICKENERS	GARNISHES
▶ Green beans, 10-oz package	▶ Evaporated milk, low-fat (2%), 1⅓ cups	▶ Tarragon, 1 tsp	▶ Instant potato flakes, 1 Tbsp	▶ Scallions, ⅓ cup thinly sliced
▶ Broccoli, 10-oz package	▶ Broth, chicken or vegetable, 1⅓ cups	▶ Thyme, ¼ tsp	▶ Cream of rice, 1 Tbsp	▶ Cashews or almonds, 2 Tbsp chopped
▶ Cauliflower, 10-oz package	▶ Milk, low-fat (1%) or fat-free, 1⅓ cups	▶ Fresh mint, ⅓ cup chopped		
▶ Asparagus, 9- or 10-oz package	▶ Soymilk, unflavored, 1⅓ cups	▶ Fresh basil, ⅓ cup chopped		▶ Sour cream, reduced-fat, 2 Tbsp
▶ Spinach or other greens, chopped, 10-oz package		▶ Cilantro, ⅓ cup chopped		▶ Grated Parmesan, 2 Tbsp
▶ Brussels sprouts, 10-oz package		▶ Marjoram or savory, ½ tsp		▶ Red bell pepper, ¼ cup minced
▶ Peas,* 10-oz package		▶ Curry powder, 1 tsp		▶ Fresh dill, 2 Tbsp chopped
▶ Lima beans,* 10-oz package				
▶ Butternut squash* puree, 12-oz package				
*starchy vegetables				

Hot & Sour Tofu-Vegetable Soup

This hot and sour soup is relatively mildly spiced. For a hotter soup, increase the black pepper to 1 teaspoon or use ½ teaspoon of red pepper flakes. **Serving suggestion:** Put together an Asian banquet, starting with this soup and then moving on to Swordfish Stir-Fry (*page 58*) or Asian-Style Micro Steamed Bass (*page 61*). Follow with Grilled Duck Salad with Soba Noodles (*page 137*) or Chicken Chow Mein (*page 116*). Then serve Cucumber Salad with Mint-Scallion Dressing (*page 202*), and for dessert, Mango-Tapioca Pudding (*page 234*).

¼ cup dried shiitake mushroom slices

2½ cups boiling water

1½ cups chicken broth, homemade (page 252) or canned

¼ cup rice vinegar

2 tablespoons reduced-sodium soy sauce

3 tablespoons minced fresh ginger

4 cloves garlic, minced

½ teaspoon pepper

¼ teaspoon salt

2 cups shredded bok choy (¼ inch wide)

8 ounces extra-firm tofu, cut into ½-inch cubes

1 tablespoon cornstarch blended with 2 tablespoons water

2 teaspoons dark sesame oil

3 scallions, thinly sliced

1 In a small heatproof bowl, combine the dried mushrooms and boiling water, and let stand for 20 minutes, or until softened. Reserving the soaking liquid, scoop out the dried mushrooms and finely chop. Strain the soaking liquid through a coffee filter or a paper towel-lined sieve.

2 In a large saucepan, combine the mushroom soaking liquid, broth, vinegar, and soy sauce, and bring to a boil. Stir in the mushrooms, ginger, garlic, pepper, and salt, and return to a boil. Reduce to a simmer, cover, and cook for 5 minutes to develop the flavors.

3 Stir in the bok choy and tofu, and cook until the bok choy is tender, about 2 minutes.

4 Stir in the cornstarch mixture and sesame oil, and cook, stirring constantly, until the mixture is slightly thickened, about 1 minute. Add the scallions and serve. *Makes 4 servings*

per serving: 149 calories, 7.4g total fat (1.1g saturated), 0mg cholesterol, 2g dietary fiber, 11g carbohydrate, 12g protein, 604mg sodium. **good source of:** calcium, selenium.

Creamy Two-Mushroom Soup

Although many cookbooks advise choosing mushrooms such as creminis with closed veils (the thin, white mushroom-y stuff that covers the dark gills), a slightly older mushroom, with gills that are showing, will probably have more flavor. When mushrooms have been sitting for awhile (but before they are over the hill and have turned slimy), they actually lose some of their moisture and their flavor begins to concentrate.

2 teaspoons olive oil

1 large onion, finely chopped

1 carrot, halved lengthwise and thinly sliced crosswise

3 cloves garlic, minced

1 pound cremini mushrooms, thinly sliced

¾ pound fresh shiitake mushrooms, stems discarded and caps thinly sliced

3 tablespoons dry sherry, white wine, or broth

2 cups chicken broth, homemade (page 252) or canned

½ cup water

½ teaspoon salt

½ teaspoon pepper

1 cup low-fat (1%) or fat-free milk

1 tablespoon cornstarch blended with 2 tablespoons water

1 In a nonstick Dutch oven or large saucepan, heat the oil over medium heat. Add the onion, carrot, and garlic, and cook, stirring frequently, until the onion is tender, about 7 minutes.

2 Stir in the cremini and shiitake mushrooms. Cover and cook, stirring frequently, until the mushrooms are softened, about 5 minutes.

3 Add the sherry, increase the heat to high, and cook until the sherry has evaporated, about 1 minute. Stir in the chicken broth, water, salt, and pepper. Bring to a boil, reduce to a simmer, cover, and cook until the soup is richly flavored, about 7 minutes.

4 Stir in the milk and bring to a boil. Add the cornstarch mixture and cook, stirring constantly, until slightly thickened, about 1 minute. *Makes 4 servings*

per serving: 166 calories, 3g total fat (0.7g saturated), 2mg cholesterol, 5g dietary fiber, 20g carbohydrate, 11g protein, 618mg sodium. good source of: beta carotene, fiber.

different *spins*

▶**Dressed-Up Black Bean Soup** Follow the directions for *Basic Black Bean Soup* and then try one of these add-ons:

• Stir 1 cup of corn into the soup just before it comes off the heat. Serve topped with a spoonful of salsa, thinly sliced scallions, and baked tortilla chips.

• Stir in 1 or 2 minced chipotle peppers packed in adobo.

• Serve topped with chopped egg white, a dollop of reduced-fat sour cream, and a sprinkling of chopped cilantro.

• Stir in 3 tablespoons of dry sherry and 3 chopped scallions just before serving.

• Serve topped with diced fresh tomato and avocado.

Basic Black Bean Soup

Like the basic black dress, this soup takes to all sorts of accessorizing. See the "Different Spins" box on this page for some ideas. To shorten the cooking time of the beans a bit, you could soak them overnight in cold water to cover by 2 inches. When you're ready to make the soup, drain off the soaking water before proceeding. The cooking time in step 2 will be cut in half. **Timing alert:** This soup takes at least 1½ hours to make, and if you choose to soak the beans ahead of time, you should expect to start the night before.

> 1 tablespoon olive oil
> 1 large onion, finely chopped
> 3 cloves garlic, minced
> 2 cups dried black beans
> 9 cups water
> 3 tablespoons tomato paste
> 1½ teaspoons oregano
> 1 teaspoon cumin
> ¾ teaspoon salt

1 In a large saucepan or Dutch oven, heat the oil over medium heat. Add the onion and garlic, and cook, stirring frequently, until the onion is tender, about 7 minutes. Add the beans and water, and bring to a boil.

2 Reduce to a simmer and skim any foam that has risen to the surface. Stir in the tomato paste, oregano, cumin, and salt. Cook, partially covered, stirring occasionally, until the beans are very tender, about 1½ hours. Check occasionally to make sure there's enough water to just cover the beans.

3 Transfer about one-fourth of the beans, with liquid, to a food processor or blender and puree. Then stir the puree back into the soup. (Or, if you have a hand blender, blend about one-fourth of the soup directly in the pot.) *Makes 4 servings*

per serving: 374 calories, 4.5g total fat (0.7g saturated), 0mg cholesterol, 24g dietary fiber, 65g carbohydrate, 21g protein, 689mg sodium. good source of: fiber, folate, magnesium, potassium, thiamin.

Caldo Verde

In this hearty Portuguese soup, the broth (*caldo*) is made green (*verde*) with lots and lots of shredded kale. An authentic caldo verde from Portugal—where it is almost the national dish—would be made with a garlicky pork sausage and a type of deep-green cabbage. This slimmed down, Americanized version uses turkey sausage and kale instead. **Serving suggestion:** Serve the soup with some Bruschetta (*page 24*).

> 2 teaspoons olive oil
>
> 1 large onion, finely chopped
>
> 3 cloves garlic, minced
>
> 2 sweet Italian-style turkey sausages (5 ounces total), casings removed, crumbled
>
> ¾ pound all-purpose potatoes, thinly sliced
>
> 6 cups shredded kale
>
> 3 cups water
>
> ¾ teaspoon salt
>
> 2 tablespoons red wine vinegar
>
> ½ teaspoon Louisiana-style hot sauce

1 In a nonstick Dutch oven or large saucepan, heat the oil over medium heat. Add the onion and garlic, and cook, stirring often, until the onion is golden brown and tender, about 10 minutes.

2 Add the turkey sausage and cook, stirring occasionally, until the sausage begins to firm up, about 5 minutes.

3 Add the potatoes and kale, stirring to coat. Add the water and salt, and bring to a boil. Reduce to a simmer, cover, and cook until the potatoes are falling apart and the kale is tender, about 15 minutes. Stir in the vinegar and hot sauce and serve. *Makes 4 servings*

per serving: 183 calories, 5.1g total fat (0.9g saturated), 23mg cholesterol, 3g dietary fiber, 26g carbohydrate, 11g protein, 698mg sodium. good source of: beta carotene, indoles, lutein, potassium, sulforaphane, thiamin, vitamin B$_6$, vitamin C, vitamin K.

Dilled Potato-Leek Soup

Although leeks are a perfectly common vegetable in many parts of the world, they have never, for some odd reason, managed to achieve that status in this country. Because the demand for leeks is low, they tend to be quite expensive and usually languish in the supermarket produce section. They deserve better than that, and here is a good recipe to start with.

> 1 tablespoon olive oil
>
> 3 leeks, thinly sliced
>
> 1 large onion, thinly sliced
>
> 3 cloves garlic, minced
>
> 1 pound all-purpose potatoes, thinly sliced
>
> 2 cups chicken broth, homemade (page 252) or canned
>
> 2 cups water
>
> ½ teaspoon salt
>
> ½ teaspoon pepper
>
> ⅔ cup minced fresh dill

1 In a nonstick Dutch oven or large saucepan, heat the oil over medium heat. Add the leeks, onion, and garlic, and cook, stirring often, until the leeks and onion are soft, about 10 minutes.

2 Add the potatoes, broth, water, salt, pepper, and ⅓ cup of the dill, and bring to a boil. Reduce to a simmer, cover, and cook until the potatoes are very tender and falling apart, about 20 minutes.

3 Stir in the remaining ⅓ cup minced dill and serve. *Makes 4 servings*

per serving: 223 calories, 5.8g total fat (1g saturated), 3mg cholesterol, 4g dietary fiber, 39g carbohydrate, 5g protein, 815mg sodium. good source of: folate, potassium, vitamin B$_6$, vitamin C.

Big-Batch Lentil-Bean Soup

This hearty soup is perfect for a big crowd. You can make the soup a day ahead, but add the macaroni shortly before serving, otherwise it will soak up a good deal of the liquid. If you are cooking the pinto beans from scratch, you can use some of the bean cooking liquid instead of the 2 cups of water called for in step 3. **Timing alert:** Start the soup the night before so you can soak the pinto beans; or if you quick-soak the beans, start at least 2 hours before you intend to serve the soup.

> 2 tablespoons olive oil
>
> 3 bunches scallions, thinly sliced (3 cups)
>
> 12 cloves garlic, minced
>
> 3 fresh jalapeño peppers, minced
>
> 5 carrots, quartered lengthwise and thinly sliced crosswise
>
> 1 pound lentils
>
> 3 cans (8 ounces each) no-salt-added tomato sauce
>
> 6 chipotle peppers in adobo, minced
>
> 2½ teaspoons salt
>
> 2 teaspoons ground coriander
>
> 1 teaspoon ground ginger
>
> 14 cups water
>
> 3½ cups cooked pinto beans (page 180) or canned (rinsed and drained)
>
> 12 ounces small elbow macaroni
>
> ½ cup chopped cilantro

1 In a stockpot, heat the oil over low heat. Add the scallions, garlic, and jalapeños, and cook, stirring frequently, until the scallions are tender, about 5 minutes. Add the carrots, cover and cook, stirring occasionally, until the carrots are crisp-tender, about 10 minutes.

2 Stir in the lentils, tomato sauce, chipotle peppers, salt, coriander, ginger, and 12 cups of the water, and bring to a boil. Reduce to a simmer, cover, and cook for 30 minutes.

3 Stir in the pinto beans and remaining 2 cups water, and cook until the lentils are tender, about 20 minutes.

4 Meanwhile, in a large pot of boiling water, cook the macaroni until tender. Drain and add to the soup along with the cilantro. *Makes 20 servings*

per serving: 219 calories, 2.2g total fat (0.3g saturated), 0mg cholesterol, 12g dietary fiber, 40g carbohydrate, 12g protein, 565mg sodium. good source of: beta carotene, fiber, folate, selenium, thiamin, vitamin C.

handling chili peppers

The substances in chili peppers that give them their distinctive heat are called capsaicinoids. The primary capsaicinoid, capsaicin, is so hot that a single drop diluted in 100,000 drops of water will actually blister the tongue.

Depending on your sensitivity to capsaicin, you will either want to wear thin rubber gloves when you handle chilies, or handle them as little as possible and then immediately wash your hands in hot soapy water. With or without gloves, do not touch your eyes while you are cutting the chilies. And don't forget to wash the utensils and cutting board after use.

The same caveats apply for dried hot peppers, with one additional caution: When grinding them (by hand or in a food processor or blender), be careful not to inhale the fumes or let them waft into your eyes.

The capsaicin is primarily concentrated in the pepper's membranous ribs (and not in the seeds as is commonly believed), so removing the ribs can help to reduce the chili pepper's bite. (Of course the seeds also impart considerable fire because they are in close contact with the ribs, so remove them, too.) With chili peppers, you will find that even those of the same type vary in hotness. So use the amounts given in a recipe as a guideline, but then add chilies a bit at a time, until the food reaches the amount of "heat" desired.

Vegetarian Split Pea Soup

Split pea soup often gets its hearty flavor from a ham hock or some smoked sausage, but in this vegetarian version, super-savory dried porcini mushrooms and a little liquid smoke (bottled essence of wood smoke) give this soup a meaty flavor without any meat (and with far less saturated fat and sodium). We used a hickory smoke-based version of liquid smoke, but you can also use mesquite.

1 package (¼ ounce) dried porcini mushrooms

1½ cups boiling water

1 tablespoon olive oil

1 medium onion, thinly sliced

2 cloves garlic, smashed and peeled

2 carrots, thinly sliced

2 cups (1 pound) split peas

3 tablespoons tomato paste

1½ teaspoons liquid smoke seasoning

1½ teaspoons salt

½ teaspoon pepper

½ teaspoon rubbed sage

6 cups water

1 In a small heatproof bowl, combine the dried mushrooms and the boiling water, and let stand for 20 minutes or until softened. Reserving the soaking liquid, scoop out the dried mushrooms. Strain the soaking liquid through a coffee filter or a paper towel-lined sieve.

2 In a nonstick Dutch oven or large saucepan, heat the oil over medium heat. Add the onion and garlic, and cook, stirring often, until the onion is golden brown and tender, about 10 minutes.

3 Add the carrots and cook until tender, about 7 minutes. Stir in the split peas, tomato paste, liquid smoke, salt, pepper, sage, mushrooms, and their soaking liquid. Add the water and bring to a boil. Reduce to a simmer, cover, and cook until the split peas are tender, about 45 minutes.

4 Working in batches, transfer the split peas to a food processor and process until smooth. (Or, if you have a hand blender, puree the soup in the pan.) Return to the saucepan and heat gently over very low heat. ***Makes 6 servings***

per serving: 274 calories, 3.2g total fat (0.4g saturated), 0mg cholesterol, 18g dietary fiber, 46g carbohydrate, 17g protein, 666mg sodium. good source of: beta carotene, fiber, folate, lutein, thiamin, potassium.

different spins

▶**Chicken Minestrone** Follow the directions for *Chicken Noodle Soup (opposite page)*, substituting 1 cup elbow macaroni for the broken vermicelli. And when cooking the carrots in step 1, add 1 cup cut green beans and 1 cup diced tomatoes. In step 3, use chopped fresh basil instead of dill, and add 1 cup cooked white beans along with the chicken.

▶**Chicken-Noodle Egg Drop Soup** Follow the directions for *Chicken Noodle Soup (opposite page)*. Before step 1, in a small bowl, stir together 3 egg whites and 1 tablespoon water. In step 3, after adding the chicken and dill, pour the egg white mixture into the boiling soup stirring constantly. Stir in 2 tablespoons lemon juice when serving.

▶**Chunky Vegetarian Split Pea Soup** Follow the directions for *Vegetarian Split Pea Soup*, and substitute 1 large peeled and sliced sweet potato for the carrots. Increase the water to 7 cups. Once the soup has been pureed, stir in 1 cup cooked brown rice, 1½ cups thawed frozen peas, ½ cup minced red onion, and ¼ cup chopped fresh basil.

Italian Cabbage, Chick-Pea & Pasta Soup

This soup is more or less a variant of a minestrone, which in Italian literally means big soup. While we've used cabbage, feel free to substitute another more unusual cooking green such as collards, beet greens, or turnip greens. The flavor will be slightly different, but the end result will still be delicious. **Serving suggestion:** For even more flavor, top the soup with a spoonful of grated Parmesan or Pesto Sauce (*page 256*).

> 1 tablespoon olive oil
>
> 2 red bell peppers, cut into ½-inch chunks
>
> 5 cloves garlic, minced
>
> 6 cups (¾ pound) shredded Savoy or green cabbage
>
> 2 cups chicken broth, homemade (page 252) or canned
>
> 2½ cups water
>
> 1 can (14½ ounces) stewed tomatoes
>
> 1 can (15½ ounces) chick-peas, rinsed and drained
>
> 2 teaspoons grated lemon zest
>
> ½ teaspoon salt
>
> ½ cup small pasta shapes, such as ditalini or elbow macaroni

1 In a nonstick Dutch oven or large saucepan, heat the oil over medium heat. Add the bell peppers and cook, stirring frequently, until soft, about 5 minutes.

2 Add the garlic and cabbage, stirring to coat. Cover and cook until the cabbage has wilted, about 5 minutes.

3 Add the broth, water, stewed tomatoes, chick-peas, 1 teaspoon of the lemon zest, and the salt, and bring to a boil. Reduce to a simmer, cover, and cook for 10 minutes.

4 Add the pasta, cover, and cook until the cabbage is tender and the pasta is al dente, about 10 minutes. Stir in the remaining 1 teaspoon lemon zest. *Makes 4 servings*

per serving: 266 calories, 5.4g total fat (0.7g saturated), 0mg cholesterol, 12g dietary fiber, 44g carbohydrate, 12g protein, 952mg sodium. good source of: beta carotene, fiber, folate, indoles, magnesium, potassium, selenium, sulforaphane, thiamin, vitamin B_6, vitamin C, vitamin E.

Chicken Noodle Soup

At its purest, chicken noodle soup is mostly chicken broth, so it pays to make your own or use a really high-quality storebought broth. Some gourmet delis even sell refrigerated "homemade" broth. This soul-soothing soup also lends itself to some simple variations: See "Different Spins" (*opposite page*).

> 6 cups chicken broth, homemade (page 252) or canned
>
> 2 carrots, thinly sliced
>
> ¼ teaspoon salt
>
> ¼ teaspoon pepper
>
> 1 cup broken vermicelli or angel hair pasta
>
> 2 cups diced cooked chicken breast
>
> ⅓ cup minced fresh dill

1 In a medium saucepan, bring the broth to a boil over medium heat. Add the carrots, salt, and pepper. Cover and cook until the carrots are tender, about 5 minutes.

2 Add the noodles to the boiling broth and cook, covered, until the noodles are tender. Drain.

3 Add the chicken and dill to the boiling soup and cook just until the chicken is heated through, about 1 minute. *Makes 4 servings*

per serving: 211 calories, 2.8g total fat (0.8g saturated), 60mg cholesterol, 2g dietary fiber, 15g carbohydrate, 28g protein, 886mg sodium. good source of: beta carotene, niacin, selenium, vitamin B_6.

did you know?

Here's a high-fiber alternative to tomato or cream sauces on pasta: Toss the cooked pasta with lentil (or other bean) soup. This is a quick version of the nutritious pasta-and-bean dishes popular in Italy. If you want a smooth sauce, puree the soup before tossing it with the pasta.

Lentil & Sausage Soup

Peppery lentils are a perfect partner for sausage—in this case turkey sausage, which has one-third the saturated fat of its pork counterpart. Not only are lentils high in flavor, fiber, and folate, but they cook in only a half hour (versus a couple of hours for most other legumes). This soup makes enough for 8 servings, so serve it to a crowd, or freeze it in 1- to 2-cup containers and have it on hand for a last-minute meal.

2 teaspoons olive oil

1 large onion, diced

4 cloves garlic, minced

3 carrots, halved lengthwise and thinly sliced crosswise

1 pound lentils

3 cans (14½ ounces each) no-salt-added stewed tomatoes, chopped with their juice

1 teaspoon salt

½ teaspoon pepper

¼ teaspoon allspice

4½ cups water

8 ounces hot Italian-style turkey sausage, casings removed, crumbled

1 In a nonstick Dutch oven or large saucepan, heat the oil over medium heat. Add the onion and garlic, and cook, stirring occasionally, until the onion is soft, about 7 minutes.

2 Stir in the carrots and cook, stirring occasionally, until the carrots are tender, about 4 minutes.

3 Add the lentils, stewed tomatoes, salt, pepper, allspice, and water, and bring to a boil. Reduce to a simmer, cover, and cook until the lentils are tender, about 30 minutes.

4 Add the sausage and simmer until cooked through, about 5 minutes. *Makes 8 servings*

per serving: 306 calories, 3.5g total fat (0.7g saturated), 20mg cholesterol, 21g dietary fiber, 46g carbohydrate, 23g protein, 512mg sodium. good source of: beta carotene, fiber, folate, potassium, thiamin, vitamin B$_6$, vitamin C, zinc.

Mushroom, Barley & Pasta Soup

This earthy soup is hearty enough for a main course. If not served right away, the barley may soak up all the liquid, but if this happens, you can eat the dish like a stew. Or, to restore it to its soup-like consistency, just thin it with a bit of water.

2 teaspoons olive oil

1 large onion, finely chopped

3 cloves garlic, minced

½ pound cremini mushrooms, thinly sliced

2 cups canned tomatoes, chopped with their juice

¾ cup pearl barley

1 teaspoon liquid smoke seasoning

¾ teaspoon salt

½ teaspoon rubbed sage

4½ cups water

½ cup small pasta shells

½ cup grated Parmesan cheese

1 In a nonstick Dutch oven or large saucepan, heat the oil over low heat. Add the onion and garlic, and cook, stirring frequently, until tender, about 7 minutes.

2 Stir in the mushrooms and cook 3 minutes. Stir in the tomatoes, barley, liquid smoke, salt, sage, and water, and bring to a boil. Reduce to a simmer, cover, and cook for 35 minutes.

3 Stir in the pasta, cover, and cook until the barley and pasta are tender, about 10 minutes. Serve the soup sprinkled with the Parmesan cheese. *Makes 4 servings*

per serving: 313 calories, 6.9g total fat (2.9g saturated), 10mg cholesterol, 9g dietary fiber, 50g carbohydrate, 15g protein, 873mg sodium. good source of: fiber, niacin, selenium.

Beet & Tomato Borscht

Though all borschts—and there are hundreds of regional versions—include beets or beet juice, this peasant soup from Eastern Europe is fundamentally a blank canvas: sort of a "stone soup." We've added lima beans and potatoes to our vegetarian rendition, but you could try Yukon Gold potatoes and black-eyed peas, or sweet potatoes and white beans, or corn and black beans. The variations are endless.

 2 teaspoons olive oil
 1 medium onion, finely chopped
 3 cloves garlic, minced
 1¼ pounds beets, peeled and cut into ½-inch chunks
 ¾ pound red potatoes, cut into 1-inch chunks
 2 cans (14½ ounces each) stewed tomatoes, chopped with their juice
 2 cups water
 1 cup frozen lima beans
 3 tablespoons no-salt-added tomato paste
 3 tablespoons red wine vinegar
 ¾ teaspoon salt

1 In a nonstick Dutch oven or large saucepan, heat the oil over medium heat. Add the onion and garlic, and cook, stirring frequently, until the onion is soft, about 7 minutes.

2 Stir in the beets, potatoes, tomatoes and their juice, water, lima beans, tomato paste, vinegar, and salt, and bring to a boil.

3 Reduce to a simmer, cover, and cook until the beets and potatoes are tender, about 1 hour. *Makes 4 servings*

per serving: 256 calories, 3.1g total fat (0.5g saturated), 0mg cholesterol, 9g dietary fiber, 53g carbohydrate, 9g protein, 882mg sodium. good source of: betacyanins, fiber, folate, magnesium, niacin, potassium, riboflavin, thiamin, vitamin B$_6$, vitamin C, vitamin E.

different spins

▶**Lentil & Chicken Soup** Follow the directions for *Lentil & Sausage Soup (opposite page)*. In step 3, stir in 1 teaspoon grated orange zest and ¼ teaspoon minced rosemary. In step 4, omit the sausage and stir in ½ pound of skinless, boneless chicken thighs cut into bite-size pieces. Cook for 10 minutes instead of 5, or until the chicken is cooked through. Stir in ¼ cup chopped mint at serving time.

▶**Chilled Borscht Garni** Follow the directions for *Beet & Tomato Borscht*, but omit the lima beans. Chill the soup after it's finished cooking. At serving time, stir in ½ cup thinly sliced radishes, ½ cup sliced scallions, and the chopped white of 1 hard-cooked egg. Top each serving with 2 tablespoons of plain fat-free yogurt and fresh dill sprigs.

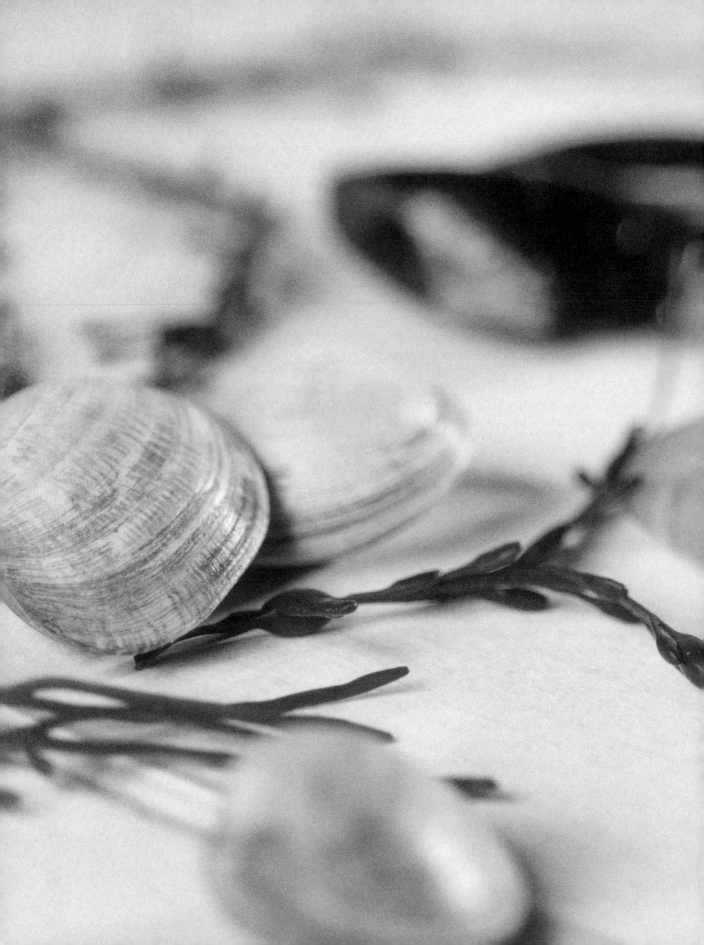

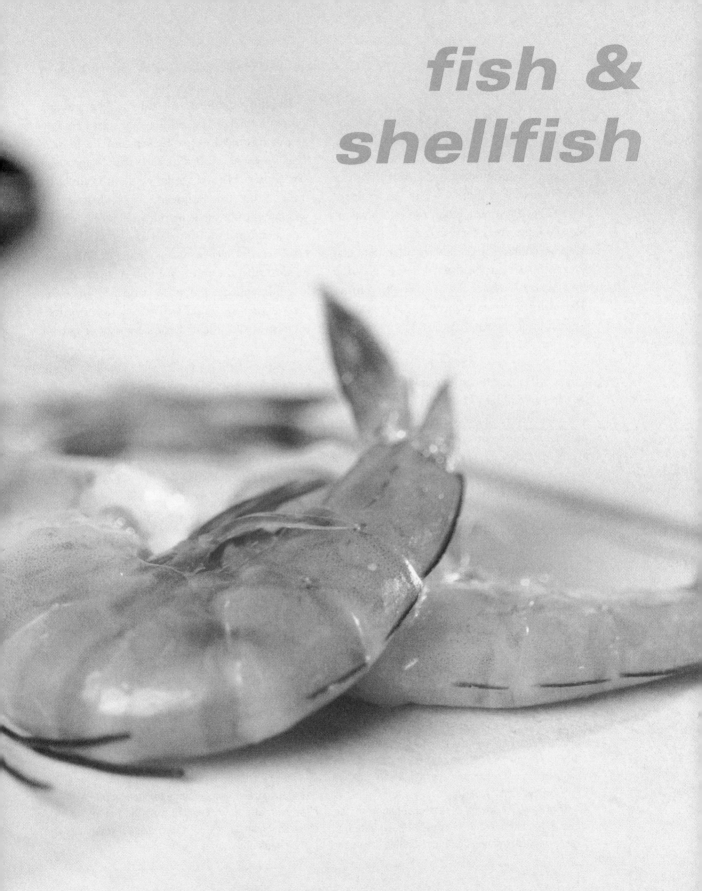

fish & shellfish

fish

Fish is delicate, and if overcooked will be dry and tough, so the trick is to find the right balance. Fish should be cooked just long enough to destroy any harmful organisms (145°F) but not beyond the point of moistness and tenderness.

Use "The 10-Minute Rule" (*below*) for calculating cooking times for fish, using any of the following cooking methods. Remember that frozen fish need not be thawed before cooking as long as you allow for the extra cooking time.

Roasting/baking Generally done at high temperatures (between 425° and 500°F), roasted fish stays moist because the high heat seals in its juices. Dry-heat methods such as roasting and baking work best with fattier fish like salmon (*see Oven-Roasted Salmon Fillets, page 46*). Leaner fish can also be cooked this way; they just need either additional moisture, or a light brushing of oil, or a protective topping (*see Walnut-Topped Baked Snapper, page 54*).

Baking in parchment paper (or foil) packets also keeps fish moist, especially if vegetables or a little liquid (such as broth or wine) are included in the packets (*see the Fish in Parchment "Recipe Creator" on page 56*).

Broiling/grilling All fish can be broiled, although thicker, fattier fillets and steaks hold up best to this method (*see Salmon Steaks with Salsa Verde, page 48, or Broiled Tuna with Mango Vinaigrette, page 51*); and while whole fish cannot be broiled, they can be grilled. Lean, delicate fish will benefit from marinating and basting to provide additional moisture (*see Broiled Halibut with Fresh Tomato-Tangerine Sauce, page 54*). There's no need to turn the fish as it broils or grills: In fact it will be moister if you don't turn it. Once the top (or the bottom, if you're grilling) is seared, the rest of the fish will cook by way of radiant heat.

Give any grill or broiler rack a liberal coating of nonstick cooking spray before grilling fish, and preheat the rack before placing the fish on it. Position the rack so the fish is 4 to 6 inches from the heat source. To eliminate the danger of the fish falling apart when you grill it, you can use a special hinged basket for whole fish or a grill topper for fillets and small steaks.

Sautéing/pan-frying Fillets of fish take well to pan-frying. A light coating of cornstarch,

the 10-minute rule

The "10-minute rule," also called the Canadian Cooking Theory, is a standard guide to fish cooking times devised by the Canadian Fisheries and Marine Service. This theory applies to all cuts—whole, fillets, and steaks—and to all methods of cooking.

Here's how it works: Simply measure the fish at its thickest point and cook it for 10 minutes per inch of thickness. For example, in cooking a fish steak that is ¾ inch thick, the total cooking time is 7½ minutes. Turn the fish (except thin fillets) halfway through the cooking time.

There are, however, a few exceptions to the rule: **1.** Measure a stuffed fish *after* it is stuffed. **2.** For frozen fish (no need to thaw), double the cooking time. **3.** Add 5 minutes if the fish is cooked in a sauce. **4.** The rule does not apply at all to microwave cooking, which is much faster than conventional methods.

Because the 10-minute rule has several exceptions, it should really be taken more as a rule of thumb. This makes it especially important to be familiar with the appearance of properly cooked fish as an additional doneness test (*see "How to Tell When Fish Is Done," opposite page*). Test for doneness well before the prescribed cooking time has elapsed: Fish will continue to cook by retained heat even after it is removed from the pan or the oven, so it may be best to stop cooking it when it is just a shade underdone.

crumbs, or flour (*see Pan-Fried Grouper with Orange-Carrot Sauce, page 55, and Red Snapper Escabeche, page 57*) will keep the fish moist, and give it a crisp crust. Make sure the pan is hot before adding the fish.

Stir-frying Chunks of fish can be stir-fried as you would poultry or meat (*see Swordfish Stir-Fry, page 58*). Watch the cooking time carefully, or the fish will overcook and dry out. As with pan-frying, the fish will benefit from a light dredging in cornstarch or flour.

Steaming Any fish that can be poached, whether whole, steak, or fillet, is also a candidate for steaming—and since the fish is not immersed in cooking liquid, it retains more of its natural flavor. There are a number of different options for steaming fish: See "Fish Steaming Methods" (*page 60*).

Microwaving The microwave is the answer for people who think cooking seafood is complicated or tricky. This method works best for cooking fish in the simplest manner possible, since any added sauces or ingredients could present some tricky microwave maneuvering. And because microwave ovens are so different, consult your manual for specific cooking times. Always check the fish for doneness before the recommended cooking time has elapsed: You can always cook it more, but nothing can be done if the fish is overcooked. Remove the fish from the oven when the edges are opaque but the center is still slightly translucent; let it stand for the indicated time after microwaving so it can continue cooking from retained heat. Test again after the standing time elapses—use the same visual clues as in "How to Tell When Fish Is Done" (*above, right*)—and return the fish to the microwave if it is not fully cooked throughout.

You can also microwave fish in parchment paper packets (but not foil). And if you need to thaw frozen fish, microwaving is an excellent way to do it.

how to tell when fish is done

Knowing what fish looks like when it's cooked properly is more important than blindly trusting cooking times. The pan you use, or the grill temperature, and a host of other factors can make the fish you are cooking behave differently than a general rule. So here are some visual clues to help you out:

When fish is done, the flesh should be just barely opaque—not translucent, but not chalky. The flesh will be firm but moist. If you take a fork and use it to pull the flesh of the fish apart, it should just barely flake apart. If it flakes too easily and seems somewhat dry, the fish is already overcooked.

Poaching This gentle cooking method can be used for almost any kind of firm-fleshed fish, and lean fish is ideal for it. Fish steaks, fillets, or whole fish can be poached by immersing the fish in a pan of simmering fish stock, a mixture of water and lemon juice or wine, or seasoned water (*see Poached Salmon with Green Mayonnaise, page 50, and Salmon, Snow Pea & Potato Salad, page 50*). Although you can improvise a poaching pan by using a roasting pan and a roasting rack, the most efficient equipment is a fish poacher—a long, narrow pan fitted with a removable rack—for large whole fish. Bring the liquid to a gentle simmer, partially cover the pan, and poach until the fish is opaque.

Stewing/braising A simple vegetable-based soup, stew, or chowder can be made into a main dish by adding chunks of fish. Since fish cooks in a relatively short amount of time, it should always be added during the final few minutes of cooking (*see Spicy Fish Chowder, page 59, and Provençal Cod Stew, page 62*).

Oven-Roasted Salmon Fillets

Salmon has so much flavor that the simplest of cooking methods are sometimes the best. The fat content of salmon (luckily it's mostly healthful omega-3 fatty acids) makes it well suited to high-temperature roasting. Be sure the oven is well preheated. When placed skin-side down on a baking sheet and baked in a hot oven, there's no need to skin the fish before roasting. Once cooked, the fish comes off the pan easily, leaving the skin behind. **Serving suggestion:** The richness of salmon pairs well with the fresh, tangy flavors of relishes and salsas. Try any of the fruit salsas in the "Recipe Creator" on page 262, or try Tomatillo Salsa (*page 261*), Papaya-Corn Salsa (*page 263*), Spicy Pear & Pepper Salsa (*page 264*), or Tomato-Melon Salsa (*page 263*).

4 salmon fillets, skin on (5 ounces each)
2 tablespoons fresh lemon juice
½ teaspoon salt

1 Preheat the oven to 450°F. Place the salmon fillets, skin-side down, in a jelly-roll pan. Sprinkle the fillets with the lemon juice and salt.

2 Roast for 10 minutes, or until the fish just barely flakes when tested with a fork. Slip a spatula between the flesh and the skin and lift, leaving the skin behind. *Makes 4 servings*

per serving: 232 calories, 12g total fat (2g saturated), 92mg cholesterol, 0g dietary fiber, 1g carbohydrate, 29g protein, 361mg sodium. good source of: niacin, omega-3 fatty acids, selenium, vitamin B_{12}, vitamin D.

Thai-Style Salmon

A fresh, uncooked salad-style vegetable sauce tops the hot baked salmon. The contrast in temperatures and textures is extremely satisfying. There is also a wonderful contrast between the richness of the salmon and the herbal, citrusy flavors of the vegetable mixture. **Serving suggestion:** For a one-dish meal, toss the vegetables with a bowl of whole-wheat linguine and serve the pasta topped with the salmon.

¼ cup fresh lime juice
4 teaspoons reduced-sodium soy sauce
1 tablespoon sugar
2 carrots, shredded
1 red bell pepper, cut into thin slivers
4 salmon fillets, skin on (5 ounces each)
1 teaspoon ground coriander
½ teaspoon salt
3 tablespoons chopped cilantro
2 tablespoons chopped fresh mint

1 Preheat the oven to 450°F. In a medium bowl, whisk together 3 tablespoons of the lime juice, the soy sauce, and sugar. Add the carrots and bell pepper, and toss to combine. Refrigerate until serving time.

2 Place the salmon fillets, skin-side down, on a baking sheet. Sprinkle the fish with the remaining 1 tablespoon lime juice, the coriander, and the salt. Roast for about 10 minutes, or until the fish just flakes when tested with a fork. Slip a spatula between the flesh and the skin and lift, leaving the skin behind.

3 Stir the cilantro and mint into the carrot-pepper mixture and spoon over the hot salmon. *Makes 4 servings*

per serving: 217 calories, 8.9g total fat (1.5g saturated), 68mg cholesterol, 2g dietary fiber, 12g carbohydrate, 23g protein, 536mg sodium. good source of: beta carotene, niacin, omega-3 fatty acids, selenium, vitamin B_{12}, vitamin C, vitamin D.

Roasted Salmon, Watercress & Lentil Salad

The watercress and lentil salad that serves as a backdrop to a simple roasted salmon is dressed with a lemony pesto-style cilantro dressing. If you're making this for company and want to get some of the preparation done ahead of time, cook the lentils, make the dressing, and toss the lentils with half of the dressing. Then closer to serving time, toss the lentils, watercress, and red onion together with the remaining dressing. And don't roast the salmon until just before serving in order to serve it warm.

2 cups chicken broth, homemade (page 252) or canned

1 cup lentils

1 cup sliced carrots

½ teaspoon salt

½ teaspoon pepper

3 tablespoons fresh lemon juice

½ cup packed cilantro sprigs

3 tablespoons water

1 tablespoon olive oil

1 clove garlic, peeled

2 bunches watercress, tough stems removed

¼ cup chopped red onion

Oven-Roasted Salmon Fillets (opposite page)

1 In a medium nonstick saucepan, combine the broth with the lentils, carrots, and ¼ teaspoon each of the salt and pepper. Cover and bring to a boil over high heat. Reduce the heat to medium-low and simmer until the lentils are tender, about 45 minutes. Drain off any excess liquid. Transfer to a large bowl and set aside to cool to lukewarm.

2 Meanwhile, in a food processor, combine the lemon juice, the remaining ¼ teaspoon each salt and pepper, the cilantro, water, oil, and garlic. Process to a smooth puree and add to the lentils.

3 Add the watercress and red onion to the lentils and toss to combine.

4 Roast the salmon. Serve the hot salmon on a bed of lentil salad. *Makes 4 servings*

per serving: 396 calories, 13g total fat (2g saturated), 68mg cholesterol, 16g dietary fiber, 34g carbohydrate, 37g protein, 593mg sodium. **good source of:** beta carotene, fiber, folate, niacin, omega-3 fatty acids, potassium, selenium, thiamin, vitamin B_{12}, vitamin B_6, vitamin D.

is fish brain food?

Fish may turn out to be brain food after all, just as grandma always claimed. Fish has already gotten the nod for its cardiovascular benefits. Now there's evidence that eating fish can play a positive role in mental health.

It may sound like a joke, but the brain is largely composed of fat. Fats, along with water, are the chief components of brain cell membranes and the specialized tissues enclosing the nerves. The anti-fat message promoted as part of heart-healthy diets makes it easy to forget that not all fats are "bad," and that some types are essential to human life.

The saturated fat that comes primarily from meat and full-fat dairy products is not what the brain cells need. They do need polyunsaturated fats, especially the long-chain omega-3 fatty acids found in fish, which are called eicosapentenoic acid (EPA) and docosahexenoic acid (DHA). Fish get them from the algae they eat.

Just exactly how (or if) these beneficial fats may promote mental health is being extensively researched. In the meantime, there are plenty of other good (and tasty) reasons to eat fish.

Barbecued Salmon with White Bean Salad

The combination of four common pantry items—ketchup, all-fruit spread, vinegar, and soy sauce—makes an instant barbecue sauce, a nice trick to know when you don't have bottled barbecue sauce on hand.

> 2 tablespoons orange all-fruit spread
> ¼ cup rice vinegar
> 1 tablespoon ketchup
> 1½ teaspoons reduced-sodium soy sauce
> ¼ teaspoon ground ginger
> 4 skinless salmon fillets (5 ounces each)
> ¼ cup chopped cilantro
> ½ teaspoon salt
> 1 Granny Smith apple, diced
> 1 cup cooked white beans (page 180) or canned (rinsed and drained)
> ¼ cup finely chopped red bell pepper
> 3 radishes (optional), thinly sliced

1 In a small bowl, combine the fruit spread, 1 tablespoon of the vinegar, the ketchup, soy sauce, and ginger. Brush the salmon with half the barbecue mixture.

2 In a medium bowl, combine the remaining 3 tablespoons vinegar, the cilantro, and salt. Add the apple, white beans, bell pepper, and radishes (if using), tossing to coat.

3 Spray a grill rack with nonstick cooking spray. Preheat the grill to medium. Grill the salmon, turning once and brushing with the remaining barbecue mixture, for 7 to 10 minutes, or until the fish just flakes when tested with a fork. Serve the salmon with the bean salad. *Makes 4 servings*

per serving: 328 calories, 11g total fat (2g saturated), 85mg cholesterol, 4g dietary fiber, 24g carbohydrate, 32g protein, 476mg sodium. good source of: niacin, omega-3 fatty acids, selenium, thiamin, vitamin B$_{12}$, vitamin D.

Salmon Steaks with Salsa Verde

Although you can get salmon fillets without their skin, salmon steaks need the skin (and the center bone) to hold them together as they cook. Just remove the skin before eating. (And in this case, where the salmon is served with a sauce, you might want to remove the skin before you plate the salmon and cover it with sauce.) **Serving suggestion:** Serve the salmon with something that will get good mileage out of the delicious green sauce, such as baked potatoes or brown rice.

> 1 green bell pepper, roasted (page 190)
> ½ cup packed cilantro sprigs
> ¼ cup orange juice
> 2 tablespoons fresh lime juice
> 1 tablespoon olive oil
> 1 canned or bottled jalapeño pepper
> 1 anchovy fillet
> ½ teaspoon salt
> 1 scallion, thinly sliced
> 4 salmon steaks (6 ounces each)
> 1 teaspoon tarragon

1 Preheat the broiler. Roast the bell pepper. (Leave the broiler on.) When the pepper is cool enough to handle, peel and transfer to a food processor or blender.

2 Add the cilantro, orange juice, lime juice, oil, jalapeño, anchovy, and ¼ teaspoon of the salt, and process to a smooth puree. Transfer the sauce to a small bowl and stir in the scallion.

3 Rub the fish with the remaining ¼ teaspoon salt and the tarragon. Broil 4 to 6 inches from the heat, turning once, for 6 minutes, or until the salmon just flakes when tested with a fork. Serve the salmon topped with the green sauce. Remove the salmon skin before eating. *Makes 4 servings*

per serving: 276 calories, 14g total fat (2.4g saturated), 93mg cholesterol, 1g dietary fiber, 6g carbohydrate, 30g protein, 418mg sodium. good source of: niacin, omega-3 fatty acids, selenium, vitamin B$_{12}$, vitamin C, vitamin D.

Herbed Salmon Burgers

When salmon is processed for canning, its bones become softened and edible, and a source of dietary calcium. Here salmon is blended with oats (for body and soluble fiber) and grated fresh apple (for moistness, soluble fiber, and a pleasing contrast to the rich salmon) to make burgers. The burger mixture is also seasoned with fresh herbs and "lite" teriyaki sauce. The "lite" on the label usually indicates that the sauce is about 50% lower in sodium than a standard teriyaki sauce. **Serving suggestion:** You can serve the burgers simply on whole-grain rolls, with tomato slices and lettuce, or up the ante and top the burgers with Red Onion Marmalade (*page 264*), Tomatillo Salsa (*page 261*), or Corn Relish (*page 264*).

1 tablespoon light mayonnaise
1 tablespoon fresh lemon juice
⅓ cup quick-cooking oats

¼ cup chopped fresh basil
2 tablespoons chopped mint
2 scallions, thinly sliced
1 small apple, peeled and grated
1 can (14¾ ounces) sockeye salmon, not drained
3 tablespoons "lite" teriyaki sauce

1 In a large bowl, combine the mayonnaise and lemon juice. Add the oats, stirring until moistened.

2 Add the basil, mint, scallions, and apple. Stir in the salmon and teriyaki sauce until evenly combined. Shape the burger mixture into four 1-inch-thick patties.

3 Spray a large nonstick skillet with nonstick cooking spray. Cook the burgers over medium heat until brown and heated through, about 4 minutes per side. *Makes 4 servings*

per serving: 236 calories, 9.6g total fat (1.9g saturated), 47mg cholesterol, 2g dietary fiber, 14g carbohydrate, 23g protein, 831mg sodium. good source of: calcium, niacin, omega-3 fatty acids, selenium, vitamin D.

canned fish

"Canned fish" usually means tuna, but there are many other canned varieties—from salmon and sardines to herring and mackerel—that are convenient ways to add heart-healthy fish to your diet. There are even canned shrimp, oysters, clams, and crabmeat. Here are some pointers:

▶**Omega-3s** These polyunsaturated fats may help lower the risk of heart disease. Canned salmon, sardines, and herring contain more omega-3s than canned tuna. A serving of sardines or herring has more than some fish-oil capsules. Canned salmon is usually packed in its own oil, which also contains omega-3s.

▶**Choose fatty fish?** Yes. Fatty fish like sardines contain more total fat, but also more of the heart-healthy omega-3 fatty acids. Just avoid canned fish containing lots of vegetable oil, if you don't want extra calories.

▶**Sardine and herring variations** Compare the labels, since brands vary greatly in their fat and calorie content. Companies may pack different

species and fish from different locales (those from colder water will have more fat), as well as add various ingredients.

▶**Cholesterol** This usually isn't an issue with canned fish. Most contain 20 to 50 mg in 3 ounces—less than meat or poultry. Sardines are an exception, with 100 mg or more in 3 ounces of some types, and shrimp usually have about 150 mg in 3 ounces, but they're still healthful choices.

▶**Boning up** If you're trying to consume more calcium, eat the bones in canned sardines, salmon, and mackerel. The bones are softened during processing. A 3-ounce serving generally supplies nearly as much calcium as a glass of milk.

▶**More salt than the sea** Canned fish is usually high in added salt, containing up to 10 times as much sodium as fresh fish. If you're trying to cut down on sodium, choose "low-salt" or "no added salt" varieties. Draining the water and rinsing the fish in a colander removes a fair amount of salt; draining the oil removes less.

Poached Salmon with Green Mayonnaise

The classic accompaniment to a poached salmon is what the French call a *mayonnaise verte*, or green mayonnaise. An authentic green mayonnaise would be made with raw egg yolks and lots of olive oil. This is fraught with health risks, so our "mayonnaise" is made with fat-free yogurt and a bit of prepared mayonnaise. Fresh spinach adds the body that would ordinarily have been provided by the emulsion of oil and egg yolks. If you can't get all of the fresh herbs called for, you can use just one or two; but if you choose dill or chives, don't use more than ¼ cup total, or the sauce will be too strongly flavored. **Timing alert:** The salmon needs to chill for about 1 hour before serving.

> 3 cups water
>
> 1 carrot, thinly sliced
>
> 1 teaspoon coriander seeds
>
> 1 bay leaf
>
> ¾ teaspoon salt
>
> 1¼ pounds salmon fillet, in 1 piece, skinless
>
> 2 cups fresh spinach leaves
>
> ⅔ cup plain fat-free yogurt
>
> 1 tablespoon light mayonnaise
>
> 1 tablespoon fresh lemon juice
>
> 2 tablespoons chopped fresh tarragon
>
> 2 tablespoons minced chives
>
> 2 tablespoons minced dill

1 In a large skillet, bring the water, carrot, coriander seeds, bay leaf, and ½ teaspoon of the salt to a boil over medium heat.

2 Add the salmon and reduce the heat to a bare simmer. Cover and cook until the fish just flakes when tested with a fork, about 10 minutes.

3 With a slotted spatula, transfer the salmon to a plate and set aside to cool. Strain the poaching liquid and reserve 2 tablespoons. Cover the salmon and refrigerate until chilled, at least 1 hour. Discard the remaining poaching liquid and the solids.

4 In a medium pan of boiling water, cook the spinach 10 seconds to blanch. Squeeze dry and transfer to a food processor. Add the reserved poaching liquid, the yogurt, mayonnaise, and lemon juice, and process to a smooth puree. Transfer to a medium bowl and stir in the remaining ¼ teaspoon salt, the tarragon, chives, and dill. Refrigerate until serving time.

5 At serving time, cut the fillet into 4 portions. Serve the salmon with the sauce spooned on top. *Makes 4 servings*

per serving: 288 calories, 14g total fat (2.3g saturated), 90mg cholesterol, 1g dietary fiber, 7g carbohydrate, 33g protein, 579mg sodium. good source of: beta carotene, niacin, omega-3 fatty acids, potassium, riboflavin, selenium, thiamin, vitamin B$_{12}$, vitamin D.

Salmon, Snow Pea & Potato Salad

Lemongrass has an aromatic citrusy flavor—like lemon but intriguingly different—and is used here in the poaching liquid for the salmon fillet. However, if you don't want to scurry around finding lemongrass (*see "About Lemongrass," opposite page*), lemon zest will do fine.

> 1 pound red potatoes, cut into bite-size chunks
>
> 6 ounces snow peas, strings removed
>
> ¾ cup water
>
> 1 stalk lemongrass, thinly sliced, or 3 strips of lemon zest
>
> ¾ pound skinless salmon fillet, in 1 piece
>
> 2 tablespoons light mayonnaise
>
> 2 tablespoons fresh lemon juice
>
> 1 tablespoon reduced-sodium soy sauce
>
> ¼ teaspoon salt
>
> ¼ cup minced dill
>
> 1 package (10 ounces) frozen corn kernels, thawed
>
> 6 cups torn mixed salad greens

1 In a vegetable steamer, steam the potatoes until firm-tender, 7 to 10 minutes. Add the snow peas during the last 1 minute of cooking time.

2 Meanwhile, in a small skillet, bring the water and lemongrass to a boil over medium heat. Add the salmon, reduce to a simmer, cover, and cook until the fish just flakes when tested with a fork, about 7 minutes.

3 With a slotted spatula, transfer the salmon to a plate and set aside to cool. Strain the poaching liquid and reserve ½ cup. When cool enough to handle, pull off and discard the salmon skin and cut the flesh into bite-size chunks.

4 In a large bowl, whisk together the reserved poaching liquid, the mayonnaise, lemon juice, soy sauce, and salt. Stir in the dill.

5 Add the potatoes, snow peas, and corn, tossing to coat with the dressing. Gently fold in the salmon. Serve the salmon salad on a bed of greens. The salad can be warm, at room temperature, or chilled. *Makes 4 servings*

per serving: 349 calories, 11g total fat (1.7g saturated), 55mg cholesterol, 6g dietary fiber, 42g carbohydrate, 35g protein, 400mg sodium. good source of: folate, niacin, omega-3 fatty acids, potassium, selenium, thiamin, vitamin B$_{12}$, vitamin B$_6$, vitamin C, vitamin D.

about lemongrass

Lemongrass, a common ingredient in Thai cooking, looks like tall, woody scallions. Although dried lemongrass is generally available at Asian markets, especially those that specialize in Southeast Asian cuisines, you can sometimes find fresh lemongrass at certain Asian markets and some farmers' markets. When choosing fresh lemongrass, look for bulbs that are soft, rather than hard and dried out. To prepare lemongrass for cooking, peel off one or two of the tough outer layers to expose the softer inside, and then thinly slice the thick bulb and about ½ inch of the stalk. Crush the pieces slightly with the flat side of a knife to release more of the flavor.

Broiled Tuna with Mango Vinaigrette

A nectar is a fruit juice that includes the fruit pulp and is invariably sweetened. It makes a nice basis for a quick, low-fat salad dressing. The yellow bell pepper is here because it has a mild, sweet flavor and contributes nice color to this dish, but you could just as easily use a red pepper.

> ¾ pound tuna steak
>
> ¾ teaspoon salt
>
> 2 cloves garlic
>
> ½ cup mango nectar
>
> 2 tablespoons red wine vinegar
>
> 1 tablespoon olive oil
>
> 3 tablespoons chopped fresh mint
>
> 1½ cups cooked pinto beans (page 180) or canned (rinsed and drained)
>
> 1 yellow bell pepper, diced
>
> 1 cup halved cherry tomatoes
>
> 3 scallions, thinly sliced

1 Preheat the broiler. Sprinkle the tuna with ¼ teaspoon of the salt. Broil the tuna 4 inches from the heat, turning once, for 7 minutes, or until the fish just flakes when tested with a fork. Set aside to cool, then cut into bite-size pieces.

2 In a small pot of boiling water, cook the garlic for 2 minutes to blanch. Drain and finely chop.

3 In a large bowl, combine the remaining ½ teaspoon salt, the garlic, mango nectar, vinegar, oil, and mint. Stir in the beans, bell pepper, tomatoes, and scallions, tossing to combine.

4 Gently fold in the tuna and serve warm, at room temperature, or chilled. *Makes 4 servings*

per serving: 261 calories, 4.9g total fat (0.8g saturated), 41mg cholesterol, 7g dietary fiber, 27g carbohydrate, 28g protein, 479mg sodium. good source of: fiber, folate, niacin, omega-3 fatty acids, potassium, selenium, thiamin, vitamin B$_6$, vitamin C.

Grilled Tuna Salad

Salade composée is the French term for a salad whose components are arranged in separate piles rather than being tossed together (the classic example being salade niçoise). Though this looks artful on the plate, it isn't much of a salad experience. So here is our version of an uncomposed salade niçoise, a combination of Yukon Gold potatoes, grilled tuna steak, and Italian green beans tossed with a mustard–lime vinaigrette.

> 1 teaspoon cumin
>
> 1 teaspoon ground coriander
>
> ¾ teaspoon salt
>
> ½ teaspoon sugar
>
> 1 pound tuna steak
>
> 1 pound Yukon Gold potatoes, cut into ¾-inch cubes
>
> ½ pound Italian flat green beans, halved crosswise
>
> 3 tablespoons fresh lime juice
>
> 1 tablespoon olive oil
>
> 1½ teaspoons Dijon mustard
>
> 8 leaves mixed salad greens
>
> 1 cup frozen corn kernels, thawed
>
> 1 small red onion, halved and thinly sliced

1 In a small bowl, stir together the cumin, coriander, ½ teaspoon of the salt, and the sugar. Rub the mixture into both sides of the tuna steak.

2 In a vegetable steamer, steam the potatoes for 7 minutes. Add the green beans and cook until the vegetables are firm-tender, about 3 minutes.

3 Meanwhile, in a large bowl, whisk together the remaining ¼ teaspoon salt, the lime juice, oil, and mustard. Add the warm potatoes and green beans to the dressing and toss to coat.

4 Spray a grill rack with nonstick cooking spray. Preheat the grill to medium. Place the tuna on the grill, close the cover, and grill for 6 to 8 minutes, or until the fish just flakes when tested with a fork. Let stand for 10 minutes before thinly slicing the tuna on the diagonal.

5 Add the mixed greens, corn, and red onion to the bowl with the potatoes and toss to combine. Add the tuna and toss gently. *Makes 4 servings*

per serving: 362 calories, 9.9g total fat (2g saturated), 42mg cholesterol, 7g dietary fiber, 39g carbohydrate, 32g protein, 564mg sodium. good source of: fiber, folate, magnesium, niacin, omega-3 fatty acids, potassium, riboflavin, selenium, thiamin, vitamin B$_{12}$, vitamin B$_6$, vitamin C, vitamin D.

Sesame-Crusted Tuna Steaks

This simple recipe could also work with salmon, halibut, or swordfish. If you're shopping for fresh tuna in the supermarket, it will most likely be cut about ¾ inch thick. This thinner cut allows the tuna to be cooked quickly.

> 3 tablespoons ketchup
>
> 4 teaspoons reduced-sodium soy sauce
>
> 2 tablespoons grated fresh ginger
>
> 1 clove garlic, minced
>
> 1 teaspoon brown sugar
>
> 4 tuna steaks, ¾ inch thick (6 ounces each)
>
> 2 teaspoons sesame seeds

1 In a small bowl, stir together the ketchup, soy sauce, ginger, garlic, and brown sugar.

2 Spray a broiler pan with nonstick cooking spray. Place the tuna on the broiler pan and brush with the ketchup mixture.

3 Preheat the broiler. Broil the tuna 4 to 6 inches from the heat for 4 minutes, or until medium-rare.

4 Sprinkle the sesame seeds over the tuna and broil for 1 minute, or until the seeds are lightly crisped. *Makes 4 servings*

per serving: 266 calories, 8.9g total fat (2.2g saturated), 63mg cholesterol, 0g dietary fiber, 6g carbohydrate, 39g protein, 379mg sodium. good source of: niacin, omega-3 fatty acids, riboflavin, selenium, thiamin, vitamin B$_{12}$, vitamin B$_6$, vitamin D.

Roasted Bluefish with Lemon-Basil Sauce

Spanish mackerel can easily be substituted for bluefish in this recipe as they are both rich-tasting fish. Look for the freshest bluefish you can find and you'll be surprised at how sweet and "not oily" it will taste.

¼ cup chopped fresh basil

1½ teaspoons grated lemon zest

¼ cup fresh lemon juice

3 tablespoons water

2 tablespoons Dijon mustard

2 teaspoons olive oil

½ teaspoon salt

1 red bell pepper, diced

1 tablespoon capers, chopped if large

1 pound skinless bluefish fillet

1 Preheat the oven to 500°F.

2 In a blender, combine the basil, lemon zest, lemon juice, water, mustard, oil, and ¼ teaspoon of the salt, and process to a smooth puree. Transfer to a bowl and add the bell pepper and capers.

3 Spray a jelly-roll pan with nonstick cooking spray. Place the bluefish on the pan and sprinkle the fish with the remaining ¼ teaspoon salt.

4 Roast the bluefish for about 10 minutes, or until the fish just flakes when tested with a fork. With a large spatula, lift the bluefish off the baking sheet. Divide into 4 portions and spoon the sauce over the top. *Makes 4 servings*

per serving: 172 calories, 7.4g total fat (1.3g saturated), 61mg cholesterol, 1g dietary fiber, 5g carbohydrate, 22g protein, 622mg sodium. good source of: niacin, omega-3 fatty acids, selenium, vitamin B_{12}, vitamin B_6, vitamin C.

Citrus-Roasted Snapper

Lime juice and orange juice season this simple baked fish dish. This type of treatment would work well for firm-fleshed fish as well as fatty types of fish: Try grouper, mackerel, or bluefish. **Serving suggestion:** Serve with Sushi Rice Salad (*page 207*), Fresh Fennel Salad (*page 203*), and, for dessert, Cranberry-Ginger Applesauce (*page 227*).

4 red snapper fillets (5 ounces each)

1 tablespoon fresh lime juice

1 tablespoon orange juice

½ teaspoon sugar

¼ teaspoon salt

2 tablespoons chopped fresh mint (optional)

1 Preheat the oven to 425°F. Spray a small baking sheet with nonstick cooking spray.

2 Sprinkle the snapper first with the lime and orange juices, then with the sugar and salt. Top with the mint, if using. Roast until the fish just flakes when tested with a fork, about 10 minutes. *Makes 4 servings*

per serving: 151 calories, 2g total fat (0.4g saturated), 53mg cholesterol, 0g dietary fiber, 2g carbohydrate, 30g protein, 211mg sodium. good source of: omega-3 fatty acids, selenium, vitamin B_{12}, vitamin B_6.

different spins

▶**Tuna-Asparagus Salad** Follow the directions for *Grilled Tuna Salad (opposite page)*, but substitute asparagus cut into 2-inch lengths for the green beans. Substitute 1 cup cooked white beans for the corn and 3 thinly sliced scallions for the red onion.

▶**Grilled Salmon Salad** Follow the directions for *Grilled Tuna Salad (opposite page)*, but substitute salmon steak for the tuna. Omit the corn and red onion, and add 2 cups halved cherry tomatoes and 4 sliced scallions.

Broiled Halibut with Fresh Tomato-Tangerine Sauce

Fresh basil, chives, and tarragon add wonderful herbal tones to this quick, uncooked sauce made with chopped fresh tomatoes and tangerine juice. Though the sauce is best with fresh herbs, you could use ½ teaspoon of dried tarragon instead of fresh. Other good options for fish in this dish are: striped bass, grouper, tilefish, bluefish, or swordfish. **Timing alert:** The fish needs to marinate for at least 1 hour before broiling.

½ cup tangerine or orange juice

2 teaspoons olive oil

2 cloves garlic, sliced

1 teaspoon hot pepper sauce

2 halibut steaks (10 ounces each), halved crosswise

2 medium tomatoes, diced

¼ cup chopped fresh basil

¼ cup minced chives or sliced scallions

2 teaspoons chopped fresh tarragon

½ teaspoon salt

1 In a nonaluminum pan, combine ¼ cup of the tangerine juice, 1 teaspoon of the oil, the garlic, and hot pepper sauce. Add the halibut, turning to coat. Marinate in the refrigerator for at least 1 hour, or up to 8 hours, turning the fish once.

2 In a medium bowl, combine the remaining ¼ cup tangerine juice, the remaining 1 teaspoon oil, the tomatoes, basil, chives, tarragon, and salt.

3 Preheat the broiler. Lift the halibut from the marinade and place on a broiler pan. Spoon the marinade over the fish. Broil 4 to 6 inches from the heat for 5 minutes, or until the fish just flakes when tested with a fork. Serve the fish with the fresh tomato sauce on top. *Makes 4 servings*

per serving: 209 calories, 5.9g total fat (5.9g saturated), 47mg cholesterol, 1g dietary fiber, 7g carbohydrate, 31g protein, 406mg sodium. **good source of:** magnesium, niacin, omega-3 fatty acids, potassium, vitamin B$_{12}$, vitamin B$_6$, vitamin C.

Walnut-Topped Baked Snapper

Red snapper generally comes with the skin on. Ask the fish store to remove it, or do it yourself: Run a thin-bladed knife under the skin at one end and, with the blade parallel to the work surface, slide the knife the full length of the fillet. Good options for other fish here are: tilapia, bluefish, or grouper.

1 teaspoon oregano

½ teaspoon salt

¼ teaspoon pepper

4 red snapper fillets (6 ounces each), skinned

2 tablespoons light mayonnaise

1 tablespoon white horseradish

1 tablespoon ketchup

1 teaspoon fresh lemon juice

¼ cup walnut halves

2 tablespoons plain dried breadcrumbs

2 tablespoons grated Parmesan cheese

2 tablespoons chopped parsley

1 Preheat the oven to 450°F. Spray a baking sheet with nonstick cooking spray.

2 In a small bowl, combine the oregano, salt, and pepper. Rub into both sides of the fish.

3 In another small bowl, combine the mayonnaise, horseradish, ketchup, and lemon juice. Place

did you know?

Canned sardines are a rich source of vitamin D: Three ounces have 63% of the RDA for this important vitamin—found in concentrated amounts in only a few foods (such as sardines, salmon, mackerel, fortified milk, and egg yolks). We need vitamin D for maintaining normal calcium in the blood and for bone health and metabolic, muscle, cardiac, and neurological functions. Vitamin D is often called the "sunshine vitamin," because 10 to 15 minutes of sun exposure several times a week will help to generate vitamin D in the body. However, those living in areas of limited sunshine, and people over 50, can benefit from vitamin D-rich foods.

the fillets on the baking sheet. Spread the mayonnaise mixture over the skinned side of the fish.

4 In a food processor, process the walnuts, breadcrumbs, Parmesan, and parsley until finely ground. Sprinkle the mixture over the fish, patting it on. Bake until the fish just flakes when tested with a fork, about 10 minutes. *Makes 4 servings*

per serving: 246 calories, 9.6g total fat (1.6g saturated), 59mg cholesterol, 1g dietary fiber, 6g carbohydrate, 33g protein, 543mg sodium. good source of: omega-3 fatty acids, selenium, vitamin B_{12}, vitamin B_6.

Greek Salad with Sardines

High in omega-3 fatty acids, sardines are a good choice for a quick, heart-healthy meal.

> 1/3 cup fresh lemon or lime juice
> 2½ teaspoons olive oil
> ¼ cup fresh dill
> ¼ cup fresh mint leaves
> ½ teaspoon salt
> ¼ teaspoon pepper
> 1 large cucumber, peeled, seeded, and thinly sliced
> 2 cups cherry tomatoes, halved
> 1 small red onion, chopped
> 6 cups mixed salad greens
> 2 cans (3¾ ounces each) sardines packed in water, drained
> 1/3 cup crumbled feta cheese

1 In a food processor, combine the lemon juice, oil, dill, mint, salt, and pepper. Puree until smooth.

2 Transfer the dressing to a large bowl. Add the cucumbers, tomatoes, and onion. Toss to combine.

3 Spoon the cucumber mixture and dressing over the salad greens. Scatter the sardines and feta on top. *Makes 4 servings*

per serving: 210 calories, 11g total fat (2.5g saturated), 46mg cholesterol, 4g dietary fiber, 13g carbohydrate, 17g protein, 902mg sodium. good source of: folate, omega-3 fatty acids, potassium, vitamin B_{12}, vitamin B_6, vitamin C, vitamin D, vitamin E.

Pan-Fried Grouper with Orange-Carrot Sauce

Grouper is a flavorful, meaty-textured fish and is well worth a trip to a fish market, because you're unlikely to find this fish in supermarkets. If grouper isn't available, substitute red snapper, sea bass, tilapia, or tilefish.

> 1 tablespoon olive oil
> 4 skinless grouper fillets (6 ounces each)
> 1 tablespoon plus 1 teaspoon cornstarch
> 3 cloves garlic, minced
> ½ cup dry white wine
> ⅔ cup orange juice
> 1/3 cup carrot juice
> ½ teaspoon salt
> ¼ teaspoon cayenne pepper
> 1 tablespoon water

1 In a large skillet, heat the oil over medium heat. Dredge the grouper in 1 tablespoon of the cornstarch, shaking off the excess. Add the grouper to the skillet and cook until the fish just flakes when tested with a fork, about 2 minutes per side. With a slotted spatula, transfer the fish to a platter and keep warm.

2 Add the garlic to the pan and cook for 30 seconds. Add the wine, increase the heat to high, and bring to a boil. Boil until the wine has evaporated by half, about 2 minutes

3 Add the orange juice, carrot juice, salt, and cayenne. Bring to a boil and cook for 2 minutes.

4 Meanwhile, in a small bowl, stir together the remaining 1 teaspoon cornstarch and the water. Stir the cornstarch mixture into the pan and cook, stirring, until the sauce is slightly thickened, about 1 minute. Spoon the sauce over the fish. *Makes 4 servings*

per serving: 240 calories, 5.2g total fat (0.9g saturated), 60mg cholesterol, 0g dietary fiber, 9g carbohydrate, 32g protein, 366mg sodium. good source of: omega-3 fatty acids, potassium, selenium, vitamin B_{12}, vitamin B_6.

recipe creator
fish in parchment

Baking fish in a parchment paper or foil packet has several advantages. You can cook with no added fat; cleanup is easy; and the permutations are endless. As an added bonus, if you're concerned with weight loss or management, this cooking method provides built-in portion control.

Pick ingredients from each of the five categories and follow these basic instructions (note that the quantities given for the ingredients are *per packet*): Cut 4 pieces (12 x 18 inches) of parchment paper or foil. With a short side of the parchment or foil facing you, place a STARCH about 3 inches from the bottom edge. Place a FISH fillet on top and cover the fish with 2 thin slices of lemon or orange. Top with 1 or 2 VEGETABLES, 1 or 2 SEASONINGS, ¼ teaspoon salt, and 1or 2 AROMATICS. Fold the parchment over the ingredients and fold in the edges to seal (if using parchment, be sure to leave a bit of headroom for the steam). Place the packets on a baking sheet and bake for 10 minutes in a 450°F oven.

The ordinary test for doneness—checking to see if the fish flesh pulls apart in flakes but is still moist—is not practical when you're cooking in a sealed packet. As a rule of thumb, if the packet is parchment, by the time it puffs up, the fish is undoubtedly done. Foil, on the other hand, does not puff, so you'll have to open the packet (watch out for the steam) to check for doneness. If the fish is almost done, the residual heat will probably cook it the rest of the way. However, if it's *really* underdone, then reseal the packet and cook another 5 minutes before checking. ***Makes 4 servings***

STARCHES	FISH	VEGETABLES	SEASONINGS	AROMATICS
▸ Potatoes, ½ cup thinly sliced, cooked	▸ Halibut, 6-oz skinless fillet	▸ Carrots + leeks, ½ cup matchsticks	▸ Reduced-sodium soy sauce, 1 Tbsp	▸ Fresh basil, 2 Tbsp chopped
▸ White or brown rice, ½ cup cooked	▸ Mackerel, 6-oz skinless fillet	▸ Mushrooms, ½ cup chopped	▸ Fresh lemon juice or lime juice, 1 Tbsp	▸ Fresh dill, 2 Tbsp chopped
▸ Sweet potatoes, ½ cup thinly sliced, cooked	▸ Bluefish, 6-oz skinless fillet	▸ Tomatoes, ½ cup chopped	▸ Salsa, 2 Tbsp	▸ Fresh parsley, 2 Tbsp chopped
▸ Couscous, ½ cup cooked	▸ Flounder, 6-oz skinless fillet	▸ Broccoli, shredded + red bell pepper matchsticks, ¼ cup each	▸ Louisiana-style hot pepper sauce, ½ tsp	▸ Fresh mint, 2 Tbsp chopped
▸ Bulgur, ½ cup cooked	▸ Tilapia, 6-oz skinless fillet	▸ Zucchini and/or yellow squash, ½ cup shredded	▸ Balsamic vinegar, 1 Tbsp	▸ Cilantro, 2 Tbsp chopped
▸ Small pasta shapes, ½ cup cooked	▸ Snapper, 6-oz skinless fillet	▸ Snow peas or sugar snap peas, ½ cup halved crosswise	▸ Olives, 1 Tbsp minced	▸ Garlic, 1 clove minced
	▸ Striped bass, 6-oz skinless fillet		▸ White wine, 2 Tbsp	
			▸ Capers, 1 tsp minced	

Red Snapper Escabeche

From the verb *escabechar* ("to pickle"), escabeche means marinade in Spanish, and there are numerous versions of this style of dish throughout Latin America and the Caribbean (in Jamaica, for example, it's called escovitch). Feel free to substitute another fish for the snapper. Bluefish and mackerel—both full-flavored fish—take well to this preparation. **Timing alert:** The snapper needs to marinate for at least 2 hours.

- 4 red snapper fillets (6 ounces each), skinned
- 1 tablespoon chili powder
- ¾ teaspoon salt
- 3 tablespoons flour
- 2 tablespoons olive oil
- 1 large red onion, halved and thinly sliced
- 1 red bell pepper, thinly sliced
- 3 cloves garlic, slivered
- 1 tablespoon sugar
- ½ cup cider vinegar
- ½ teaspoon thyme
- ⅔ cup orange juice
- ⅓ cup dried currants or raisins
- ¼ teaspoon black pepper

1 Sprinkle the snapper with the chili powder and ½ teaspoon of the salt. Dredge the snapper in the flour, shaking off the excess.

2 In a large nonstick skillet, heat 1 tablespoon of the oil over medium heat. Add 2 of the snapper fillets and cook until golden brown and the fish just flakes when tested with a fork, about 3 minutes per side. With a slotted spatula, transfer the fish to a shallow glass dish large enough to hold all 4 of the fillets in a single layer. Repeat with the remaining oil and fillets.

3 Add the onion, bell pepper, and garlic to the dish, sprinkle the sugar over the vegetables and cook, stirring frequently, until the onion is crisp-tender, about 5 minutes.

4 Add the vinegar to the skillet and bring to a boil. Add the remaining ¼ teaspoon salt, the thyme, orange juice, currants, and black pepper.

Bring to a boil and boil until slightly reduced and syrupy, about 4 minutes.

5 Pour the sauce over the fish, cover, and refrigerate, occasionally spooning the sauce over the fish, for at least 2 hours or up to overnight. Serve chilled or at room temperature. *Makes 4 servings*

per serving: 349 calories, 9.6g total fat (1.5g saturated), 60mg cholesterol, 3g dietary fiber, 30g carbohydrate, 36g protein, 534mg sodium. good source of: omega-3 fatty acids, potassium, selenium, vitamin B_{12}, vitamin B_6, vitamin C.

Grilled Mackerel

A little bit of sugar in the spice rub that goes on the mackerel helps deepen the flavor of the grilled fish. This preparation also works well with bluefish. Though the mackerel is delicious on its own, it goes particularly well with a sweet and tangy chutney, such as Tomato–Orange Chutney (*page 267*).

- 2 teaspoons paprika
- 2 teaspoons cumin
- 1 teaspoon sugar
- ½ teaspoon salt
- ½ teaspoon pepper
- 4 skinless mackerel fillets (5 ounces each)

1 In a small bowl, combine the paprika, cumin, sugar, salt, and pepper. Rub the mixture into both sides of the mackerel fillets.

2 Preheat the broiler. Place the mackerel on a broiler pan and broil 4 inches from the heat until the fish just flakes when tested with a fork, about 5 minutes. Serve the fish with the chutney. *Makes 4 servings*

per serving: 180 calories, 7.1g total fat (2g saturated), 78mg cholesterol, 0g dietary fiber, 2g carbohydrate, 25g protein, 363mg sodium. good source of: niacin, omega-3 fatty acids, selenium, vitamin B_{12}, vitamin B_6, vitamin D.

different spins

▶Southwestern Cod Cakes Follow the directions for *Curried Cod Cakes*, but substitute 1 teaspoon each ground cumin and ground coriander for the curry powder. Omit the mango chutney and add 1 diced plum tomato. Substitute yellow cornmeal for the breadcrumbs.

Curried Cod Cakes

The magic ingredient in these cod cakes is instant mashed potato flakes. They help the cod cakes hold together, and also add moistness, flavor, and some B vitamins. Be sure to find a brand that is nothing but dehydrated potatoes, without any added seasonings, sodium, or fat. Other good options for fish in this dish are: scrod, salmon, snapper, grouper. **Serving suggestion:** Top the cakes with Fresh Pineapple-Jícama Relish (*page 265*) or Hot & Spicy Cocktail Sauce (*page 256*), and serve Cucumber Salad (*page 202*) alongside.

> 1¼ pounds skinless cod fillets
>
> 2 tablespoons instant mashed potato flakes
>
> 3 tablespoons mango chutney, finely chopped
>
> ¼ cup diced red bell pepper
>
> 1 tablespoon Dijon mustard
>
> 2 teaspoons Louisiana-style hot pepper sauce
>
> 2 teaspoons curry powder
>
> ½ teaspoon salt
>
> ½ teaspoon black pepper
>
> 1 large egg white
>
> ½ cup plain dried breadcrumbs
>
> 2 tablespoons olive oil

1 Place the cod in a vegetable steamer. Cover and steam until the fish just flakes when tested with a fork, about 10 minutes. Let cool to room temperature. When cool enough to handle, flake the fish into a large bowl.

2 Add the potato flakes, chutney, bell pepper, mustard, hot pepper sauce, curry powder, salt, and black pepper to the cod and stir to combine.

3 In a small bowl, with an electric mixer, beat the egg white to stiff peaks. Gently fold the egg white into the cod mixture.

4 Shape the cod mixture into 8 cakes. Dredge the cakes in the breadcrumbs, patting the crumbs onto the cakes.

5 In a large nonstick skillet, heat 1 tablespoon of the oil over medium heat. Add 4 of the cakes and cook until crisp and golden, about 3 minutes per side. Repeat with the remaining oil and cakes. *Makes 4 servings*

per serving: 202 calories, 6.2g total fat (0.8g saturated), 37mg cholesterol, 1g dietary fiber, 18g carbohydrate, 18g protein, 748mg sodium. good source of: selenium, vitamin B_{12}.

Swordfish Stir-Fry

Though the term stir-fry conjures up Chinese ingredients and flavors, the concept of quickly cooking cut-up food in a small amount of oil can be applied to all sorts of delicious sautés. Here swordfish (which is sturdy enough to stand up to being tossed around) is stir-fried with ingredients reminiscent of Mediterranean dishes: fresh fennel, garlic, orange juice, and olives. Coating the swordfish in cornstarch to keep it moist and tender is another trick borrowed from Chinese cooking. **Serving suggestion:** Serve with a bowl of couscous, and for dessert offer Triple Chocolate Pudding (*page 233*).

> 4 teaspoons olive oil
>
> ½ small fennel bulb, cut into matchsticks
>
> 3 cloves garlic, minced
>
> 2 scallions, cut into 1-inch lengths
>
> 1 pound skinless swordfish steak, cut into 1-inch chunks
>
> 2 tablespoons cornstarch
>
> 1½ cups grape tomatoes, halved

¼ cup Calamata olives, pitted and
coarsely chopped

¼ cup orange juice

½ teaspoon salt

1 In a large nonstick skillet, heat 2 teaspoons of the oil over medium-high heat. Add the fennel matchsticks and stir-fry until lightly browned, about 3 minutes.

2 Add the garlic and scallions, and stir-fry until the scallions have wilted, about 2 minutes. Transfer the vegetables to a plate.

3 Dredge the swordfish in the cornstarch, shaking off the excess. Add the remaining 2 teaspoons of oil to the pan. Add the swordfish to the pan and stir-fry until golden brown, about 3 minutes.

4 Return the fennel mixture to the pan along with the tomatoes, olives, orange juice, and salt, and cook, stirring, until the tomatoes have softened and the fish is cooked through, about 3 minutes. *Makes 4 servings*

per serving: 270 calories, 12g total fat (2.3g saturated), 56mg cholesterol, 2g dietary fiber, 11g carbohydrate, 30g protein, 486mg sodium. good source of: niacin, selenium, vitamin B$_{12}$, vitamin B$_6$.

---

a quick trick for pitting olives

In the world of olives, there are some that cling ferociously to their pits (like tiny Niçoise olives), and some that are relatively easy to pit. The unpittable olives are generally added to recipes with the pits still in; but bigger, meatier olives (such as Calamata or Gaeta) are easily pitted, using this trick: Place the olives (you can do a few at a time) on a work surface and cover them with the flat side of a chef's knife. With the palm of your hand, apply a small amount of downward pressure: You'll feel the olives crack open. Then you can easily remove the pits.

Spicy Fish Chowder

Cod is a great choice for chowders and fish stews. Not only is it low in fat, but it has a sturdy texture that can stand up to being "stewed." It also comes in large steaks, so you can cut it into satisfying chunks. If you live near a Hispanic market, you should be able to find batatas, which are dry-fleshed sweet potatoes with a mottled red-purple skin. Batatas are a favorite in Puerto Rican and other Latin American cuisines. Naturally, a regular orange-fleshed sweet potato will work just as well.

¾ pound batata or sweet potato, peeled and cut into ½-inch chunks

2 teaspoons olive oil

2 slices (1 ounce) turkey bacon, coarsely chopped

2 green bell peppers, cut into 1-inch squares

1 chipotle pepper in adobo, finely chopped

3 cloves garlic, minced

½ teaspoon salt

2 tablespoons flour

1½ cups low-fat (1%) milk

1 pound skinless, boneless cod steak, cut into 8 chunks

1 In a medium pot of boiling water, cook the batata until just tender, about 8 minutes.

2 Meanwhile, in a large nonstick skillet, heat the oil over medium heat. Add the turkey bacon, bell peppers, chipotle pepper, garlic, and salt, and cook, stirring frequently, until the bell peppers are crisp-tender, about 5 minutes.

3 Sprinkle the flour over the peppers, stirring to coat. Gradually stir in the milk. Stir in the batata. Bring the mixture to a boil, place the cod on top, reduce to a simmer, cover, and cook until the cod just flakes when tested with a fork, about 5 minutes. *Makes 4 servings*

per serving: 267 calories, 5.7g total fat (1.5g saturated), 58mg cholesterol, 3g dietary fiber, 27g carbohydrate, 26g protein, 515mg sodium. good source of: beta carotene, potassium, riboflavin, selenium, vitamin B$_{12}$, vitamin B$_6$, vitamin C.

Steamed Fish on a Bed of Cabbage & Potatoes

Bacon, cabbage, and apples are a classic combination. Here, a very small amount of bacon is cooked, the fat is drained, and the pan is wiped dry, leaving crisp bacon bits to accent the vegetables without much fat. Meaty-flavored tilapia holds up well to the cabbage-apple flavor, but other good options are: grouper, red snapper, or halibut fillets.

¼ cup water

1 slice bacon (¾ ounce), coarsely chopped

2 teaspoons olive oil

2 onions, finely chopped

4 cups shredded cabbage (12 ounces)

¾ pound all-purpose potatoes, thinly sliced

¾ cup apple juice

1 teaspoon salt

4 tilapia fillets (6 ounces each)

½ cup chopped fresh dill

1 In a large nonstick skillet, heat the water over medium heat. Add the bacon and cook until the bacon has rendered its fat, the water has evaporated, and the bacon is lightly crisped, about 5 minutes. Remove the bacon with a slotted spoon. Pour off the fat from the skillet and wipe the fat out with paper towels (it's okay to leave a film of fat in the pan).

2 Add the oil to the skillet and heat over medium heat. Add the onions and cook, stirring frequently, until golden brown, about 10 minutes.

3 Add the cabbage and cook, stirring frequently, until lightly browned, about 10 minutes. Stir in the reserved bacon, the potatoes, apple juice, and ½ teaspoon of the salt. Cover and cook until the potatoes are tender, about 10 minutes.

4 Sprinkle the fish with the remaining ½ teaspoon salt and scatter the dill over one side of the

fish steaming methods

There are a number of different options for steaming fish, some involving specialized equipment and some not. Regardless of the equipment being used, there are a few simple rules for fish-steaming:
 1. The water in the steamer bottom should not touch the steamer basket (or insert). **2.** Bring the water to a boil before you add the fish; the timing should not start until the water is boiling. **3.** Remove the fish from the steamer as soon as it's done to keep it from overcooking.

▶ **In a Chinese bamboo steamer** The Chinese are masters at steaming, and a multitiered bamboo steamer is the best piece of equipment for steaming fish. In the larger sizes of steamer, you can fit 4 fillets, steaks, or a small whole fish in one layer. Line the steamer with a cabbage or lettuce leaf, or place the fish on a plate in the steamer. If you are steaming on a plate, you should remove the fish a bit before it's completely done, because the residual heat in the plate will continue to cook the fish. This is especially important for thin fillets.

▶ **In a skillet on a cake rack** If you've got a cake rack that will fit in a skillet and a heatproof plate or pie plate, you're all set. Place the rack in the skillet. Place the plate on the rack and the fish on the plate. Cover and steam. Depending upon the size of the rack, skillet, and plate, you can steam flat or folded fillets, steaks, and small whole fish.

▶ **In a steamer insert** Many pasta pots come with a steamer insert, which works well for steaming vegetables. But they are often not big enough to accommodate a number of fish fillets. However, you can fold the fillets in half and then they will fit quite well in this type of steamer.

▶ **In a skillet on a bed of vegetables** Soft, tender vegetables provide a bed on which to steam fish. Cover the skillet and the moisture from the vegetables will cook the fish.

▶ **In the oven** Fish can also be oven-steamed on a bed of thinly sliced vegetables. Put the vegetables in a roasting pan and place the fish on top. Cover the pan and the fish will steam in its own juices.

fish. Fold the fillets in half over the dill. Place the folded fish on top of the vegetables. Cover and cook until the fish just flakes when tested with a fork, about 5 minutes. *Makes 4 servings*

per serving: 355 calories, 8.2g total fat (2.1g saturated), 94mg cholesterol, 4g dietary fiber, 31g carbohydrate, 39g protein, 779mg sodium. **good source of:** niacin, potassium, selenium, thiamin, vitamin B_{12}, vitamin B_6, vitamin C, vitamin D, vitamin E.

Skillet-Steamed Cod with Squash & Tomatoes

If you make this dish during tomato season and heirloom tomatoes are available in your area, choose them for this fresh tomato sauce. Other good options for fish to use in this dish are: red snapper, mackerel, bluefish, or tilapia.

2 teaspoons olive oil

2 yellow summer squash, quartered lengthwise and thinly sliced crosswise

2 large tomatoes, coarsely chopped

1½ teaspoons grated lemon zest

¼ cup chopped fresh basil

3 tablespoons minced chives or scallions

½ teaspoon salt

4 cod fillets (5 ounces each)

1 In a large skillet, heat the oil over medium heat. Add the squash and cook until tender, about 7 minutes.

2 Add the tomatoes, lemon zest, basil, chives, and salt, and bring to a boil. Reduce to a simmer.

3 Add the fish, cover, and cook until the fish just flakes when tested with a fork, about 7 minutes. *Makes 4 servings*

per serving: 128 calories, 3.3g total fat (0.5g saturated), 37mg cholesterol, 3g dietary fiber, 8g carbohydrate, 17g protein, 353mg sodium. **good source of:** selenium, vitamin B_{12}, vitamin C.

Asian-Style Micro-Steamed Bass

Try this quick and easy microwave preparation for any firm-textured fish, such as snapper, grouper, sea bass, or halibut. The small amount of dark sesame oil in the sauce goes a long way and lends a deep flavor to the fish.

¼ cup minced cilantro or parsley

2 scallions, thinly sliced

1 tablespoon minced fresh ginger

1 clove garlic, minced

2 tablespoons reduced-sodium soy sauce

2 teaspoons dark sesame oil

4 skinless striped bass fillets (6 ounces each)

½ teaspoon salt

1 In a small bowl, combine the cilantro, scallions, ginger, and garlic. In another small bowl, stir together the soy sauce and sesame oil.

2 Place the fish in a large, microwave-safe dish and sprinkle with the salt. Cover loosely with plastic wrap. Microwave on high for 3 minutes. Rotate the plate and cook for 3 minutes more, or until the fish just flakes when tested with a fork.

3 Transfer the fish to serving plates. Pour any juices from the cooking plate into the soy sauce mixture and stir to combine. Sprinkle the scallion-ginger mixture over the fish and spoon the sauce on top. *Makes 4 servings*

per serving: 194 calories, 4.6g total fat (0.8g saturated), 60mg cholesterol, 0g dietary fiber, 2g carbohydrate, 34g protein, 634mg sodium. **good source of:** omega-3 fatty acids, selenium, vitamin B_{12}, vitamin B_6.

Provençal Cod Stew

Rouille, the spicy garlic mayonnaise that is the classic accompaniment to a Provençale fish stew, is usually served on top of the dish, but you could also use it to spread lightly on thin pieces of toasted sourdough to serve alongside the stew. Or, you could leave the rouille out altogether.

Rouille:
1 large red bell pepper, roasted (page 190)
2 tablespoons light mayonnaise
1 garlic clove, peeled
¼ teaspoon cayenne pepper

Fish Stew:
1 tablespoon olive oil
1 large red bell pepper, thinly sliced
1 yellow summer squash, halved
*　lengthwise and thinly sliced*
1 medium onion, halved and thinly sliced
3 cloves garlic, slivered
½ teaspoon fennel seeds
½ teaspoon salt
¼ cup water
2 cans (14½ ounces each) no-salt-added
*　stewed tomatoes*
1 pound cod steaks, skinned, boned and
*　cut into 1-inch pieces*

1 Make the rouille: Preheat the broiler. Roast the pepper. When it's cool enough to handle, peel and transfer to a food processor. Add the mayonnaise, garlic, and cayenne, and process to a smooth puree. Transfer the rouille to a small bowl and refrigerate until serving time.

2 Make the fish stew: In a nonstick Dutch oven or flameproof casserole, heat the oil over medium-high heat. Stir in the bell pepper, squash, onion, garlic, fennel seeds, and salt. Cook, stirring, until the vegetables start to soften, 2 to 3 minutes.

3 Add the water. Reduce the heat to medium, cover, and cook, stirring occasionally, until the vegetables are tender, about 5 minutes.

4 Add the tomatoes to the pan and cook, uncovered, stirring occasionally, until the mixture is the consistency of tomato sauce, about 10 minutes.

5 Add the fish to the pan and reduce the heat to a gentle simmer. Cover and cook until the fish just flakes when tested with a fork, 3 to 5 minutes. Ladle the stew into bowls and top with some of rouille. *Makes 4 servings*

per serving: 277 calories, 7.2g total fat (0.9g saturated), 55mg cholesterol, 7g dietary fiber, 23g carbohydrate, 29g protein, 463mg sodium. good source of: beta carotene, potassium, selenium, vitamin B_{12}, vitamin B_6, vitamin C.

shellfish

Shellfish is a broad category that includes some seemingly unrelated animals. Clams and octopus are both considered shellfish, for example. The various members of this category have equally disparate flavors (ranging from sweet to briny) and textures (ranging from "meaty" to soft and delicate). These differences, naturally, affect their cooking methods. But the one thing they have in common is that they are generally lean (with no intramuscular fat like meat or poultry), and so can toughen very easily. The trick is to heat shellfish sufficiently to destroy harmful organisms, but not so long as to toughen their flesh; shellfish can overcook in a matter of seconds.

shrimp

Roasting/baking Shrimp, especially large ones, take well to these dry-heat methods. They can simply be tossed with olive oil and herbs and cooked in their shells, or shelled and roasted with vegetables (*see Roasted Shrimp & Asparagus Salad, page 67*).

Boiling If you're cooking mass quantities of shrimp, then boiling is a good option. Otherwise, poach them.

Broiling/grilling Large shrimp, in or out of the shell, can be grilled (on skewers or on a grill topper), broiled (on skewers or on a broiler pan), or pan-grilled in a stovetop grill pan. They can be marinated in a wet mixture or tossed in a dry rub (*see Zesty Lime-Broiled Shrimp, page 68*). Either way, they cook in a matter of minutes, leaving little or no time for basting, and should be watched carefully to prevent overcooking.

Sautéing/stir-frying Shrimp should be quickly cooked to prevent their getting tough, so moving them around in a skillet over medium to medium-high heat works well. For a healthful sauté, use a nonstick pan and a small amount of oil. Get the oil hot, but not smoking, before adding the shrimp. Shrimp can be sautéed on their own or with vegetables (*see Shrimp Scampi, page 67, or Sautéed Shrimp with Basil & Cherry Tomatoes, page 68*). Be sure to remove the shrimp from the pan as soon as they are done

Steaming Steaming provides a gentle, fat-free method for cooking shrimp. Steam them in a steamer insert, on a steaming rack, in a bamboo steamer, or on a bed of moist vegetables (*see*

"Fish Steaming Methods," page 60). Shrimp also turn out moist if baked in parchment or foil packets (actually a form of oven-steaming).

Microwaving This is a good method for cooking shrimp (in the shell): They stay moist and there's certainly no faster way to cook them. Because microwave ovens are so different, consult your manual for specific cooking times.

Poaching If you're cooking shrimp to be served cold or to use in another recipe, you can poach them in water or fish stock; or use a mixture of water and lemon juice or wine. Flavor the cooking liquid with herbs, if you like. The advantage to this method over boiling is that you'll also have a flavorful liquid that can be used to make a sauce or be added to a soup or salad dressing.

Stewing/braising Shrimp can be added to chowders, soups, and stews providing that they are added during the final stages of cooking (*see Shrimp Jambalaya, page 69*).

how to tell when shellfish are done

Shellfish undergo characteristic changes when cooked, which can help you judge doneness.

▶**Shrimp** Shrimp will feel firm to the touch and their flesh with turn opaque. If they are in the shell, their color will change from grayish-green to bright pink or orange.

▶**Scallops** Small bay scallops and larger sea scallops cook at different rates, but the visual test for doneness is the same for both: They will firm up and become opaque throughout.

▶**Crabs** The shells of live crabs will turn from green or blue to scarlet, and the flesh will turn from translucent to opaque. In addition, the apron (a triangular flap of shell on the crab's belly) will loosen when the flesh is cooked. Soft-shell crabs will turn light red or brown and feel firm to the touch.

▶**Lobster** A lobster shell will turn from green or blue to scarlet, and its flesh will turn from translucent to opaque. (You can also test lobster for doneness by tugging on one of the small legs—it should pull off easily.)

▶**Clams** Clams cooked in the shell will open when they are done. Any clams that do not open should be discarded as this is an indication that they were not alive when they went into the pot. Shucked clam meats will turn opaque and firm-textured, and their edges will curl slightly.

▶**Mussels** Mussels are done when their shells open. Any mussels that do not open should be discarded as this is an indication that they were not alive when they went into the pot.

▶**Oysters** Whole oyster meats will become slightly opaque when they're done, but the real clue to their doneness is that their edges will begin to curl.

▶**Squid & octopus** Squid and octopus will turn opaque and be fork-tender. This can be hard to judge with thin rings of squid, but biting a piece will help.

scallops

Roasting/baking It's difficult to successfully roast or bake scallops by themselves, because the surround-heat of this method toughens them quickly. It helps to protect the food from the full intensity of the dry heat with a sauce or coating.

Broiling/grilling Quick-cooking scallops take well to these high-heat methods; coating them with a bit of oil or a marinade helps keep them moist (*see Simple Grilled Scallops, page 71, and Broiled Scallops with Baby Spinach, page 70*).

Sautéing/stir-frying Both sea scallops and bay scallops can be stir-fried or sautéed. Because they tend to be large and thick, sea scallops should be halved horizontally to facilitate quick cooking (*see Scallop Stir-Fry, page 71, and Sautéed Bay Scallops with Citrus Sauce, page 70*).

Steaming Steaming provides a gentle, fat-free method for cooking scallops. Steam them in a steamer insert, on a steaming rack, in a bamboo steamer, or on a bed of moist vegetables (*see "Fish Steaming Methods," page 60*). Scallops also turn out moist if baked in parchment or foil packets (actually a form of oven-steaming).

Microwaving Because microwave ovens can be so different, consult your manual for specific cooking times.

Poaching Poach scallops in fish stock, or a mixture of water and lemon juice or wine (flavor the poaching liquid with herbs, if you like). Bring the liquid to a gentle simmer, add the scallops, partially cover the pan, and poach until done.

Stewing/braising Scallops can be added to stews, soups, and chowders. Add the scallops at the last minute or two of cooking to keep them moist and tender (*see Manhattan Shellfish Chowder, page 77*).

crabs

When you buy lump crabmeat or crab legs at the market, you will be buying already cooked crab, so cooking it is basically reheating it. Unlike

> ### soft-shell crabs
>
> In the life of a blue crab, there comes a time when it sheds its old shell to grow a larger shell. When caught during the few short days before it grows the new shell, this so-called soft-shell crab is completely edible. Soft-shell crabs are sold alive and need to be cleaned (killed) before cooking. The most common cooking method is sautéing, with the crabs being dredged in flour or cornstarch first. A small amount of oil in a hot nonstick pan should do the trick.

other shellfish, crabmeat doesn't get too tough with this second cooking. Live crabs come in two basic forms, hard-shell and soft-shell (*see box, above*).

Boiling Drop well-scrubbed, live hard-shell crabs into a large pot of boiling water. Once the water has returned to a boil, turn it down to a simmer and cook until the shells have turned bright red. For extra flavor you can season the water with herbs and spices or a special mixture called crab boil (*see "Crab Boil," page 73*).

Pan-steaming Hard-shell crabs can be steamed, not in a rack over boiling water, but in a small amount of liquid: Place them in a pot with about 1 to 2 inches of boiling liquid (water, wine, or seasoned broth), cover, and steam over high heat until they turn red. If desired, season the steaming liquid with thyme, ginger, and any other herbs and spices that appeal to you.

lobster

The most common method of cooking lobster is alive, in a large pot of boiling water. For other cooking methods, the lobster may need to be killed first. If you want the fish seller to perform this task for you, be sure to make your purchase the same day you plan to cook the shellfish.

Baking Lobsters can be baked and in fact it is a very good way of cooking them. They will remain succulent and moist, will get neither waterlogged nor dried out. Plunge one at a time into a pot of boiling water and boil for 1 minute.

Transfer to a pan large enough to hold them in a single layer and bake at 450°F until done.

Broiling/grilling In order to broil or grill lobsters, they first have to be split in half lengthwise. Once split, clean and remove the stomach. Place the lobsters on foil to catch any juices. Brush the lobster flesh with some oil and broil until the flesh is just opaque. Spoon the collected juices over the lobster when serving.

Pan-steaming Live lobsters can be steamed whole. Bring about 2 inches of seasoned liquid to a boil in the bottom of a large pot. Add the lobsters, cover, and steam until done. Serve the cooked lobsters with the pan juices.

Boiling Live lobsters are boiled in a large quantity of boiling water (*see Lobster with Dipping Sauces, page 74*).

mussels

Pan-steaming This is the most common way of cooking mussels. About 1 to 2 inches of liquid (water, wine, or seasoned broth) is brought to a boil, the mussels are added, the pot is covered, and the mussels are cooked over high heat until their shells open. Any mussels that do not open should be discarded. You can use this method to cook the mussels before removing them from the shells and incorporating into a dish that needs no further cooking (like a salad). Or you can steam them in their shells, and serve them hot along with the broth that's created as they cook (*see Hot & Spicy Mussels, page 75*).

clams

Broiling/grilling Clams in their shells can be cooked on a grill until the shells open. Shucked clams can be oven-broiled if given a crumb coating to protect them from the intense heat—a good alternative to frying them.

Sautéing This method for cooking shucked clams traditionally requires quite a bit of butter or oil, both for flavor and to keep the delicate shellfish from sticking to the pan and breaking

apart. For a healthier low-fat sauté, be sure to use a nonstick pan and just a little bit of oil. A light dredging in flour or breadcrumbs will also help keep the clams from breaking up.

Pan-steaming Clams in their shells are steamed not over boiling water but in a small amount of liquid. About 1 to 2 inches of liquid (water, wine, or seasoned broth) is brought to a boil, the clams are added, the pot is covered, and the clams are cooked over high heat until their shells open (*see Littleneck Clams with Carrot-Ginger Sauce, page 76, and Steamer Clams in Fennel Broth, page 78*). Any clams that do not open should be discarded. Clams can also be wrapped in foil packets and either "steamed" in the oven or on top of a grill.

Stewing/braising Shucked clams can be added to soups, stews, and chowders. They should be added during the final minute or two of cooking (*see Creamy New England Clam Chowder, page 75*). Steamed clams that are then shucked can also be added to soups, stews, and chowders, but just at the last minute to reheat (*see Manhattan Shellfish Chowder, page 77*).

clams & mussels, alive, alive-o

Clams and mussels must be alive when you cook them. So, the first thing you do before cooking them is make sure they are alive. Here's how you do it:

▶ **Mussels** A mussel that is closed is alive. However, mussel shells will open slightly when exposed to temperature changes. To see if an opened mussel is still alive, try to slide the top shell laterally across the bottom shell. A live mussel will stay rigid.

▶ **Clams** Clams, too, may gape open but still be alive. Just give them a sharp rap on the counter. A live clam will clam up.

oysters

Broiling/grilling Shucked oysters can be oven-broiled if given a crumb coating to protect them from the intense heat—a good alternative to frying them.

Sautéing This method for cooking shucked oysters traditionally requires quite a bit of butter or oil, both for flavor and to keep the delicate oysters from sticking to the pan and breaking apart. For a healthier low-fat sauté, be sure to use a nonstick pan and just a little bit of oil. A light dredging in flour, cornmeal, or breadcrumbs will also help keep the oysters from breaking up (*see Pan-Fried Oysters, page 79*).

Stewing/braising Shucked oysters can be added to soups, stews, and chowders (*see Oyster Stew with Garlic Toast, page 79*), providing they are added during the final cooking stage.

squid & octopus

Squid and octopus are, curiously, classed as shellfish. They belong to a class of mollusks called cephalopods, whose pliable body consists of a beaked head, an internal shell (in some species), and tentacles sprouting directly from the head (cephalopod is derived from the Greek meaning "headed foot"). Squid and octopus are the most popular edible cephalopods.

For tender squid, it needs to be cooked either very quickly, or very slowly. There is no in-between.

Octopus, on the other hand is tough and needs to be precooked before using it in a prepared dish. Place the cleaned octopus into boiling, salted water and simmer until the skin can be peeled off. This may take anywhere from 15 to 60 minutes, depending on the age and size of the octopus. Some cooks feel that octopus must be pounded to tenderize it before cooking; others find that cooking alone is sufficient.

Broiling/grilling Squid bodies can be opened up, brushed with oil, and grilled for just a few minutes.

Sautéing/stir-frying Squid bodies cut crosswise into rings can be sautéed or stir-fried in oil in a nonstick skillet.

Braising/stewing On the other end of the cooking spectrum for squid, slow-cooking in liquid will also make them tender. Squid can be braised either cut in pieces or whole. Often, whole squid is stuffed and then braised in a well-seasoned broth or sauce. To prepare stuffed squid, fill the bodies three-fourths full with a favorite stuffing and secure them with toothpicks to keep the stuffing inside. Squid can be braised in a skillet or in a 350°F oven.

cleaning shrimp

Shrimp purchased shelled and deveined are ready to be cooked, though this makes the shrimp more expensive. The less expensive option is to shell and devein them yourself. It's not difficult to do once you know how. You can shell the shrimp before cooking, or cook them with the shells on, which some people feel adds flavor to the dish.

To prepare uncooked shrimp, use a small sharp knife to make a shallow cut down the back (outer curved side) of each shrimp, then pull off the shell and legs. (Remove the tail portion of the shell, or leave it on for decoration.) Use the knife tip or a metal skewer to pick out the black intestinal vein at the back; working under cold running water will help free the vein. (For shrimp cooked in the shell, peel the shell with your fingers and devein as described above.)

A sharp pair of scissors makes the task even easier. Use the scissors to cut through the shell on the back side of the shrimp, pushing the tip of the scissor into the vein at the same time. When you pull off the shell the vein will be removed with it.

There are also specialized shrimp-deveining tools on the market.

Roasted Shrimp & Asparagus Salad

Cutting asparagus on the diagonal is not absolutely necessary, but it makes for a more attractive presentation in a salad.

2½ teaspoons olive oil

¼ cup fresh lemon juice

1 tablespoon Dijon mustard

½ teaspoon salt

⅓ cup finely diced red bell pepper

½ teaspoon tarragon

3 tablespoons water

1 pound asparagus, cut on the diagonal into 2-inch lengths

1 pound large shrimp, shelled and deveined

1 Preheat the oven to 450°F. In a large bowl, whisk together 1½ teaspoons of the oil, the lemon juice, mustard, and salt. Measure out 2 tablespoons of this mixture and set aside. To the dressing remaining in the bowl, add the bell pepper and tarragon.

2 In a small bowl, stir together the water and remaining 1 teaspoon oil. Place the asparagus in a roasting pan, pour the water-oil mixture over the asparagus, and toss to coat. Roast the asparagus, shaking the pan occasionally, until the asparagus are piping hot, about 5 minutes.

3 Add the shrimp and the reserved 2 tablespoons lemon dressing to the roasting pan with the asparagus. Toss to combine.

4 Return the pan to the oven and roast until the asparagus are crisp-tender and the shrimp are opaque throughout, about 6 minutes. Transfer the shrimp and asparagus to the bowl with the dressing and bell pepper, and toss to combine. *Makes 4 servings*

per serving: 119 calories, 4.1g total fat (0.6g saturated), 135mg cholesterol, 1g dietary fiber, 5g carbohydrate, 16g protein, 547mg sodium. **good source of:** selenium, vitamin B_{12}, vitamin C, vitamin D.

---

different *spins*

▶ **Lime Scampi** Follow the directions for *Shrimp Scampi*, but use lime zest and juice instead of lemon zest and juice, and cilantro instead of parsley. Add ½ teaspoon ground coriander in step 2.

▶ **Orange Scampi** Follow the directions for *Shrimp Scampi*, but use orange zest instead of lemon zest and ¼ cup orange juice plus 1 tablespoon vinegar instead of lemon juice. Add 1½ teaspoons tarragon and ¼ teaspoon pepper in step 2.

Shrimp Scampi

In Italian, a *scampo* is any of several small lobster-like crustaceans, including, most notably, prawns. *Scampi* (the plural) are often prepared very simply with garlic and olive oil (or butter), and Americans have borrowed the word scampi to indicate this cooking style. Thus Shrimp Scampi is shrimp that are prepared with oil and garlic, even though the literal translation would be "Shrimp Prawns."

1 tablespoon olive oil

5 cloves garlic, minced

1½ pounds large shrimp, shelled and deveined

¾ teaspoon salt

⅓ cup chopped parsley

¾ teaspoon grated lemon zest

¼ cup fresh lemon juice

1 In a large nonstick skillet, heat the oil over medium-high heat. Add the garlic and cook 1 minute. Add the shrimp and salt, and cook until the shrimp are not quite opaque throughout, about 2 minutes.

2 Add the parsley and lemon zest, and cook 1 minute. Add the lemon juice, swirling to combine. *Makes 4 servings*

per serving: 144 calories, 4.6g total fat (0.8g saturated), 202mg cholesterol, 0g dietary fiber, 3g carbohydrate, 22g protein, 671mg sodium. **good source of:** omega-3 fatty acids, selenium, vitamin B_{12}, vitamin D.

Zesty Lime-Broiled Shrimp

This dish is pretty, elegant, and simple to make. **Serving suggestion:** Though these shrimp are delicious by themselves, you might want to try a fresh salsa or relish to go with them. Tart flavors would be a nice contrast. Try Tomatillo Salsa (*page 261*), Fresh Pineapple-Jícama Relish (*page 265*), or Mixed Fruit Chutney (*page 266*).

> ½ teaspoon grated lime zest
>
> 2 tablespoons fresh lime juice
>
> 2 tablespoons reduced-sodium soy sauce
>
> 2 teaspoons light brown sugar
>
> ⅛ teaspoon cayenne pepper
>
> 1 pound large shrimp, shelled and deveined

1 In a large bowl, stir together the lime zest, lime juice, soy sauce, brown sugar, and cayenne. Add the shrimp, tossing to coat, and let marinate while you preheat the broiler.

2 Preheat the broiler. Place the shrimp on a broiler pan, drizzle the marinade over them, and broil 4 to 5 inches from the heat for 4 minutes, or until lightly browned and opaque throughout. *Makes 4 servings*

per serving: 85 calories, 0.8g total fat (0.2g saturated), 135mg cholesterol, 0g dietary fiber, 4g carbohydrate, 15g protein, 422mg sodium. good source of: selenium, vitamin B$_{12}$, vitamin D.

---

did you know?

Size designations for shrimp (or prawns) are based on loose industry standards, not rules. For example, so-called "jumbo" shrimp will have as few as 16 to 20 shrimp per pound; "large" shrimp will have 21 to 25; "medium" will be more like 30 to 35 per pound. So when buying shrimp, if you go for a smaller size (which are somewhat cheaper), you need to keep in mind that more pieces of shrimp per pound means more time spent shelling and deveining.

Sautéed Shrimp with Basil & Cherry Tomatoes

Serving suggestion: If you like, turn this into a one-dish dinner by tossing the shrimp and its sauce with a bowl of pasta. Serve a salad on the side.

> 2 teaspoons olive oil
>
> 2 scallions, thinly sliced
>
> 3 cloves garlic, slivered
>
> 1 pound large shrimp, shelled and deveined
>
> 2 cups halved cherry tomatoes (red and yellow)
>
> ¼ cup chopped fresh basil
>
> ½ teaspoon salt
>
> ¼ cup chopped fresh mint

1 In a large nonstick skillet, heat the oil over medium heat. Add the scallions and garlic, and cook until the scallions are slightly softened, about 1 minute.

2 Add the shrimp and cook until opaque on the outside but still a bit translucent in the center, about 3 minutes. With a slotted spoon, transfer the shrimp to a plate.

3 Add the cherry tomatoes, basil, and salt to the skillet and cook until the tomatoes are softened and begin to get juicy, about 4 minutes.

4 Return the shrimp to the skillet. Stir until opaque throughout, about 1 minute. Stir in the mint and serve. *Makes 4 servings*

per serving: 108 calories, 3.3g total fat (0.6g saturated), 135mg cholesterol, 1g dietary fiber, 4g carbohydrate, 15g protein, 454mg sodium. good source of: selenium, vitamin B$_{12}$, vitamin D.

Radiatore with Fennel, Oranges & Shrimp

Blood oranges, like fennel and Calamata olives, are native to the Mediterranean (though they are now grown in this country) and work happily together in this shrimp and pasta dish.

2 blood oranges or navel oranges

8 ounces radiatore pasta

1 tablespoon olive oil

1 medium red onion, halved and thinly sliced

2 cups thinly sliced fennel

¾ pound medium shrimp, shelled and deveined

¼ cup dry white wine or chicken broth

½ teaspoon salt

½ teaspoon pepper

6 Calamata or other brine-cured black olives, pitted and coarsely chopped

1 Grate 1 teaspoon of zest from one of the oranges and set aside. Peel both oranges, removing all of the spongy white pith. Working over a bowl, cut out the sections from in between the membranes, letting the sections drop into the bowl. Squeeze the juice from the membranes into the bowl. Cover and set aside.

2 In a large pot of boiling water, cook the pasta according to package directions. Drain.

3 Meanwhile, in a large nonstick skillet, heat the oil over high heat. Add the onion and fennel, and cook, stirring, until the fennel is tender, about 7 minutes.

4 Add the shrimp, wine, salt, and pepper, and cook until the shrimp are just opaque throughout, 3 to 4 minutes. Remove from the heat.

5 In a large serving bowl, toss the pasta with the shrimp mixture. Add the oranges (and juice), orange zest, and olives, and toss again. *Makes 4 servings*

per serving: 348 calories, 6.5g total fat (0.9g saturated), 101mg cholesterol, 5g dietary fiber, 51g carbohydrate, 19g protein, 525mg sodium. **good source of:** folate, niacin, selenium, thiamin, vitamin B$_{12}$, vitamin C.

Shrimp Jambalaya

There are two types of spicy pork sausage called chorizo: The Mexican version is made with fresh pork; the Spanish version is a hard, cured sausage. We've used the Spanish version here, because it is full flavored and a little goes a long way. In a pinch, you could use pepperoni instead.

1 tablespoon olive oil

1 red onion, finely chopped

3 cloves garlic, minced

2 green bell peppers, cut into ½ -inch squares

1 stalk celery, thinly sliced

1 ounce Spanish chorizo sausage, diced

1¼ cups Texmati or pecan rice

1¾ cups chicken broth, homemade (page 252) or canned

1 cup water

½ teaspoon thyme

½ teaspoon salt

¼ teaspoon red pepper flakes

1 pound large shrimp, shelled and deveined

1 In a large saucepan, heat the oil over medium heat. Add the onion and garlic, and cook, stirring frequently, until the onion is soft, about 7 minutes.

2 Add the bell peppers and celery, and cook until the peppers are crisp-tender, about 5 minutes. Stir in the chorizo.

3 Add the rice, stirring to coat. Add the broth, water, thyme, salt, and red pepper flakes, and bring to a boil. Reduce to a simmer, cover, and cook for 17 minutes or until the rice is tender.

4 Stir in the shrimp, cover, and cook until the shrimp are opaque throughout, about 4 minutes. *Makes 4 servings*

per serving: 412 calories, 7.2g total fat (1.8g saturated), 174mg cholesterol, 3g dietary fiber, 55g carbohydrate, 26g protein, 779mg sodium. **good source of:** selenium, vitamin B$_{12}$, vitamin C, vitamin D.

Broiled Scallops with Baby Spinach

Cutting large sea scallops in half horizontally makes them go further and also increases their surface area for coating with the creamy lemon-mustard dressing. Although baby spinach has become quite common in produce markets (along with other baby greens, such as mesclun), you could use regular spinach, torn into bite-size pieces, instead.

> 1¼ pounds sea scallops, halved horizontally
>
> 2 tablespoons fresh lemon juice
>
> 2 cloves garlic, minced
>
> ½ teaspoon pepper
>
> ¼ teaspoon salt
>
> 1 tablespoon olive oil
>
> 8 cups loosely packed baby spinach
>
> ¼ cup reduced-fat sour cream
>
> 2 tablespoons plain fat-free yogurt
>
> 1 tablespoon Dijon mustard

1 Preheat the broiler. Place the scallops on a jelly-roll pan. Sprinkle with 1 tablespoon of the lemon juice, the garlic, ¼ teaspoon of the pepper, and the salt. Drizzle the oil over the scallops. Toss well, then spread out in a single layer. Broil 4 to 6 inches from the heat for 2 to 3 minutes, or until the scallops are just barely opaque in the center.

2 Divide the spinach among 4 dinner plates. Reserving the pan juices, place the broiled scallops on top of the spinach.

3 In a small bowl, combine the scallop cooking juices, the remaining 1 tablespoon lemon juice, the remaining ¼ teaspoon pepper, the sour cream, yogurt, and mustard. Drizzle the dressing over the scallops and serve. *Makes 4 servings*

per serving: 210 calories, 6.5g total fat (1.9g saturated), 54mg cholesterol, 3g dietary fiber, 10g carbohydrate, 28g protein, 567mg sodium. **good source of:** beta carotene, folate, magnesium, omega-3 fatty acids, potassium, selenium, vitamin B_{12}, vitamin B_6, vitamin E.

Bay Scallops with Citrus Sauce

The tart refreshing flavors of orange and grapefruit juices play well against the sweet richness of scallops. Dry vermouth adds an herbal undertone to the sauce, accentuating the sweet-herbal flavor of the tarragon.

> 2 tablespoons flour
>
> ½ teaspoon salt
>
> 1 pound bay scallops or quartered sea scallops
>
> 4 teaspoons olive oil
>
> 1 red bell pepper, diced
>
> 3 shallots, minced, or 2 scallions, thinly sliced
>
> ½ cup dry vermouth or dry white wine
>
> ½ cup orange juice
>
> ¼ cup pink grapefruit juice
>
> ¾ teaspoon tarragon
>
> 1 teaspoon cornstarch blended with 1 tablespoon water

1 On a large plate, combine the flour and ¼ teaspoon of the salt. Dredge the scallops in the flour mixture, shaking off the excess.

2 In a large nonstick skillet, heat the oil over medium heat. Add the scallops and cook until just opaque in the center, about 1 minute. With a slotted spoon, transfer the scallops to a plate.

3 Add the bell pepper and shallots to the skillet and cook until the pepper is crisp-tender, about 3 minutes. Add the vermouth, increase the heat to high, and cook, stirring, until the liquid is reduced by half, about 1 minute.

4 Add the orange juice, grapefruit juice, tarragon, and remaining ¼ teaspoon salt, and bring to a boil. Boil for 2 minutes to reduce the liquid slightly. Add the cornstarch mixture and cook, stirring, until slightly thickened, about 1 minute.

5 Reduce the heat to low, return the scallops to the pan, and cook just until the scallops are heated through, about 30 seconds. *Makes 4 servings*

per serving: 215 calories, 5.6g total fat (0.7g saturated), 37mg cholesterol, 1g dietary fiber, 16g carbohydrate, 20g protein, 478mg sodium. **good source of:** selenium, vitamin B_{12}, vitamin C.

Scallop Stir-Fry

Jícama, a root vegetable available at many super-markets and Latin American markets, provides added crunch and sweetness to this stir-fry. To cut jícama into matchsticks, first peel it, then halve it through the stem end so that it will lay flat on the work surface. Thinly slice into half rounds then stack the slices and cut them into matchsticks.

> 4 teaspoons olive oil
>
> 1 zucchini, cut into matchsticks
>
> 1 cup jícama matchsticks
>
> 1 red bell pepper, cut into matchsticks
>
> 2 cloves garlic, minced
>
> 1 tablespoon minced fresh ginger
>
> ½ teaspoon salt
>
> ¾ pound sea scallops, halved horizontally
>
> 2 tablespoons cornstarch
>
> 3 scallions, cut on the diagonal into 1-inch lengths
>
> ¼ cup water

1 In a large nonstick skillet, heat 2 teaspoons of the oil over medium heat. Add the zucchini, jíca-ma, and bell pepper, and cook, stirring frequently, until crisp-tender, about 4 minutes.

2 Add the garlic, ginger, and ¼ teaspoon of the salt, and cook for 30 seconds. Transfer the veg-etable mixture to a platter.

3 Add the remaining 2 teaspoons oil to the pan. Dredge the scallops in the cornstarch, shaking off the excess. Add the scallops, scallions, and the remaining ¼ teaspoon salt to the skillet and cook, stirring frequently, until the scallops are crisp on the outside and opaque on the inside, about 2 minutes.

4 Return the vegetables to the pan along with the water and toss to combine. *Makes 4 servings*

per serving: 165 calories, 5.4g total fat (0.7g saturated), 28mg cholesterol, 3g dietary fiber, 14g carbohydrate, 16g protein, 434mg sodium. good source of: selenium, vitamin B$_{12}$, vitamin C.

Simple Grilled Scallops

Serve these simple grilled scallops as is, or dress them up by serving one of these sauces or salsas on the side: Papaya-Corn Salsa (*page 263*), Salsa Verde (*page 258*), or Chimichurri Sauce (*page 258*).

> 2 teaspoons olive oil
>
> ½ teaspoon salt
>
> ½ teaspoon rosemary, minced
>
> 1 pound sea scallops

1 Spray a grill topper (or stovetop grill pan) with nonstick cooking spray. Preheat the grill (or grill pan, over medium heat).

2 In a large bowl, stir together the oil, sea salt, and rosemary. Blot the scallops dry if they are weeping any liquid and transfer them to the bowl. Toss with the oil mixture.

3 Place the scallops on the grill topper (or grill pan) and cook, turning the scallops once, until just opaque, about 3 minutes. *Makes 4 servings*

per serving: 153 calories, 6.2g total fat (1g saturated), 39mg cholesterol, 0g dietary fiber, 3g carbohydrate, 21g protein, 520mg sodium. good source of: magne-sium, omega-3 fatty acids, vitamin B$_{12}$.

different spins

▶**Scallops Chow Fun** To imitate a Chinese noodle dish called chow fun, cook 4 lasagna noodles in a pot of boiling water. Cut the cooked noodles crosswise into ½-inch-wide pieces. Then follow the directions for *Scallop Stir-Fry*, through step 3. Remove the scallops from the pan and set aside. Add the lasagna pieces and 2 more teaspoons of oil to the skillet and cook, stirring, until the pasta is hot, about 2 minutes. Return the vegetables and scallops to the pan and con-tinue as in step 4.

Chilled Calamari & Scallop Salad

After skillet-steaming the scallops and squid in a small amount of seasoned water, the cooking liquid is reduced by about half and used as the basis of the lemony salad dressing. **Timing alert:** The salad should chill for about 2 hours before serving.

½ cup water

2 cloves garlic, minced

2 teaspoons fennel seeds

1½ teaspoons grated lemon zest

½ teaspoon salt

½ teaspoon red pepper flakes

½ pound clean squid bodies (no tentacles), cut into ½-inch-wide rings

½ pound sea scallops, halved horizontally

4 teaspoons olive oil

⅓ cup fresh lemon juice

2 celery stalks, halved lengthwise and thinly sliced crosswise

1 yellow bell pepper, cut into thin strips

½ cup diced red onion

1 In a large skillet, combine the water, garlic, fennel seeds, lemon zest, salt, and red pepper flakes.

2 Bring to a simmer over low heat. Add the squid and scallops, and cook, uncovered, until the squid are tender and the scallops are opaque throughout, about 3 minutes. With a slotted spoon, transfer the shellfish to a bowl.

3 Bring the liquid remaining in the skillet to a boil over high heat. Add the olive oil, return to a boil, and boil until the mixture is reduced to ¼ cup, 2 to 3 minutes. Strain into a large bowl. Whisk in the lemon juice.

4 Add the celery, bell pepper, and red onion. Add the squid and scallops and toss to combine. Cover and refrigerate until the seafood is well chilled, about 2 hours. *Makes 4 servings*

per serving: 188 calories, 7.4g total fat (1.2g saturated), 150mg cholesterol, 2g dietary fiber, 11g carbohydrate, 19g protein, 587mg sodium. good source of: omega-3 fatty acids, selenium, vitamin B$_{12}$, vitamin C.

how to section a grapefruit

The easiest way to remove the membrane from individual grapefruit sections is to actually cut the sections away from the membranes. Begin by peeling the grapefruit, leaving it whole. Then use a sharp knife to peel the membrane off the outside of the fruit. Holding the grapefruit over a bowl to catch the juices, cut toward the center of the fruit, along the inner membranes, to release the sections. If the recipe calls for the juice, squeeze the membranes—you'll get a surprising amount of juice.

Crab, Grapefruit & Avocado Salad

This main-course salad is similar to a classic dish called Crab Louis. The origins of the dish are disputed (several West Coast chefs have been credited with the invention), but all renditions of it involve crabmeat, avocado, and a creamy tomato chili-based dressing.

½ cup plain fat-free yogurt

3 tablespoons ketchup

1 tablespoon light mayonnaise

1 tablespoon fresh lemon juice

½ teaspoon tarragon

½ teaspoon salt

¼ teaspoon cayenne pepper

6 cups bite-size pieces romaine lettuce

1 pound lump crabmeat, picked over to remove any cartilage

2 cups cherry tomatoes, halved

2 pink grapefruits, peeled and sectioned

½ cup diced Hass avocado

1 In a large bowl, combine the yogurt, ketchup, mayonnaise, lemon juice, tarragon, salt, and cayenne. Add the romaine, crabmeat, and tomatoes, tossing to combine.

2 Divide the crabmeat mixture among 4 plates and scatter the grapefruit sections and avocado on top. *Makes 4 servings*

per serving: 256 calories, 4.9g total fat (0.5g saturated), 122mg cholesterol, 5g dietary fiber, 22g carbohydrate, 32g protein, 891mg sodium. good source of: folate, lycopene, potassium, vitamin C.

Parmesan-Crusted Crab Cakes

A squeeze of fresh lemon juice is all these chunky, scallion-flecked crab cakes really need. But if you'd like to convert them to dinner party fare, you could make a fresh relish or salsa to go with them. Try Corn Relish (*page 264*), Tomato-Melon Salsa (*page 263*), or Hot & Spicy Cocktail Sauce (*page 256*).

1 pound lump crabmeat, picked over to remove any cartilage

4 scallions, thinly sliced

¼ cup chopped cilantro

2 teaspoons Dijon mustard

½ teaspoon salt

2 large egg whites

⅔ cup plain dried breadcrumbs

4 teaspoons grated Parmesan cheese

4 teaspoons olive oil

Lemon wedges, for serving

1 In a large bowl, combine the crabmeat, scallions, cilantro, mustard, and salt. In a small bowl, with an electric mixer, beat the egg whites until stiff peaks form. Gently fold into the crabmeat mixture. Shape into 8 crab cakes.

2 In a shallow bowl, stir together the breadcrumbs and Parmesan. Dip the cakes in the breadcrumb mixture. Gently pat the breadcrumb mixture onto the crab cakes.

3 In a large nonstick skillet, heat 2 teaspoons of the oil over medium heat. Add half the crab cakes, and cook for 2 to 3 minutes per side, or until hot and cooked through. Repeat with the remaining oil and crab cakes. Serve with lemon wedges. *Makes 4 servings*

per serving: 230 calories, 6.1g total fat (1.2g saturated), 115mg cholesterol, 1g dietary fiber, 14g carbohydrate, 28g protein, 893mg sodium. good source of: niacin, omega-3 fatty acids, selenium, vitamin B$_{12}$, zinc.

crab boil

Live crabs are often cooked in what is called "crab boil," which is simply boiling water seasoned with a traditional combination of herbs and spices. Crab boil mix can be purchased in any area where live crabs are sold (or by mail order). The mixture can include allspice, mustard seed, cayenne, dill seed, bay leaf, coriander seed, thyme, pepper, and salt, but it will vary from manufacturer to manufacturer. You can also make your own (*recipe follows*).

Crab boil mix can be added directly to the cooking water, or, for easy removal, placed in a square of cheesecloth and tied with a piece of string. Add a squeeze of lemon juice or lemon slices to the water as well. The same mixture can be used to season the cooking water for lobster, crayfish, or shrimp. Use about ¼ cup of crab boil for 4 quarts of water and 3 pounds of shellfish.

▶**Crab boil** Combine 2 tablespoons each of black peppercorns, mustard seeds, and coriander seeds with 1 tablespoon each of ground cloves, allspice, dill seeds, thyme, and red pepper flakes. Add 12 bay leaves. Makes about ¾ cup

Linguine with Thai-Style Crab Sauce

The signature ingredients in Thai-style cooking are lime juice, fresh basil, and fresh mint. The combination of fresh flavors plays well against the richness of crabmeat. The cornstarch-thickened sauce lends a silkiness that in most sauces would be provided by fat.

> 10 ounces linguine
>
> 1 tablespoon olive oil
>
> 1 red bell pepper, cut into ¼-inch-wide strips
>
> 6 scallions, thinly sliced
>
> 4 cloves garlic, minced
>
> ½ pound lump crabmeat, picked over to remove any cartilage
>
> 1 teaspoon cornstarch
>
> ¼ teaspoon salt
>
> 3 tablespoons reduced-sodium soy sauce
>
> 3 tablespoons fresh lime juice
>
> ½ cup chopped fresh basil
>
> ¼ cup chopped fresh mint

1 In a large pot of boiling water, cook the pasta according to package directions. Drain, reserving ½ cup of the pasta cooking water. Transfer the pasta to a large bowl.

2 Meanwhile, in a large nonstick skillet, heat the oil over medium heat. Add the bell pepper, scallions, and garlic, and cook, stirring frequently, until the bell pepper is tender, about 5 minutes.

3 Add the crabmeat and cook, stirring, until heated through, about 3 minutes.

4 Place the cornstarch and salt in a small bowl. Stir in the reserved pasta cooking water, soy sauce, and lime juice until smooth. Pour the mixture into the skillet and bring to a boil. Cook, stirring constantly, until the sauce is slightly thickened, about 1 minute.

5 Pour the sauce over the pasta, add the basil and mint, and toss to combine. *Makes 4 servings*

per serving: 385 calories, 5.7g total fat (0.8g saturated), 57mg cholesterol, 4g dietary fiber, 61g carbohydrate, 22g protein, 714mg sodium. good source of: omega-3 fatty acids, selenium, vitamin B$_{12}$, vitamin C, zinc.

Lobster with Dipping Sauces

Lobster—without melted butter—is the ultimate low-fat (and low-cholesterol) splurge. Try one (or all) of the sauces suggested below. (The nutritional analysis does not include the dipping sauces.) We've added some fresh herbs to the lobster cooking water, but they are not absolutely necessary.

> 2 tablespoons coarse sea salt or kosher salt
>
> ½ cup basil leaves
>
> ½ cup parsley leaves
>
> 4 live lobsters (1¼ to 1½ pounds each)
>
> Dipping Sauces (recipes follow)

1 Bring a lobster pot (or a large spaghetti pot) of water to a rolling boil. Add the salt, basil, and parsley, and return to a boil. Slip 2 of the lobsters into the boiling water. Cover and return to a boil. Uncover and boil for 6 minutes or until the shells are red-orange. With tongs, remove the lobsters and transfer them to a large colander to drain. Repeat with the remaining 2 lobsters.

2 Meanwhile, make one (or all) of the dipping sauces. Serve the lobsters hot, at room temperature, or chilled, with the dipping sauces on the side. *Makes 4 servings*

per serving: 46 calories, 0.3g total fat (0.1g saturated), 32mg cholesterol, 0g dietary fiber, 1g carbohydrate, 9g protein, 171mg sodium. good source of: selenium, vitamin B$_{12}$.

Thai-Style Dipping Sauce In a small saucepan, combine 2 tablespoons soy sauce and 2 tablespoons sugar, and stir over low heat until the sugar has melted. Transfer to a bowl and stir in ⅓ cup fresh lime juice and 1 teaspoon dark sesame oil.

Tomato-Jalapeño Dipping Sauce In a small bowl, stir together ½ cup ketchup, 1 minced canned or bottled jalapeño, and 2 teaspoons balsamic vinegar.

Herbed Lemon Dipping Sauce In a small bowl, whisk together ¼ cup fresh lemon juice, 1 tablespoon olive oil, and ½ teaspoon salt. Stir in 2 tablespoons chopped fresh basil and 2 teaspoons minced chives.

Creamy New England Clam Chowder

Bacon lends an inimitable flavor to this New England clam stew. Although bacon certainly has some strikes against it—such as saturated fat and sodium—you don't have to forgo it if it's used as a seasoning instead of a main ingredient. Luckily, bacon freezes beautifully so you can buy a half-pound and just cut off small amounts when you need it.

1 slice bacon (¾ ounce), finely chopped

1¾ cups water

1 red bell pepper, cut into ½-inch squares

3 cloves garlic, minced

¾ pound red potatoes, cut into ½-inch chunks

1 cup bottled clam juice or chicken broth

½ teaspoon salt

½ teaspoon black pepper

1 can (14½ ounces) creamed corn

½ cup milk

1 cup shucked clams (from 2 dozen littlenecks), coarsely chopped

1 In a large saucepan, cook the bacon and ¼ cup of the water over low heat until the bacon is lightly crisped, about 3 minutes. Add the bell pepper and garlic, and cook, stirring frequently, until the bell pepper is crisp-tender, about 5 minutes. Add the potatoes, tossing to coat.

2 Stir in the remaining 1½ cups water, the clam juice, salt, and black pepper, and bring to a boil. Reduce to a simmer, cover, and cook until the potatoes are tender, about 10 minutes.

3 Stir in the creamed corn and milk, and bring to a boil. Add the clams, reduce to a simmer, and cook just until the clams are cooked through, about 2 minutes. ***Makes 4 servings***

per serving: 265 calories, 3.6g total fat (1.2g saturated), 44mg cholesterol, 3g dietary fiber, 41g carbohydrate, 20g protein, 816mg sodium. good source of: niacin, potassium, riboflavin, selenium, thiamin, vitamin B$_{12}$, vitamin B$_6$, vitamin C.

Hot & Spicy Mussels

Beautiful blue-black mussels pan-steamed over a heady mixture of white wine, garlic, and onions is one of the best—and simplest—shellfish dishes you can make. As the mussels steam, they open up and release flavorful juices into the pan. A chunk of good peasant bread for sopping up the juices is an essential accompaniment to this dish.

1 tablespoon olive oil

1 small onion, finely chopped

6 cloves garlic, minced

½ teaspoon red pepper flakes

1 cup dry white wine

2 tablespoons fresh lime juice

4 pounds mussels, scrubbed and debearded

¼ cup chopped cilantro

¼ cup chopped parsley

1 In a Dutch oven or flameproof casserole, heat the oil over medium heat. Add the onion, garlic, and red pepper flakes, and cook, stirring frequently, until the onion is soft, about 7 minutes.

2 Add the wine and lime juice, and bring to a boil. Add the mussels, cover, and cook, shaking the pan occasionally, until all the mussels have opened, 8 to 10 minutes. Remove the pan from the heat. Discard any mussels that have not opened. Stir in the cilantro and parsley. ***Makes 4 servings***

per serving: 235 calories, 7.3g total fat (1.2g saturated), 48mg cholesterol, 1g dietary fiber, 11g carbohydrate, 21g protein, 322mg sodium. good source of: omega-3 fatty acids, riboflavin, selenium, thiamin, vitamin B$_{12}$.

Fettuccine with Mussels & Spinach

The mussel's so-called beard (also called the byssus) is made of threads that the mussel manufactures in order to attach itself to rocks and pilings. The beards need to be removed before cooking.

8 ounces fettuccine

½ cup dry white wine

½ teaspoon thyme

2 dozen mussels, scrubbed and debearded

1 tablespoon olive oil

4 garlic cloves, thinly sliced

12 cups loosely packed spinach leaves

½ teaspoon pepper

¼ teaspoon salt

1 In a large pot of boiling water, cook the pasta according to package directions. Drain.

2 Meanwhile, in a large saucepan, combine the wine and thyme. Cover and bring to a boil over high heat. Add the mussels, reduce the heat to medium-high, cover, and cook, shaking the pan occasionally, until all the mussels have opened, 4 to 6 minutes. Remove the pan from the heat. Discard any mussels that have not opened.

3 After draining the pasta, add the oil and garlic to the pasta cooking pot. Cook over high heat, stirring constantly, until the garlic is golden, 1 to 2 minutes. Add the spinach, pepper, and salt, and cook, stirring, until the spinach is just wilted, 3 to 4 minutes.

how to debeard a mussel

To prepare mussels for cooking (they are most commonly cooked in their shells), scrub the shells (with a stiff brush, if necessary) and rinse under cold running water. Scrape any tough encrustations from the shells with a sturdy knife. Pull the stringy "beards"—the fibrous dark tufts protruding from the shells—out of the mussels before rinsing them. They will not pull out easily, so just be insistent.

4 Return the drained pasta to the pot with the spinach mixture and toss just until heated through. Remove from the heat.

5 Shell the mussels and add to the pasta. Strain the mussel cooking juices through a fine-mesh strainer into the pasta pot and toss to mix well. *Makes 4 servings*

per serving: 385 calories, 7.1g total fat (3.3g saturated), 27mg cholesterol, 6g dietary fiber, 23g protein, 550mg sodium. **good source of:** beta carotene, folate, lutein, magnesium, potassium, riboflavin, selenium, vitamin B_{12}, vitamin C.

Littleneck Clams with Carrot-Ginger Sauce

The smallest amount of butter added at the end of cooking gives the carrot-ginger sauce a silky texture. **Serving suggestion:** Serve the clams and the sauce over brown rice or linguine.

2 teaspoons olive oil

3 shallots, minced

5 cloves garlic, minced

1 tablespoon minced fresh ginger

1¼ cups carrot juice

2 dozen littleneck clams, well scrubbed

1¼ cups frozen corn kernels

¼ teaspoon salt

¼ cup chopped fresh basil

2 teaspoons unsalted butter

1 In a large skillet, heat the oil over low heat. Add the shallots, garlic, and ginger, and cook, stirring frequently, until the shallots are tender, about 5 minutes.

2 Add the carrot juice, increase the heat to medium-high, and bring to a boil. Add the clams, cover, and cook, shaking the pan occasionally, for 5 to 10 minutes, or until all the clams have opened. Remove the skillet from the heat. (Discard any clams that do not open.) When cool enough to handle, remove the clam meat from the shells, coarsely chop, and set aside. Discard the shells.

different spins

▶**Spicy Mussel & Shrimp Chowder** Follow the directions for *Manhattan Shellfish Chowder*, but substitute an equal amount of mussels for the clams, and shelled and deveined shrimp for the scallops. Increase the garlic to 5 cloves and substitute 2 cans (14½ ounces each) of diced tomatoes with jalapeño for the stewed tomatoes.

▶**Clam & Calamari Chowder** Follow the directions for *Manhattan Shellfish Chowder*, but substitute ½ pound of cleaned squid (sliced crosswise into rings) for the scallops. Add the squid when you would add the scallops, in step 4.

3 Return the carrot mixture to a boil. Stir in the corn and salt, and cook until the corn is heated through, about 1 minute. Off the heat, add the clams, basil, and butter, and swirl to combine. *Makes 4 servings*

per serving: 212 calories, 5.8g total fat (1.7g saturated), 43mg cholesterol, 2g dietary fiber, 24g carbohydrate, 18g protein, 235mg sodium. good source of: beta carotene, potassium, riboflavin, selenium, vitamin B$_{12}$, vitamin B$_6$.

Manhattan Shellfish Chowder

James Beard once called Manhattan clam chowder "a vegetable soup that accidentally had some clams dumped into it." Indeed many Manhattan chowders seem to be just that. Here we start with fresh littleneck clams in the shell and sea scallops and let them dominate in an herbed tomato and white wine broth.

>   1 small onion, finely chopped
>
>   3 cloves garlic, minced
>
>   ¾ cup dry white wine or water
>
>   1 dozen littleneck clams, well scrubbed
>
>   ¾ pound all-purpose potatoes, peeled and cut into ½-inch cubes
>
>   2 cups water

>   2 cans (14½ ounces each) no-salt-added stewed tomatoes, chopped with their juice
>
>   ½ teaspoon oregano
>
>   ½ teaspoon salt
>
>   ¾ pound sea scallops, halved horizontally

1 In a Dutch oven or flameproof casserole, combine the onion, garlic, wine, and clams. Bring to a boil over moderate heat, cover, and cook, shaking the pan occasionally, for 5 to 10 minutes, or until all the clams have opened. Remove the skillet from the heat. (Discard any clams that do not open.) Remove the clams from the pan. When cool enough to handle, remove the clam meat from the shells, coarsely chop, and set aside. Discard the shells.

2 Add the potatoes and water to the pan and bring to a boil. Reduce to a simmer, cover, and cook until the potatoes are firm-tender, about 5 minutes.

3 Add the tomatoes and their juice, the oregano, and salt, and return to a boil. Reduce the heat to a simmer, cover, and cook for 15 minutes or until the potatoes are tender.

4 Add the scallops to the pan, cover, and cook for 2 minutes, or until they are almost cooked through. Return the clam meats to the pan and cook just until heated through, about 30 seconds. *Makes 4 servings*

per serving: 258 calories, 1.1g total fat (0.1g saturated), 37mg cholesterol, 5g dietary fiber, 32g carbohydrate, 21g protein, 474mg sodium. good source of: potassium, selenium, vitamin B$_{12}$, vitamin B$_6$, vitamin C.

Clams in Red Sauce over Couscous

Although clams in red sauce is more commonly served with a strand pasta (like spaghetti), couscous provides a better way to get every drop of the delicious sauce.

> 2 teaspoons olive oil
>
> ¼ cup finely chopped onion
>
> 3 cloves garlic, minced
>
> 1 can (14½ ounces) diced tomatoes with basil
>
> ¼ teaspoon red pepper flakes
>
> 2 dozen littleneck or other hard-shelled clams, well scrubbed
>
> 1½ cups boiling water
>
> 1 cup couscous (7½ ounces)

1 In a large nonstick skillet, heat the oil over low heat. Add the onion and garlic, and cook, stirring frequently, until tender, about 7 minutes.

2 Add the tomatoes and red pepper flakes, increase the heat to medium, and bring to a boil. Add the clams, cover, and cook, shaking the pan occasionally, for 5 to 10 minutes, or until all the clams have opened. Remove the skillet from the heat. (Discard any clams that do not open.)

the clam purge

All clams should be rinsed—and preferably swirled about—in several changes of cold water to loosen the grit they accumulate. But some people like to take this a step further and purge the grit by soaking clams in salt water—usually a gallon of cold water to which 2 teaspoons of salt have been added. Let the clams sit in this solution in the refrigerator for 2 to 3 hours. The theory is that the live clams will filter new, clean water through their systems and at the same time expel any grit they may have had in them when they were harvested. You can also try using a cup of cornmeal instead of, or in addition to, the salt.

3 Meanwhile, in a medium heatproof bowl, pour the boiling water over the couscous. Cover and let stand 5 minutes, until the couscous has absorbed the water and is tender.

4 When cool enough to handle, remove the clam meat from the shells and stir the clams back into the sauce. Serve the clams and sauce over the couscous. ***Makes 4 servings***

per serving: 332 calories, 3.7g total fat (0.5g saturated), 38mg cholesterol, 4g dietary fiber, 50g carbohydrate, 22g protein, 245mg sodium. **good source of:** selenium, vitamin B_{12}.

Steamer Clams in Fennel Broth

This shoreline favorite is generally served by the bucketful along with a bowl of melted butter for dipping. We've skipped the butter and suggested a number of dipping sauces, though you could stay simple and use the flavorful cooking broth as the dipping sauce. Steamer clams tend to be sandy, so rinse them well.

> 4 pounds steamer clams
>
> 2 cups water
>
> 2 teaspoons lemon zest
>
> 1½ teaspoons fennel seeds
>
> ¼ teaspoon red pepper flakes
>
> Salsa Verde (page 258), Fresh Ginger & Lime Dressing (page 254), or Chimichurri Sauce (page 258), optional

1 Scrub the clams with a brush until no longer muddy then soak in several changes of cold water until the water runs clear.

2 In a large pot, combine the water, lemon zest, fennel seeds, and red pepper flakes. Add the clams. Cover the pot and bring to a boil. Cook, shaking the pan occasionally, for 5 to 10 minutes, or until all the clams have opened. Remove the pan from the heat. Discard any clams that do not open.

3 With a slotted spoon, transfer the clams to individual serving bowls. Strain the broth through cheesecloth or a fine-mesh sieve and divide the broth among 4 small bowls or cups.

4 To eat the steamers, peel the black skin off the protruding siphon (called the "neck"). Hold the clam by the neck and swish it around in the broth to rinse it. Then dip it into the dipping sauce (if using), biting it off at the neck (the neck is edible, but tends to be chewy). *Makes 4 servings*

per serving: 101 calories, 1.3g total fat (0.1g saturated), 46mg cholesterol, 0g dietary fiber, 4g carbohydrate, 17g protein, 76mg sodium. good source of: iron, selenium, vitamin B_{12}.

Pan-Fried Oysters

Browned in just 2 teaspoons of oil, these delicate crusty oysters barely fit the definition of "fried."

> 4 teaspoons Dijon mustard
>
> 1 tablespoon chili sauce
>
> 1 teaspoon fresh lemon juice
>
> ¼ teaspoon Louisiana-style hot sauce
>
> ¼ teaspoon tarragon
>
> ¼ cup flour
>
> 2 tablespoons yellow cornmeal
>
> ¼ teaspoon baking powder
>
> ¼ teaspoon salt
>
> 1 large egg white
>
> 1 tablespoon water
>
> 1 dozen oysters, shucked
>
> 2 teaspoons olive oil

1 In a small bowl, combine the mustard, chili sauce, lemon juice, hot sauce, and tarragon. Set aside.

2 In a shallow bowl, combine the flour, cornmeal, baking powder, and salt. In another shallow bowl, beat the egg white with the water. Dip the oysters first in the egg white, then in the flour mixture.

3 In a large nonstick skillet, heat the oil over medium–high heat. Add the oysters and cook until golden brown and crisp, about 2 minutes per side. Serve with the mustard sauce spooned alongside. *Makes 4 servings*

per serving: 105 calories, 3.5g total fat (0.5g saturated), 11mg cholesterol, 1g dietary fiber, 14g carbohydrate, 5g protein, 440mg sodium. good source of: selenium, vitamin B12, zinc.

Oyster Stew with Garlic Toast

Unless you have experience shucking live oysters, it's safer and faster to have this service performed by the fish seller. Fortunately, fish stores and the seafood departments of supermarkets sell already shucked oysters in their own liquor (which is what the liquid that comes out of oysters is called). If your shucked oysters don't have the ½ cup of liquor called for in the recipe, add bottled clam juice or chicken broth to make up the difference.

> 4 large slices (2 ounces) whole-wheat Italian bread, without seeds
>
> 1 clove garlic, halved
>
> ¼ cup nonfat dry milk powder
>
> 3 tablespoons flour
>
> 3 cups low-fat (1%) milk
>
> ½ teaspoon salt
>
> ¼ teaspoon cayenne pepper
>
> 3 dozen shucked oysters, with their liquor
>
> 3 tablespoons minced chives

1 Toast the bread under the broiler or in a toaster oven. Rub the bread with the cut garlic clove. Discard the garlic.

2 In a large bowl, combine the dry milk and flour. Whisk in ½ cup of the liquid milk until smooth. Whisk in the remaining 2½ cups milk. Transfer to a large skillet. Add the salt and cayenne, and cook, stirring frequently, until the sauce is slightly thickened and the consistency of heavy cream, about 3 minutes.

3 Stir in ½ cup of oyster liquor. Bring the mixture to a simmer over low heat. Add the oysters, cover, and cook just until the edges of the oysters begin to curl, about 2 minutes. Stir in the chives.

4 Place a garlic toast in the bottom of each of 4 soup bowls and spoon the stew on top. *Makes 4 servings*

per serving: 229 calories, 4.5g total fat (1.9g saturated), 39mg cholesterol, 1g dietary fiber, 30g carbohydrate, 16g protein, 716mg sodium. good source of: calcium, omega-3 fatty acids, riboflavin, selenium, thiamin, vitamin B_{12}, zinc.

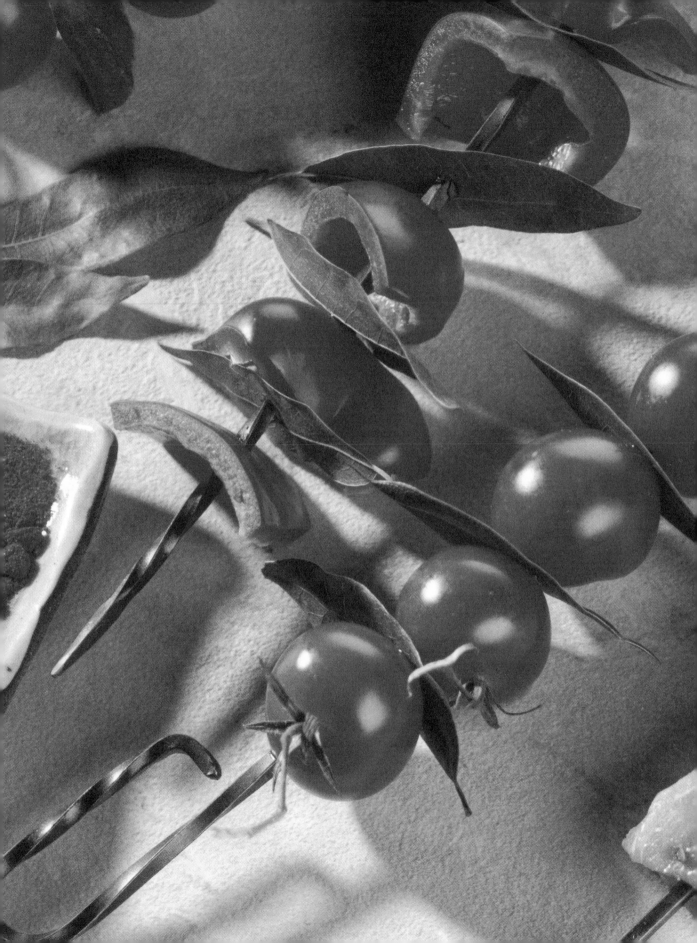

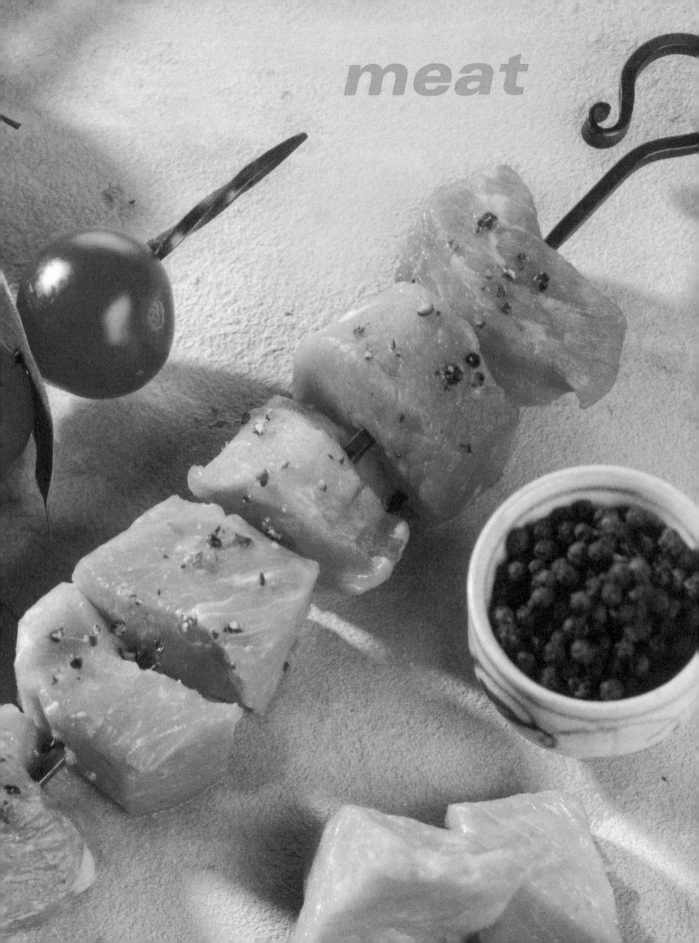

Though there are many reasons to cut back on meat in the diet, there are several ways you can have your meat and eat it, too: **1)** Learn how to cook with lean cuts. **2)** Eat smaller portions—about 3 ounces cooked per person. **3)** Use small amounts of meat in dishes with other components (stir-fries, soups, and salads, for example).

The flavors we appreciate in meat evolve during the cooking process. Heat causes certain compounds in the meat to develop the familiar taste and characteristic smell that we associate with it. In addition, high temperatures bring about complex "browning reactions" that make the outer crust of meats, such as roast beef and broiled chops, intensely savory.

Cooking meat successfully demands careful timing and temperature control. The goal is to cook the food just until the connective tissue is softened, but not so long that the muscle fibers turn tough, which can happen quickly with the leaner cuts, as they have less intramuscular fat to keep them moist and tender. With lean meat, you're better off with very fast, high-heat cooking to keep the juices in.

For all meats, you should trim the external fat before cooking, since this is one of the biggest sources of fat in meat. Trimming external fat before cooking results in a 19% reduction in fat content, and has no negative effect on flavor, tenderness, or juiciness.

the leanest cuts

Cooking lean meats presents certain challenges, and it should be noted that all of the recipes in this book (including all of the cooking charts) have focused on these cuts, which are:

Pork Center-cut loin (either whole or cut into chops) and pork tenderloin are the leanest cuts of pork around. Loin has about 7 grams of fat per 3-ounce serving cooked, and tenderloin has just over 4 grams. Surprisingly, ham, too, is a fairly lean cut, especially if you can find an extra-lean ham with no external fat. Of course it can have quite a bit of sodium (choose reduced-sodium types), but it has only 5 grams of fat per 3-ounce serving.

Beef Eye round, top round, bottom round, sirloin, flank steak, and tenderloin are the leanest cuts, and the best choices for low-fat cooking. They range from 4.6 grams of fat (eye round) to 12 grams (tenderloin) for 3 ounces cooked.

Lamb The leanest cuts of lamb are leg and loin, with 7 to 8 grams of fat for 3 ounces cooked. Shoulder—slightly higher at just over 9 grams per 3 ounces—is also a good choice.

pork

Because of many warnings over the years about pork and trichinosis, many cooks think it is necessary to cook pork to the well-done stage to eliminate this risk. Today, however, trichinosis has been virtually eliminated. According to the Food Safety and Inspection Service, as little as 0.1% of the pork supply nowadays may be infected with *Trichinella spiralis*, the parasite that causes trichinosis. In addition, this parasite is destroyed at 137°F, and the recommended internal temperature of cooked pork is 160°F, providing a handsome margin of safety. At that internal temperature, the meat is still juicy, with slight traces of pink.

Roasting As with other meats, cooking times for pork depend on the size and thickness of the cut and whether the meat is boneless or boned. Pork should be roasted without any liquid in the pan and the pan should be uncovered, otherwise the meat will steam rather than roast (*see Orange-Glazed Roast Pork, page 84, and Roast Pork Salad with Mushrooms & Watercress, page 85*).

Baking Chops and tenderloin can be baked along with vegetables for a one-dish meal. Lean tenderloin can also be ground and used to make meatballs or meatloaf (*see Southwestern Meatloaf, page 90*).

pork cooking chart

Always check for doneness about 15 minutes before the first time listed in the range of times. For pork that is juicy and tender, stop the cooking when the temperature registers 155°F on a meat thermometer (*see "How to Use a Meat Thermometer," page 107*). Let the pork stand for 15 minutes; during that time, the meat will continue to "cook" and the temperature will rise another 5 degrees, to 160°F.

CUT	AMOUNT	METHOD
CENTER-CUT LOIN	bone-in, 3 to 5 lbs	**Roasting** 325°F for 1¼ to 2 hours, or until meat thermometer reads 160°F
	boneless, 2 to 4 lbs	**Roasting** 325°F for 45 minutes to 1½ hours, or until meat thermometer reads 160°F
	cut for stir-fry	**Stir-frying** *See Meat Stir-Fries "Recipe Creator" on page 95*
CENTER-CUT LOIN CHOPS	bone-in, 1 inch thick	**Baking** 350°F for 20–25 minutes
	bone-in, ½ inch thick	**Broiling/grilling** 4 to 6 inches from heat, 3–4 minutes per side
	boneless, ½ to 1 inch thick	**Broiling/grilling** 4 to 6 inches from heat, 3–4 minutes per side
TENDERLOIN	whole, ¾ to 1 lb	**Roasting** 400°F for 25–30 minutes, or until meat thermometer reads 160°F
	cut into 1-inch chunks	**Broiling/grilling** Thread on skewers, cook 4 to 6 inches from heat, turning as they cook, about 8 minutes
	sliced ½ inch thick	**Pan-frying** In lightly oiled nonstick skillet, over medium heat, 1½–2 minutes per side
	sliced and pounded to a ¼-inch thickness	**Pan-frying** In lightly oiled nonstick skillet, over medium heat, 1 minute per side
	cut for stir-fry	**Stir-frying** *See Meat Stir-Fries "Recipe Creator" on page 95*
HAM, BAKED	fully cooked, bone-in, 14 to 16 lbs	**Baking** 325°F for 15–18 minutes per pound, or until meat thermometer reads 140°F

Broiling/grilling Pork loin, chops, and cubes of loin or tenderloin threaded on skewers can be broiled or grilled (*see Broiled Herb-Rubbed Pork Chops and Jerk Pork Kebabs, both on page 86*).

Pan-frying You can successfully pan-fry thin slices of pork, such as scallopine and cutlets, with a small amount of fat if you use a nonstick skillet, dredge the pork in a coating mixture, and get the pan good and hot before adding the pork (*see Pork Scallops Piccata, page 88*).

Stir-frying The key to stir-frying is to cut the meat very thin (about ¼ x ½-inch strips) so it cooks quickly (*see the Meat-Stir-Fries "Recipe Creator," page 95*).

Stewing/braising Usually reserved for fattier cuts of pork, you can still stew lean cuts if you use one of two tricks. You can sear the meat, remove it from the pan, stew the other ingredients, and add the pork back in toward the end of the cooking (*see Green Pork Chili, page 89*). Or you can make a quick-cooking stew so the pork does not get tough (*see Pork Vindaloo, page 87*).

Orange-Glazed Roast Pork

Pork tenderloin is the leanest cut: For 3 ounces of cooked, it has only 4.1 g fat (1.4 g saturated), compared with, for example, pork shoulder, which has 11 g fat (3.7 g saturated). Pork tenderloins are often packed 2 to a vacuum-sealed plastic package. Use the one you need, wrap the other and freeze it for a later date. You can serve the pork on its own (see below for a menu suggestion), slice it for sandwiches, add it to a salad, or toss in a pasta sauce. **Serving suggestions:** Serve slices of the roast pork with Couscous Salad (*page 207*), Lemon-Dill Beans & Peas (*page 181*), and Carrot-Pistachio Biscotti (*page 249*) for dessert.

> 1 tablespoon reduced-sodium soy sauce
> 1 tablespoon frozen orange juice concentrate
> 1¼ teaspoons dark brown sugar
> 1½ teaspoons mustard
> ¼ teaspoon pepper
> ¾ pound pork tenderloin

1 Preheat the oven to 425°F. In a small bowl, stir together the soy sauce, orange juice concentrate, brown sugar, mustard, and pepper.

2 Place the tenderloin on a rack in a roasting pan and brush with the soy sauce mixture. Roast for 25 minutes, or until the pork is cooked through and a meat thermometer reads 160°F.

---

different spins

▶ **Pineapple-Glazed Pork** Follow the directions for *Orange-Glazed Roast Pork*, but use pineapple juice concentrate instead of orange juice. Add ½ teaspoon rosemary.

3 Transfer the pork to a plate and let stand for 10 minutes before slicing. Slice the pork slightly on the diagonal into ¼-inch-thick slices, reserving any juices that collect on the plate. Serve the pork with the pan juices. *Makes 4 servings*

per serving: 119 calories, 3.1g total fat (1g saturated), 55mg cholesterol, 0g dietary fiber, 4g carbohydrate, 18g protein, 224mg sodium. good source of: niacin, selenium, thiamin, vitamin B_{12}, vitamin B_6.

Roast Pork & Sweet Potato Salad

Sweet potatoes and plums are naturally sweet counterpoints to roast pork. If fresh plums aren't in season, substitute ½ cup of bite-size pitted dried plums (prunes).

> Orange-Glazed Roast Pork (at left)
> ¼ cup cider vinegar
> 2 tablespoons reduced-sodium soy sauce
> 2 tablespoons frozen orange juice concentrate
> 2 teaspoons olive oil
> 1 teaspoon light brown sugar
> ¼ teaspoon ground ginger
> ¼ teaspoon salt
> 1 pound sweet potatoes, peeled and cut into 1-inch chunks
> ½ pound Italian prune plums, cut into ½-inch-thick wedges
> 1 stalk celery, halved lengthwise and thinly sliced crosswise
> 2 scallions, thinly sliced

1 Roast the pork as directed. When cool enough to handle, thinly slice and cut the slices into ½-inch-wide strips.

2 Meanwhile, in a large bowl, whisk together the vinegar, soy sauce, orange juice concentrate, oil, brown sugar, ginger, and salt. Stir in any juices that have collected on the plate with the pork.

3 In a vegetable steamer, steam the sweet potatoes until tender, about 10 minutes. Add to the bowl with the dressing.

4 Add the plums, celery, pork, and scallions to the bowl and toss. *Makes 4 servings*

per serving: 264 calories, 5.7g total fat (1.4g saturated), 47mg cholesterol, 4g dietary fiber, 34g carbohydrate, 20g protein, 622mg sodium. good source of: beta carotene, niacin, potassium, riboflavin, selenium, thiamin, vitamin B_6, vitamin C.

Roast Pork Salad with Mushrooms & Watercress

One of the virtues of pork tenderloin—in addition to the fact that it's lean—is that it comes as a ¾- to 1-pound "roast," a size convenient for only 4 servings. This means it cooks quickly, and you won't be stuck with pounds of leftover meat.

> 3 cloves garlic, minced
> 1½ teaspoons rosemary, minced
> 1 teaspoon fennel seeds, crushed
> ¾ teaspoon salt

½ teaspoon pepper
¾ pound pork tenderloin
⅓ cup frozen apple juice concentrate, thawed
2 tablespoons fresh lemon juice
1 tablespoon olive oil
2 cups sliced mushrooms
2 cups packed watercress
2 Granny Smith apples, cut into thin wedges

1 Preheat the oven to 425°F. In a medium bowl, combine the garlic, rosemary, fennel, ¼ teaspoon of the salt, and the pepper. Measure out 2 teaspoons of the herb mixture and rub it into the pork.

2 Roast the pork for 25 minutes, or until it is cooked through but still juicy and a meat thermometer reads 160°F. Let the pork stand for 10 minutes before slicing. Cut the pork into ½-inch-thick slices, reserving any juices on the plate.

3 Meanwhile, to the herb mixture remaining in the bowl, add the remaining ½ teaspoon salt, the apple juice concentrate, lemon juice, and oil.

4 Add the pork and cooking juices to the dressing. Add the mushrooms, watercress, and apples, tossing to coat. Serve warm or at room temperature. *Makes 4 servings*

per serving: 223 calories, 6.9g total fat (1.6g saturated), 50mg cholesterol, 3g dietary fiber, 22g carbohydrate, 20g protein, 488mg sodium. good source of: niacin, riboflavin, selenium, thiamin.

how to tell when meat is done

In addition to the objective test of meat's doneness made with a meat thermometer (*see "How to Use a Meat Thermometer," page 107*), there are some visual clues that cooks use to see if meat is done.

▶ **Pork** Pork loin and chops will feel almost firm with a slight give to the touch (your finger should not bounce off the meat). If you insert a fork into the center of the loin, the tines will be very hot and the juices will run clear with a tinge of yellow. Pork tenderloin will feel almost firm to the touch, but slightly less so than pork loin. Poked, the juices will run clear with a tinge of yellow.

▶ **Beef** The two main ways of judging beef's doneness—which can range from medium-rare to well-done—are texture and color. The longer beef cooks, the firmer its texture. Beef cooked to medium-rare will give slightly when pressed, and a well-done piece will have no give at all. As to color, a medium-rare piece of meat will be pink, not rosy red. Meat cooked to medium will be slightly pink, and well-done meat will be uniformly brown.

▶ **Lamb** Lamb can be cooked to varying degrees of doneness, and the tests for doneness for both texture and color are identical to beef.

Jerk Pork Kebabs

Cubes of pork tenderloin are cooked in a spicy Jamaican-style jerk marinade until richly browned and tender. **Serving suggestion:** Serve the kebabs with a fruit salsa (*see "Recipe Creator," page 262*).

  1½ teaspoons thyme

  1 teaspoon pepper

  ¾ teaspoon salt

  ¾ teaspoon allspice

  ½ teaspoon ground ginger

  2 tablespoons red wine vinegar or balsamic vinegar

  2 tablespoons light brown sugar

  4 scallions, thinly sliced

  4 cloves garlic, minced

  1 pound pork tenderloin, cut into ½-inch chunks

1 Spray a broiler pan with nonstick cooking spray. Preheat the broiler. In a large bowl, stir together the thyme, pepper, salt, allspice, and ginger until well combined.

2 Stir in the vinegar, brown sugar, scallions, and garlic. Add the pork and toss well to coat.

3 Thread the pork on four 10-inch skewers. Broil the pork 4 to 6 inches from the heat for 8 minutes, turning the skewers occasionally, until the pork is richly browned and cooked through (but still juicy). *Makes 4 servings*

per serving: 177 calories, 4.2g total fat (1.5g saturated), 67mg cholesterol, 1g dietary fiber, 9g carbohydrate, 24g protein, 489mg sodium. **good source of:** niacin, riboflavin, selenium, thiamin.

Broiled Herb-Rubbed Pork Chops

You could also make this with so-called boneless chops (sometimes sold as medallions or cutlets). Or make your own boneless chops by buying 1¼ pounds of a boneless center-cut loin roast and cutting it into ¾-inch slices. **Serving suggestion:** The simple, rich flavor of these chops would match well with a slightly sweet condiment. Try Fresh Vidalia Onion Relish (*page 265*), Corn Relish (*page 264*), or Lemon-Honey Quince (*page 229*).

  ¾ teaspoon rubbed sage

  ½ teaspoon rosemary, minced

  ½ teaspoon salt

  ½ teaspoon pepper

  ½ teaspoon sugar

  1 bay leaf, very finely crumbled

  2 cloves garlic, minced

  4 well-trimmed center-cut loin pork chops (about ½ inch thick, 6 ounces each)

1 In a small bowl, stir together the sage, rosemary, salt, pepper, sugar, and bay leaf. Add the garlic and stir to combine.

---

different spins

▶**Jerk Pork Salad** Cook the *Jerk Pork Kebabs* as directed. Add the cooked pork to 6 cups of mixed salad greens, 1 cup pineapple chunks, and 1 diced red bell pepper. Toss with Orange-Balsamic Dressing (*page 254*).

▶**Broiled Herb-Rubbed Shrimp** Follow the directions for *Broiled Herb-Rubbed Pork Chops*, but use 1 pound large shrimp instead of the pork. In step 2, broil the shrimp for only 2 minutes, or until opaque throughout. Serve with Hot & Spicy Cocktail Sauce (*page 256*).

▶**Jerked Chicken** Follow the directions for *Jerk Pork Kebabs*, but use skinless, boneless chicken thighs instead of pork.

▶**Broiled Herb-Rubbed Chicken Breast** Follow the directions for *Broiled Herb-Rubbed Pork Chops*, but use 4 skinless, boneless chicken breast halves (5 ounces each) instead of the pork.

rubs & marinades

There are two traditional methods of adding flavor to meat: rubs and marinades.

▶ **Rubs** Rubs are blends of herbs and/or spices that are applied all over the surface of meat before cooking. They can either be "dry rubs" or "wet rubs" (where the herbs and spices are mixed with a bit of liquid to form a paste). For a more pronounced flavor, coat the meat several hours before cooking and refrigerate.

▶ **Marinades** A marinade is a liquid flavoring mixture that usually contains acidic ingredients, such as wine or vinegar. It should be used to add flavor, but not to tenderize meat. The amount of time that

lean meat has to sit in a marinade to "tenderize" also turns the surface of the meat mushy. Make enough marinade to completely cover the meat, and place in a covered nonreactive container in the refrigerator. (Or, place the marinade and the meat in a tightly sealed plastic bag, turning it occasionally to cover all sides.) The meat only needs to marinate for 15 minutes to 2 hours to add flavor.

▶ **Caution:** Uncooked marinade becomes contaminated from raw meat sitting in it and is therefore not safe to consume as is. If you want to use the marinade as a sauce, cook it at a rolling boil for several minutes before serving.

2 Spray a broiler pan with nonstick cooking spray. Preheat the broiler. Rub the spice mixture into both sides of the chops and place on the broiler pan. Broil 4 to 6 inches from the heat for 3 to 4 minutes per side or until cooked through but still juicy. *Makes 4 servings*

per serving: 237 calories, 8.9g total fat (3.1g saturated), 91mg cholesterol, 0g dietary fiber, 1g carbohydrate, 35g protein, 365mg sodium. good source of: niacin, riboflavin, selenium, thiamin, vitamin B$_{12}$, vitamin B$_6$, zinc.

Pork Vindaloo

Vindaloo is a dish that originated in Goa, a former Portuguese colony and now a state on the west coast of India. Vindaloo started life as a Portuguese concoction of pork, wine (*vinho*), and garlic (*alho*), but evolved over time into one of the hottest dishes in Indian cuisine. **Timing alert:** The pork needs to marinate for at least 1 hour.

⅓ cup raisins

¼ cup water

3 tablespoons fresh lime juice

3 canned or bottled jalapeño peppers

1 teaspoon cumin

1 teaspoon coriander

½ teaspoon ground ginger

½ teaspoon fennel seeds

1 pound pork tenderloin, cut into ½-inch chunks

1 tablespoon olive oil

⅔ cup chicken broth, homemade (page 252) or canned

¼ teaspoon salt

1 cup frozen peas

1 teaspoon cornstarch blended with 1 tablespoon water

1 In a food processor, combine the raisins, water, lime juice, jalapeños, cumin, coriander, ginger, and fennel, and process until smooth. Transfer to a bowl and add the pork, tossing to combine. Cover and let marinate for at least 1 hour or up to overnight in the refrigerator.

2 In a large nonstick skillet, heat the oil over medium heat. Reserving the marinade, add the pork to the pan and cook, stirring, until lightly browned, about 5 minutes.

3 Add the reserved marinade, the broth, and salt, and bring to a boil. Reduce to a simmer, cover, and cook until the pork is tender, about 5 minutes.

4 Add the peas and cook until heated through, about 2 minutes. Return to a boil, stir in the cornstarch mixture, and cook, stirring constantly, until the stew is slightly thickened, about 1 minute. *Makes 4 servings*

per serving: 256 calories, 8.4g total fat (2g saturated), 75mg cholesterol, 3g dietary fiber, 19g carbohydrate, 27g protein, 456mg sodium. good source of: niacin, riboflavin, selenium, thiamin, vitamin B$_{12}$, vitamin B$_6$, zinc.

Pork Scallops Piccata

If pork scallops (thin cutlets) are hard to find, make your own by slicing pork loin or tenderloin and pounding it thin. Tenderloin has a very soft texture and is very easy to pound with either the flat side of a meat pounder or the bottom of a small skillet. Once pounded, cutlets cook up in no time at all.

1 pound pork tenderloin

1 tablespoon flour

1 teaspoon ground ginger

¾ teaspoon salt

½ teaspoon pepper

1 tablespoon olive oil

2 cloves garlic, minced

¾ cup chicken broth, homemade (page 252) or canned

¼ cup fresh lemon juice

2 teaspoons cornstarch

2 tablespoons chopped fresh basil

1 Cut the pork into 8 pieces. Place the pieces between 2 sheets of wax paper and with the flat side of a small skillet or meat pounder, pound the pork slices to a ⅛-inch thickness.

2 On a large plate, combine the flour, ginger, ½ teaspoon of the salt, and the pepper. Dredge the pork in the spice mixture.

3 In a large nonstick skillet, heat the oil over medium heat. Add the pork cutlets and cook until browned and cooked through, about 2 minutes per side. Transfer to a platter and keep warm.

4 Add the garlic and ¼ cup of the broth to the pan and stir to scrape up any browned bits clinging to the pan. In a small bowl, whisk the remaining ½ cup broth and the lemon juice into the cornstarch. Add the mixture to the pan along with the remaining ¼ teaspoon salt. Bring to a boil over medium heat, and boil until the sauce is lightly thickened, about 1 minute. Stir in the basil. Spoon the sauce over the pork. *Makes 4 servings*

per serving: 213 calories, 8.8g total fat (2.4g saturated), 80mg cholesterol, 0g dietary fiber, 5g carbohydrate, 27g protein, 577mg sodium. **good source of:** niacin, riboflavin, selenium, thiamin, vitamin B$_{12}$, vitamin B$_6$.

Shells with Picadillo Sauce

There is a Cuban rendition of picadillo as well as one from Mexico. And there are undoubtedly as many home versions of this warming, spicy ground meat combination as there are dedicated picadillo cooks. Though traditionally served on its own or over rice, here the picadillo is used as a pasta sauce.

½ pound pork tenderloin, cut into large chunks

2 teaspoons olive oil

1 large onion, diced

3 garlic cloves, minced

1 large green bell pepper, diced

1 canned or bottled jalapeño pepper, minced

1 can (15 ounces) crushed tomatoes

⅓ cup raisins

3 tablespoons minced green olives

½ teaspoon oregano

½ teaspoon salt

10 ounces pasta shells

1 In a food processor, pulse the pork until finely ground.

2 In a large nonstick skillet, heat the oil over medium heat. Add the onion and garlic, and cook, stirring occasionally, until tender, about 7 minutes. Add the bell pepper and jalapeño, and cook until the bell pepper is tender, about 5 minutes.

3 Stir in the pork and cook until no longer pink, about 4 minutes.

4 Add the tomatoes, raisins, olives, oregano, and salt, and bring to a boil. Reduce to a simmer, cover, and cook until the sauce is flavorful and slightly thickened, about 15 minutes.

5 Meanwhile, in a large pot of boiling water, cook the pasta according to package directions. Drain. Transfer to a large bowl and toss with the sauce. *Makes 4 servings*

per serving: 428 calories, 6.3g total fat (1.3g saturated), 37mg cholesterol, 6g dietary fiber, 72g carbohydrate, 23g protein, 574mg sodium. good source of: folate, niacin, potassium, riboflavin, selenium, thiamin, vitamin B$_6$, vitamin C.

Green Pork Chili

No tomatoes and no beans in this traditional Southwestern pork-based version of chili. And the green in the title comes from a combination of herbs and chili peppers: in this case, scallions, mild chilies, jalapeños, and cilantro. Look for cans of hominy in the Latin American section of your supermarket, usually close to the beans. Although the flavor and texture won't be quite the same, you can use 1½ cups of frozen corn kernels if you can't find hominy. Add the corn during the final 5 minutes of cooking time.

- 1 tablespoon olive oil
- 1 pound pork tenderloin, cut into 1-inch chunks
- 5 scallions, thinly sliced
- 4 cloves garlic, minced
- 1 can (4½ ounces) chopped mild green chilies
- 2 canned or bottled jalapeño peppers, minced
- 2 teaspoons ground coriander
- 1 teaspoon oregano
- ½ teaspoon salt
- 1 cup water
- 1 can (15 ounces) hominy, rinsed and drained
- ½ cup chopped cilantro
- 2 tablespoons fresh lime juice

1 In a nonstick Dutch oven or flameproof casserole, heat the oil over medium-high heat. Add the pork and cook until browned, about 4 minutes. With a slotted spoon, transfer the pork to a plate.

2 Reduce the heat to medium. Add the scallions and garlic and cook until the scallions are tender, about 2 minutes. Stir in the mild green chilies and jalapeños, and cook 1 minute.

3 Return the pork to the pan. Add the coriander, oregano, and salt, stirring to coat. Add the water and bring to a boil. Add the hominy and ¼ cup of the cilantro. Reduce to a simmer, cover, and cook until the pork is tender, about 20 minutes.

4 Stir in the remaining ¼ cup cilantro and the lime juice just before serving. *Makes 4 servings*

per serving: 265 calories, 8.5g total fat (2g saturated), 74mg cholesterol, 5g dietary fiber, 20g carbohydrate, 26g protein, 711mg sodium. good source of: niacin, riboflavin, selenium, thiamin, vitamin B$_{12}$, vitamin B$_6$, zinc.

different spins

▶**Pineapple Pork Piccata** Follow the directions for *Pork Scallops Piccata (opposite page)*, but reduce the lemon juice to 2 tablespoons and add ¼ cup thawed pineapple juice concentrate when adding the lemon juice. Add ¼ cup finely diced red bell pepper when adding the garlic to the pan. Substitute chopped fresh mint for the basil.

▶**Turkey Picadillo** Follow the directions for *Shells with Picadillo Sauce (opposite page)*, but substitute skinless, boneless turkey breast for the pork. Increase the olive oil to 1 tablespoon and add 1 red bell pepper along with the green in step 2. Use radiatore instead of shells. Add ¼ cup chopped cilantro when tossing.

Southwestern Meatloaf

Pork is often the meat of choice (over beef) for many Southwestern dishes (*see Green Pork Chili, page 89*). Here we've used it in a meatloaf (lightened with some lean turkey breast) that has other Southwestern components, such as cilantro, chili powder, corn, and salsa. Although you can buy both turkey and pork preground, grinding your own ensures the leanest mix possible.

> 1 pound pork tenderloin, cut into chunks
>
> ½ pound skinless, boneless turkey breast, cut into chunks
>
> 1 cup frozen corn kernels, thawed
>
> 1 green bell pepper, finely chopped
>
> ½ cup chopped cilantro
>
> 1½ teaspoons chili powder
>
> ¾ teaspoon salt
>
> 3 slices (1 ounce each) firm whole-wheat sandwich bread, crumbled
>
> ½ cup fat-free or low-fat (1%) milk
>
> ½ cup bottled medium to hot salsa
>
> 3 large egg whites

1 In a food processor, combine the pork and turkey, and process until finely ground, about 30 seconds. Transfer to a large bowl and stir in the corn, bell pepper, cilantro, chili powder, and salt.

2 In a small bowl, combine the bread and milk until evenly moistened. Add to the pork and turkey mixture along with the salsa and egg whites, mixing until well combined.

3 Preheat the oven to 350°F. Spoon the mixture into a 9 x 5-inch loaf pan. Bake for 35 to 45 minutes, or until the juices run clear.

4 Remove from the oven, let stand for 10 minutes in the pan, then turn out of the pan onto a platter. Serve warm or chilled. *Makes 6 servings*

per serving: 253 calories, 4.7g total fat (1.4g saturated), 83mg cholesterol, 3g dietary fiber, 16g carbohydrate, 36g protein, 557mg sodium. good source of: niacin, riboflavin, selenium, thiamin, vitamin B_{12}, vitamin B_6, vitamin C, zinc.

Ham, Lentil & Rice Salad

The sweet-tart flavors of pineapple go well with the salty-rich flavors of ham, which is why they are so often put together. So, why fix it if it ain't broke? We've used a modest amount of good smoked ham, just enough to appreciate its flavor without overwhelming the dish with it.

> 2 cups chicken broth, homemade (page 252) or canned
>
> 1 cup water
>
> 4 cloves garlic, minced
>
> 1 cup lentils
>
> ½ cup aromatic rice, such as basmati, jasmine, or Texmati
>
> ⅓ cup fresh lemon juice
>
> 4 teaspoons olive oil
>
> ¼ teaspoon salt
>
> ½ teaspoon pepper
>
> 1 can (20 ounces) juice-packed pineapple chunks, drained
>
> 1 small red onion, minced
>
> ½ pound reduced-sodium smoked ham, cut into thin matchsticks

1 In a medium saucepan, bring the broth, water, and garlic to a boil over medium heat. Add the lentils and reduce to a simmer. Cover, and cook for 10 minutes. Add the rice and cook until the rice and lentils are tender, about 20 minutes.

2 Meanwhile, in a large bowl, combine the lemon juice, oil, salt, and pepper.

3 Add the warm lentil mixture, the pineapple, and red onion to the dressing and toss to combine. Let cool to room temperature.

4 Add the ham, toss to combine, and serve at room temperature or chilled. *Makes 4 servings*

per serving: 456 calories, 8.3g total fat (1.8g saturated), 30mg cholesterol, 18g dietary fiber, 6g carbohydrate, 30g protein, 927mg sodium. good source of: fiber, folate, niacin, potassium, selenium, thiamin, vitamin B_6, vitamin C, zinc.

beef

Roasting Large cuts of meat, like roasts, are cooked whole in an oven ranging from 325°F to 425°F, depending upon the cut (*see "Beef Cooking Chart," page 93*).

Broiling/grilling Cubes of beef on skewers, ground meat patties, and steaks (*see Simple Broiled Flank Steak, page 92*) can be broiled or grilled. Broil or grill 4 to 6 inches from the heat until the meat is the desired degree of doneness.

Pan-frying Many cuts of steak can be successfully pan-fried if you use a nonstick pan sprayed with nonstick cooking spray, and if you get the pan good and hot before adding the steak.

Stir-frying The key to stir-frying is to cut the meat into very thin strips so it cooks quickly. For low-fat beef stir-fries, use flank steak or sirloin steak (*see Meat Stir-Fries "Recipe Creator," page 95*).

Braising/stewing Thin cuts of lean meat can be rolled around a stuffing and braised (*see Beef Braciole, at right*). Larger pieces of lean meat can also be stewed but not in the traditional way. Lean beef needs to be coated in flour or cornstarch, cooked briefly until browned, and returned to the stew pot just to reheat (*see Beer-Braised Beef Stew, page 94, and West African-Style Beef Stew, page 96*).

---

making your own braciole

One of the ways to cope with lean (*i.e.*, not-so-tender) cuts of meat is to pound them lightly with a mallet or meat pounder. This technique breaks up the connective tissue, tenderizing the meat. A classic example of a dish that uses pounded beef is braciole. You can buy the beef from the butcher already pounded, or you can do it yourself. If you don't have a meat pounder or mallet, use a small heavy skillet.

Beef Braciole

Braciole is actually a specific meat cut (very thin slices), but it has come to mean a dish in which this cut is commonly used: stuffed meat rolls (also called *involtini* in Italian). In this example, the meat is wrapped around a mixture of broccoli and Parmesan and then braised in an herbed tomato sauce. If you can't find braciole, you can pound slices of top round to make your own (*see "Making Your Own Braciole, below left*). **Serving suggestion:** Serve these rolls over brown rice or pasta and top with some shaved Parmesan cheese.

> 1 cup frozen chopped broccoli, thawed, well drained, and squeezed dry
> ¼ cup plain dried breadcrumbs
> ¼ cup dried currants
> 2 tablespoons grated Parmesan cheese
> 8 thin slices (10 ounces) top round for braciole
> 3 tablespoons flour
> 2 teaspoons olive oil
> 1 can (28 ounces) crushed tomatoes
> 2 tablespoons tomato paste
> ½ teaspoon oregano
> ½ teaspoon salt

1 In a small bowl, combine the broccoli, breadcrumbs, currants, and Parmesan. Spread the broccoli mixture on the beef slices and roll them up from one short end. Secure with a toothpick.

2 Dredge the beef rolls in the flour, shaking off the excess. In a large nonstick skillet, heat the oil over medium-high heat. Add the beef rolls and cook 3 to 4 minutes, turning them as they brown.

3 Add the crushed tomatoes, tomato paste, oregano, and salt. Bring to a boil. Reduce to a simmer, cover, and cook until the beef is tender, about 15 minutes. *Makes 4 servings*

per serving: 357 calories, 12g total fat (3.8g saturated), 66mg cholesterol, 6g dietary fiber, 34g carbohydrate, 32g protein, 776mg sodium. good source of: niacin, potassium, riboflavin, thiamin, vitamin B_{12}, vitamin B_6, vitamin C, zinc.

Simple Broiled Flank Steak

The simplest of seasonings is all you need for lean flank steak, in this case a sweet-tart glaze of currant jelly and lemon juice. Cook the steak quickly under the broiler so it will stay juicy, and then carve it across the grain into thin slices. This helps make the pieces of steak tender. **Serving suggestion:** This simple broiled steak would partner well with a whole range of high-flavored sauces. Try one of these: Chimichurri Sauce (*page 258*), Spicy Cranberry Sauce (*page 259*), or Red Onion Marmalade (*page 264*).

2 tablespoons red currant jelly
½ teaspoon grated lemon zest
1 tablespoon fresh lemon juice
1 teaspoon dillweed
½ teaspoon salt
¼ teaspoon pepper
1 pound flank steak

1 In a small bowl, stir together the jelly, lemon zest, lemon juice, dillweed, salt, and pepper. Brush the mixture on both sides of the flank steak.

2 Preheat the broiler. Broil the flank steak 4 to 6 inches from the heat for 4 to 5 minutes per side for medium. Let stand for 10 minutes, then thinly slice across the grain. *Makes 4 servings*

> ## how to carve a flank steak
>
> Flank steak is a pretty lean cut, with long muscle fibers running its length. If you were to cut the steak "with the grain," that is in the same direction as the muscle fibers, the slices would be difficult to chew. But if you cut the steak "across the grain," perpendicular to the direction of the muscle fibers, you will be shortening the fibers, resulting in much more tender slices. Although this may sound mysterious, once you see a flank steak, the so-called "grain" will be quite obvious.

per serving: 197 calories, 8.2g total fat (3.5g saturated), 54mg cholesterol, 0g dietary fiber, 7g carbohydrate, 22g protein, 361mg sodium. **good source of:** niacin, selenium, vitamin B_{12}, zinc.

Ginger-Grilled Sirloin Salad with Watercress

A rainbow of colors in this salad is a sure sign that you are getting a healthy helping of vitamins, minerals, and phytochemicals. And by using a relatively lean cut of beef, you can have a meat dish that has a modest amount of saturated fat. To get the most mileage out of the grilled steak, slice it as thin as possible.

1 tablespoon sesame seeds
2 tablespoons reduced-sodium soy sauce
1 tablespoon coarsely chopped fresh ginger
2 cloves garlic, peeled
⅛ teaspoon red pepper flakes
10 ounces boneless sirloin steak
2 tablespoons rice vinegar
4 cups loosely packed watercress sprigs, tough stems removed
1½ cups frozen corn kernels, thawed
1 large red bell pepper, thinly sliced
2 scallions, thinly sliced

1 In a small dry skillet, toast the sesame seeds over low heat until lightly toasted, about 3 minutes. Remove from the skillet and set aside.

2 Preheat the broiler. In a mini-food processor, combine the soy sauce, ginger, garlic, and red pepper flakes, and process until very finely chopped.

3 Rub half of the soy sauce mixture over both sides of the steak and broil 4 to 6 inches from the heat for 4 to 5 minutes per side for medium. Transfer the steak to a plate and set aside.

4 Transfer the remaining soy sauce mixture to a salad bowl. Mix in the vinegar and any steak juices that have collected on the plate. Add the water-

beef cooking chart

Always check for doneness about 15 minutes before the first time listed in the range of times. Stop cooking when the internal temperature (*see "How to Use a Meat Thermometer," page 107*) registers about 5 degrees less than the desired doneness. Let the meat stand 15 minutes; during that time, the meat will continue to "cook" and the temperature will rise another 5 degrees.

CUT	AMOUNT	METHOD
SIRLOIN	boneless tip roast, 3 to 4 lbs	**Roasting** 325°F for 2¼ to 2½ hours, or until meat thermometer reads 135°F for medium-rare, or 145°F for medium
	boneless tip roast, 6 to 8 lbs	**Roasting** 325°F for 3 to 4 hours, or until meat thermometer reads 135°F for medium-rare, or 145°F for medium
	steak, 1 inch thick	**Broiling/grilling** 4 to 6 inches from heat, 3–4 minutes per side for medium-rare **Pan-frying** In lightly oiled nonstick skillet, over medium heat, 3–4 minutes per side for medium-rare
	cut for stir-fry	**Stir-frying** *See Meat Stir-Fries "Recipe Creator" on page 95*
TENDERLOIN	whole, 4 to 6 lbs	**Roasting** 425°F for 45–60 minutes, or until meat thermometer reads 135°F for medium-rare, or 145°F for medium
	steaks, 1 inch thick	**Broiling/grilling** 4 to 6 inches from heat, 3–4 minutes per side for medium-rare **Pan-frying** In lightly oiled nonstick skillet, over medium heat, 3–4 minutes per side for medium-rare
EYE ROUND, ROAST	2 to 3 lbs	**Roasting** 325°F for 40–60 minutes, or until meat thermometer reads 135°F for medium-rare, or 145°F for medium
TOP ROUND, ROAST	3 to 5 lbs	**Roasting** 325°F for 1¼ to 2¼ hours, or until meat thermometer reads 135°F for medium-rare, or 145°F for medium
FLANK STEAK	1 to 2 lbs	**Broiling/grilling** 4 to 6 inches from heat, 4–5 minutes per side, or until meat thermometer reads 135°F for medium-rare, or 145°F for medium
	cut for stir-fry	**Stir-frying** *See Meat Stir-Fries "Recipe Creator" on page 95*

cress, corn, bell pepper, and scallions, and toss to combine.

5 Thinly slice the steak. Make a bed of watercress salad on 4 serving plates. Top with the steak slices. Sprinkle the salad with the toasted sesame seeds. *Makes 4 servings*

per serving: 208 calories, 7.7g total fat (2.6g saturated), 46mg cholesterol, 3g dietary fiber, 18g carbohydrate, 19g protein, 314mg sodium. good source of: selenium, vitamin B_{12}, vitamin B_6, vitamin C, zinc.

Thai-Style Beef & Noodle Salad

This beef and noodle salad is tossed in a dressing inspired by the interplay of sour, salty, and sweet flavors typical of Thai cuisine.

10 ounces well-trimmed beef sirloin

½ teaspoon salt

8 ounces spaghetti

¼ cup ketchup

3 tablespoons fresh lime juice

2 tablespoons reduced-sodium soy sauce

2 teaspoons light brown sugar

¼ teaspoon red pepper flakes

4 scallions, thinly sliced

1 large carrot, shredded

1 Granny Smith apple, cut into ⅓-inch dice

1 Preheat the broiler. Sprinkle the meat with ¼ teaspoon of the salt. Broil 4 to 6 inches from the heat for 3 to 4 minutes per side, or until medium-rare. Place the beef on a plate and let it stand for 10 minutes. Then thinly slice the beef on the diagonal, and cut the slices into bite-size pieces. Reserve any juices on the plate.

2 Meanwhile, in a large pot of boiling water, cook the spaghetti according to package directions. Drain well.

3 In a large bowl, combine the remaining ¼ teaspoon salt, the ketchup, lime juice, soy sauce, brown sugar, and red pepper flakes. Add the drained pasta and toss well.

4 Add the beef pieces and any juices from the plate, the scallions, carrot, and apple. Toss well to combine. Serve at room temperature or chilled.
Makes 4 servings

per serving: 413 calories, 9.5g total fat (3.4g saturated), 47mg cholesterol, 3g dietary fiber, 58g carbohydrate, 24g protein, 787mg sodium. good source of: beta carotene, selenium, vitamin B$_{12}$, zinc.

Beer-Braised Beef Stew

In general, stews use fatty cuts of meat that can hold up to long, slow cooking. Here we've used a lean cut of meat, dredged it in flour, and browned it to seal in its juices. It then gets removed from the pan so it won't get overdone while the other ingredients cook. It's added back at the end just to reheat.

¾ pound bottom round of beef, cut into ¾-inch cubes

3 tablespoons flour

3 teaspoons olive oil

2 Spanish onions (1 pound), halved and thinly sliced

4 cloves garlic, minced

3 carrots, halved lengthwise and thinly sliced crosswise

1½ cups dark beer

1 cup chicken broth, homemade (page 252) or canned

2 tablespoons tomato paste

¾ teaspoon thyme

¾ teaspoon salt

¼ teaspoon pepper

1 Dredge the beef in the flour, shaking off the excess. In a nonstick Dutch oven or flameproof casserole, heat 1 teaspoon of the oil over medium-high heat. Add half the beef and cook until richly browned, about 5 minutes. With a slotted spoon, transfer the beef to a plate. Repeat with 1 teaspoon of oil and the remaining beef. Set aside.

2 Reduce the heat to medium. Add the remaining 1 teaspoon oil to the pan along with the onions and garlic, and cook, stirring frequently, until golden brown, about 10 minutes.

3 Add the carrots and cook, stirring frequently, until tender, about 10 minutes.

4 Stir in the beer and cook until the beer is reduced by half, about 5 minutes.

5 Stir in the broth, tomato paste, thyme, salt, and pepper. Bring to a boil, reduce to a simmer, cover,

recipe creator
meat stir-fries

Stir-fries are a good way to eat just a little bit of meat (and a lot of vegetables). Pick ingredients from the four categories and follow these basic instructions: Cut the MEAT into ½-inch slices, and then cut the slices into strips ¼ inch wide (or buy it precut for stir-fry). In a small bowl, stir together 1 cup chicken broth, 2 teaspoons cornstarch, 1 teaspoon brown sugar, and ½ teaspoon salt to make a coating sauce; set aside. In a wok or large nonstick skillet, heat 2 teaspoons olive or canola oil over medium-high heat. Stir-fry the MEAT until cooked through, about 3 minutes. With a slotted spoon, transfer the meat to a plate. Choose 2 to 5 VEGETABLES, using a total of 5 cups. Add 1 tablespoon oil and any hard vegetables (asparagus, broccoli, cauliflower, carrots, rutabaga, or beans) to the pan; stir-fry for 3 minutes. Add any soft vegetables, 1 to 3 AROMATICS, and 1 or 2 SEASONINGS. Cook until the vegetables are crisp-tender, about 3 minutes. Stir the coating sauce to recombine. Return the meat to the pan, along with the coating sauce; cook until heated through and evenly coated, about 1 minute. *Makes 4 servings*

MEAT	VEGETABLES	AROMATICS	SEASONINGS
▶ Beef sirloin, ½ pound well-trimmed	▶ Red or green bell peppers, cut into matchsticks	▶ Scallions, 3 sliced	▶ Red pepper flakes, ½ tsp
▶ Flank steak, ½ pound	▶ Onions or leeks, cut into matchsticks	▶ Garlic, 3 cloves minced	▶ Chili powder or curry powder, 1 tsp
▶ Boneless lamb loin, ½ pound well-trimmed	▶ Asparagus, cut into 1-inch lengths	▶ Shallots, ¼ cup minced	▶ Rosemary, ½ tsp minced
▶ Boneless leg of lamb, ½ pound	▶ Broccoli florets		▶ Thyme, ½ tsp
▶ Boneless pork loin, ½ pound well-trimmed	▶ Shiitake or button mushrooms, sliced		▶ Fennel seeds, ¾ tsp crushed
▶ Pork tenderloin, ½ pound	▶ Carrots, cut into matchsticks		▶ Dark sesame oil, 1 tsp
	▶ Rutabaga, cut into matchsticks		
	▶ Green beans, cut into 1-inch lengths		

and cook until the vegetables are tender, about 10 minutes. Return the beef to the pan and cook until just heated through, about 2 minutes. *Makes 4 servings*

per serving: 291 calories, 8.3g total fat (2g saturated), 52mg cholesterol, 4g dietary fiber, 27g carbohydrate, 21g protein, 667mg sodium. **good source of:** beta carotene, selenium, vitamin B_{12}, vitamin B_6, zinc.

West African-Style Beef Stew

The two ingredients that have earned this stew its title are peanut butter and sweet potatoes—though in Africa the potatoes would more likely be yams, which are similar in taste but botanically different from sweet potatoes. The peanut butter adds a wonderful richness of flavor for a modest amount of fat: 2.7 grams per serving, and almost all of it unsaturated. **Serving suggestion:** Although it may seem unconventional, serve the stew with a stack of warm flour tortillas and a tossed salad with Fresh Ginger & Lime Dressing (*page 254*).

*¾ pound beef top round, cut into
    ½-inch chunks*

2 tablespoons flour

2 teaspoons olive oil

6 scallions, thinly sliced

5 cloves garlic, minced

*1 cup chicken broth, homemade
    (page 252) or canned*

*1¼ pounds sweet potatoes, peeled and
    cut into ½-inch chunks*

2 tablespoons tomato paste

*2 teaspoons Louisiana-style hot pepper
    sauce*

½ teaspoon salt

4 teaspoons creamy peanut butter

1 Dredge the beef in the flour, shaking off the excess. In a nonstick Dutch oven or flameproof casserole, heat the oil over medium heat. Add the beef and cook until lightly browned, about 4 minutes. With a slotted spoon, transfer the beef to a plate.

2 Add the scallions and garlic to the pan and cook until the scallions are tender, about 2 minutes.

3 Add the broth, sweet potatoes, tomato paste, hot sauce, and salt. Bring to a boil, reduce to a simmer, cover, and cook until the sweet potatoes are tender, about 10 minutes.

4 Stir in the peanut butter. Return the beef to the pan, cover, and cook until the beef is heated through, about 2 minutes. *Makes 4 servings*

per serving: 412 calories, 11g total fat (2.7g saturated), 77mg cholesterol, 4g dietary fiber, 43g carbohydrate, 36g protein, 614mg sodium. good source of: beta carotene, niacin, riboflavin, vitamin B_{12}, vitamin B_6, vitamin C, vitamin E, zinc.

making the most of meat

Using various ingredients, like grains and moist vegetables, to "stretch" ground meat dishes (such as meatloaf, meatballs, or burgers), performs three important functions: **1)** It allows you to have a satisfying and meaty serving without eating too much saturated fat. **2)** It provides another opportunity for getting some all-important nutrients into your diet. **3)** It helps to moisturize lean cuts of meat.

Here are some good ingredients to add to ground meat:

▶**Bulgur** Cooked (or soaked) bulgur is an excellent meat stretcher. Not only is it high in fiber, but it has a good chew to it, similar to that of ground meat. You can replace up to one-third of a ground meat mixture with bulgur.

▶**Oats** Try using toasted oats in a meatloaf or burger. While raw oats might impart an uncooked flavor to the dish, toasted oats give a rich, nutty flavor and a dry, rather than gummy texture. Use 1 cup for every 4 ounces of meat.

▶**TVP (TSP)** This texturized vegetable protein is the filler to end all fillers. It is a good source of protein, its flavor is neutral (which is desirable in this case), and it has an exceptionally satisfying, meaty texture. You can replace up to one-third of a ground meat mixture with TVP. It is also good in pasta sauces, completely or partially replacing ground meat or poultry.

▶**Beans** Mashed cooked beans won't make a good filler for meat in sauces and stews, but you can use well-drained, mashed beans to replace about one-fourth of the meat in meatloaves, burgers, or meatballs.

▶**Mushrooms** Finely diced fresh mushrooms can stand in for up to one-third of the meat in burgers, meatloaves, and meatballs.

Smart Beef Meatloaf

You can get a beefy meatloaf without all the saturated fat if you use a couple of tricks: Start with a meat mixture that stretches a small amount of beef with lean turkey breast, then add sautéed mushrooms for meaty flavor and moisture, and bulgur to "beef" up the texture.

> ⅔ cup bulgur
>
> 1⅓ cups boiling water
>
> 1 tablespoon olive oil
>
> 1 medium onion, finely chopped
>
> 10 ounces mushrooms, coarsely chopped
>
> 6 ounces green beans
>
> 5 cloves garlic, minced
>
> 6 ounces top round of beef, cut into large chunks
>
> 10 ounces lean ground turkey
>
> 3 large egg whites
>
> 3 tablespoons tomato paste
>
> 1 tablespoon plus 1 teaspoon Dijon mustard
>
> 2½ teaspoons Worcestershire sauce
>
> 1 teaspoon salt

1 In a large heatproof bowl, combine the bulgur and boiling water. Let stand until the bulgur has softened, about 30 minutes. Drain and squeeze dry. Return the bulgur to the bowl.

2 Preheat the oven to 350°F. Meanwhile, in a large nonstick skillet, heat the oil over medium heat. Add the onion and cook, stirring frequently, until the onion is soft, about 7 minutes.

3 Add the mushrooms and green beans to the pan and cook, stirring frequently, until the mushrooms are richly browned, about 7 minutes. Add the garlic and ½ cup water, and cook, stirring frequently, until the vegetables are very tender and the water has evaporated, about 5 minutes.

4 Transfer the sautéed vegetables to a food processor and pulse on and off until evenly chopped (there should still be some texture, and it should *not* be a puree). Add the vegetables to the bowl with the bulgur.

5 Add the beef to the food processor (no need to clean the bowl) and pulse on and off until coarsely ground. Add to the bowl along with the turkey, egg whites, tomato paste, mustard, Worcestershire sauce, and salt. Mix until well combined. Spoon the mixture into a 9 x 5-inch loaf pan.

6 Bake until the loaf is firm and the juices run clear, about 45 minutes. Let cool 10 minutes in the pan, then turn the loaf out of the pan onto a platter. Serve the meatloaf warm or at room temperature. *Makes 6 servings*

per serving: 240 calories, 8.5g total fat (2.3g saturated), 51mg cholesterol, 5g dietary fiber, 21g carbohydrate, 22g protein, 643mg sodium. good source of: niacin, vitamin B_{12}, vitamin B_6.

lamb

While many retail cuts of lamb are sold trimmed of most external fat, some cuts, such as the leg or shoulder, may be sold with some of the fat intact. Trim the lamb carefully before cooking. Some lamb cuts may also retain pieces of the fell, a papery membrane that covers surface fat. Butchers often leave the fell intact on large cuts, since it helps the meat retain its shape and natural juices. Any fell on small cuts should be removed, as it can distort the shape of the meat during cooking.

Since most cuts of lamb are naturally tender, they don't need to be tenderized further when cooked with dry-heat methods, such as roasting, grilling, or broiling. One advantage of dry-heat methods is that they allow the fat to drip off during cooking. Firmer cuts, such as shoulder, on the other hand, will benefit from moist-heat cooking methods, such as stewing or braising. The long, slow simmering helps to tenderize the meat and allows its juices and flavors to blend with those of the other ingredients.

lamb cooking chart

Always check for doneness about 15 minutes before the first time listed in the range of times. For medium-rare, stop cooking when the internal temperature registers about 5 degrees less than the desired doneness (*see "How to Use a Meat Thermometer," page 107*). With dry-heat methods (roasting, grilling, and broiling), the meat should be cooked until it is slightly pink; cooked longer, it will lose a good deal of its flavor. Let the meat stand 15 minutes; during that time, the meat will continue to "cook" and the temperature will rise another 5 degrees.

CUT	AMOUNT	METHOD
LEG	whole, bone-in, 5 to 7 lbs	**Roasting** 325°F for 1¾ to 2¾ hours, or until meat thermometer reads 135°F for medium-rare, or 145°F for medium
	half, bone-in, 3 to 4 lbs	**Roasting** 325°F for 1½ to 1¾ hours, or until meat thermometer reads 135°F for medium-rare, or 145°F for medium
	boneless, 3 to 5 lbs	**Roasting** 325° for 1¼ to 2¼ hours, or until meat thermometer reads 135°F for medium-rare, or 145°F for medium
	butterflied, 3 lbs	**Grilling** 15–25 minutes for medium-rare
	steaks, 1 inch thick	**Pan-frying** In lightly oiled nonstick skillet, over medium heat, 4 minutes per side for medium-rare
	cut for stir-fry	**Stir-frying** *See Meat Stir-Fries "Recipe Creator" on page 95*
	1-inch chunks	**Broiling/grilling** Thread on skewers, cook 4 to 6 inches from heat, turning, about 8 minutes
LOIN	rack, 1½ to 2 lbs	**Roasting** 375°F for 45 minutes, or until meat thermometer reads 135°F for medium-rare, or 145°F for medium
	chops, 1 inch thick	**Broiling/grilling** 4 to 6 inches from heat, 4 minutes per side for medium-rare **Pan-frying** In lightly oiled nonstick skillet, over medium heat, 4 minutes per side for medium-rare
	boneless, cut for stir-fry	**Stir-frying** *See Meat Stir-Fries "Recipe Creator" on page 95*
SHOULDER	chops, 1 inch thick	**Broiling/grilling** 4 to 6 inches from heat, 4 minutes per side for medium-rare **Pan-frying** In lightly oiled nonstick skillet, over medium heat, 4 minutes per side for medium-rare

Roasting Larger cuts of lamb, such as the leg, loin, or rack, are particularly good when roasted. The lamb will be pink inside and remain juicy and tender. Longer cooking may dry it out. (*See "Lamb Cooking Chart," opposite page.*)

Broiling/grilling Smaller cuts of lamb, such as chops or cubes, can be broiled or grilled. Kebabs made from leg or shoulder can be threaded on skewers and either broiled, grilled, or pan-grilled. Larger cuts, usually boneless, such as leg of lamb, can be successfully grilled or broiled if they are butterflied (cut in half lengthwise and opened like a book) so they will cook evenly and in a shorter amount of time.

Pan-frying Chops and lamb steaks, from the loin, leg, or shoulder, can be pan-fried. Get a nonstick pan hot, add a small amount of oil, and pan-fry about 4 minutes per side for medium-rare. The timing will of course vary depending upon the thickness of the cut (*see Lamb Steak with Kasha & Wilted Scallions, page 100*).

Stir-frying While you can sometimes find lamb cut for stir-fry in your butcher case, you can also cut your own. Look for leg steaks, loin, or shoulder chops. Cut the meat into thin strips, cutting away and discarding any fat. The lamb will cook in a flash (*see Spicy Stir-Fried Lamb & Spinach, at right, and Meat Stir-Fries "Recipe Creator," page 95*).

Braising/stewing Lean chunks of lamb, such as those from the leg, can be braised for a moderate amount of time without drying out. (*see Moroccan Lamb & White Bean Stew, page 101*). Somewhat fattier cuts of lamb, such as well-trimmed shoulder, stand up to longer stewing and become very tender (*see Lamb & Turnip Curry, page 100*).

Spicy Stir-Fried Lamb & Spinach

The combination of red pepper flakes and grated fresh ginger gives this dish its heat. If you can't find hoisin sauce, a thick, sweet and spicy Chinese condiment, you can substitute red currant jelly.

⅓ cup chicken broth, homemade (page 252) or canned

1 tablespoon plus 1 teaspoon reduced-sodium soy sauce

1 tablespoon hoisin sauce

½ teaspoon red pepper flakes

1 tablespoon cornstarch

3 teaspoons olive oil

¾ pound boneless leg of lamb steak, thinly sliced and cut into ½-inch-wide strips

6 scallions, cut into 2-inch lengths

1 tablespoon grated fresh ginger

3 cloves garlic, minced

2 large red bell peppers, cut into strips

6 cups packed spinach leaves, shredded

1 In a small bowl, combine the broth, soy sauce, hoisin, red pepper flakes, and cornstarch. Set aside.

2 In a large nonstick skillet, heat 1 teaspoon of the oil over high heat. Add the lamb and stir-fry until no longer pink, 2 to 3 minutes. With a slotted spoon, transfer the lamb to a plate.

3 Add the remaining 2 teaspoons oil, the scallions, ginger, and garlic, and stir-fry for 1 minute. Add the bell peppers, reduce the heat to medium, and stir-fry until crisp-tender, about 3 minutes.

4 Add the spinach, in batches, and stir-fry until wilted, about 1 minute. Stir the broth mixture again to recombine and add it to the skillet. Bring to a boil, return the lamb to the pan, and cook, stirring, until the the sauce has thickened, about 1 minute. *Makes 4 servings*

per serving: 213 calories, 8.4g total fat (2.1g saturated), 56mg cholesterol, 4g dietary fiber, 14g carbohydrate, 22g protein, 400mg sodium. good source of: beta carotene, folate, lutein, niacin, potassium, quercetin, riboflavin, selenium, vitamin B_{12}, vitamin B_6, vitamin C, zinc.

Lamb Steak with Kasha & Wilted Scallions

Kasha—cracked roasted buckwheat groats—is traditionally prepared by tossing it with beaten egg and then quickly cooking the mixture in a dry skillet. The egg-coated grains are then cooked in boiling liquid until they are softened.

- 2 teaspoons coriander
- 1 teaspoon salt
- ½ teaspoon ground ginger
- ½ teaspoon sugar
- 4 boneless lamb steaks (4 ounces each), about 1 inch thick, cut from the leg
- 4 teaspoons olive oil
- 10 ounces mushrooms, thinly sliced
- 1 large carrot, quartered lengthwise and thinly sliced crosswise
- 1 cup kasha
- 2 large egg whites, lightly beaten
- 2 cups boiling water
- 8 scallions, cut into 1-inch lengths

1 In a small bowl, stir together 1½ teaspoons of the coriander, ¼ teaspoon of the salt, the ginger, and sugar. Rub the spice mixture into the lamb until well coated. Set aside.

2 In a large nonstick skillet, heat 2 teaspoons of the oil over medium heat. Add the mushrooms and carrot, and cook, stirring frequently, until the mushrooms are golden brown and tender, about 5 minutes. Transfer to a bowl.

3 In a small bowl, stir together the kasha and egg whites until well coated. Add to the skillet and cook over medium heat, stirring constantly, until the grains are separate.

4 Stir in the remaining ½ teaspoon coriander and ¾ teaspoon salt. Add the mushroom mixture and boiling water and return to a boil. Reduce to a simmer, cover, and cook until the kasha is tender, about 10 minutes.

5 Meanwhile, in a separate large nonstick skillet, heat the remaining 2 teaspoons oil over medium-high heat. Add the lamb and cook for 5 minutes.

6 Turn the lamb over, add the scallions, and cook until the lamb is browned on the outside and medium-rare inside, about 5 minutes. Serve the lamb and scallions on a bed of kasha. *Makes 4 servings*

per serving: 262 calories, 11g total fat (2.9g saturated), 63mg cholesterol, 3g dietary fiber, 15g carbohydrate, 26g protein, 670mg sodium. good source of: beta carotene, riboflavin, niacin, vitamin B$_{12}$, selenium, zinc.

Lamb & Turnip Curry

This unusual curry pairs lamb and turnips (two full-flavored ingredients that have a natural affinity for one another) and braises them in a coconut sauce flavored with curry spices. One of the tricks of the trade here is to use a banana to thicken the sauce and at the same time add a slight sweetness that brings out the curry flavors. **Serving suggestion:** Serve this sweet and mildly spiced curry on a bed of basmati rice.

- 2 teaspoons olive oil
- ¾ pound well-trimmed boneless lamb shoulder, cut into ½-inch chunks
- 1 large onion, finely chopped
- 1 tablespoon plus 1 teaspoon curry powder
- 1 small banana, cut into chunks
- 1½ cups water
- 1 teaspoon coconut extract
- ¾ cup plain fat-free yogurt
- 3 tablespoons tomato paste
- ¾ teaspoon salt
- 1 pound white turnips, peeled and cut into ½-inch chunks
- 1¼ cups frozen peas

1 In a nonstick Dutch oven or flameproof casserole, heat 1 teaspoon of the oil over medium-high heat. Add half the lamb and cook until browned, about 5 minutes. With a slotted spoon, transfer the lamb to a plate. Repeat with the remaining 1 teaspoon oil and the remaining lamb.

2 Reduce the heat to medium, add the onion, and cook, stirring frequently, until soft, about 7 minutes.

3 Add the curry powder and cook until fragrant, about 2 minutes. Transfer the onion mixture to a blender or food processor. Add the banana, water, and coconut extract, and process to a smooth puree.

4 Return the puree to the Dutch oven along with ¼ cup of the yogurt, the tomato paste, and salt, and bring to a simmer.

5 Return the lamb to the Dutch oven and add the turnips. Cover and simmer until the lamb is tender, about 45 minutes.

6 Add the peas and cook until heated through, about 3 minutes. Serve topped with the remaining ½ cup yogurt. *Makes 4 servings*

per serving: 290 calories, 10g total fat (3.2g saturated), 52mg cholesterol, 7g dietary fiber, 30g carbohydrate, 22g protein, 710mg sodium. good source of: niacin, potassium, riboflavin, selenium, vitamin B_{12}, vitamin B_6, vitamin C, zinc.

Moroccan Lamb & White Bean Stew

The ingredients in this stew are inspired by North African cuisine, which typically combines lamb, beans, and dried fruit with warm spices such as cinnamon and ginger. Parsnips are the somewhat unorthodox addition here, and if you don't like them or can't get them, just use an equivalent amount of carrots instead.

1½ cups chicken broth, homemade (page 252) or canned

¾ teaspoon ground ginger

½ teaspoon cinnamon

½ teaspoon pepper

1 large onion, finely chopped

2 carrots, thinly sliced

2 parsnips, thinly sliced

¾ pound leg of lamb, cut into ½-inch pieces

½ cup pitted dried plums (prunes), coarsely chopped

3 tablespoons tomato paste

1½ cups cooked white beans (page 180) or canned (rinsed and drained)

½ teaspoon salt

¼ cup chopped cilantro

1 tablespoon fresh lemon juice

1 In a Dutch oven or large saucepan, combine the broth, ginger, cinnamon, and pepper, and bring to a boil over medium heat. Add the onion, carrots, and parsnips, and cook, stirring frequently, until the vegetables have softened, about 10 minutes.

2 Stir in the lamb and cook until the lamb is no longer pink, about 5 minutes.

3 Add the dried plums, tomato paste, white beans, salt, and 2 tablespoons of the cilantro. Cover and simmer until the lamb is cooked through and tender, about 20 minutes. Stir in the remaining 2 tablespoons cilantro and the lemon juice. *Makes 4 servings*

per serving: 392 calories, 10g total fat (3.5g saturated), 81mg cholesterol, 9g dietary fiber, 43g carbohydrate, 34g protein, 628mg sodium. good source of: beta carotene, fiber, folate, niacin, potassium, selenium, vitamin B_{12}, zinc.

different spins

▶**Moroccan Lamb & Chick-Pea Stew** Follow the directions for *Moroccan Lamb & White Bean Stew*, but substitute dried apricots for the dried plums and chick-peas for the white beans. Omit the parsnips and add 2 more carrots.

▶**Herbed Lamb & White Bean Stew** Follow the directions for *Moroccan Lamb & White Bean Stew*, but substitute ½ teaspoon each of rosemary and tarragon for the ginger and cinnamon. Omit the dried plums. Substitute chopped parsley for the cilantro.

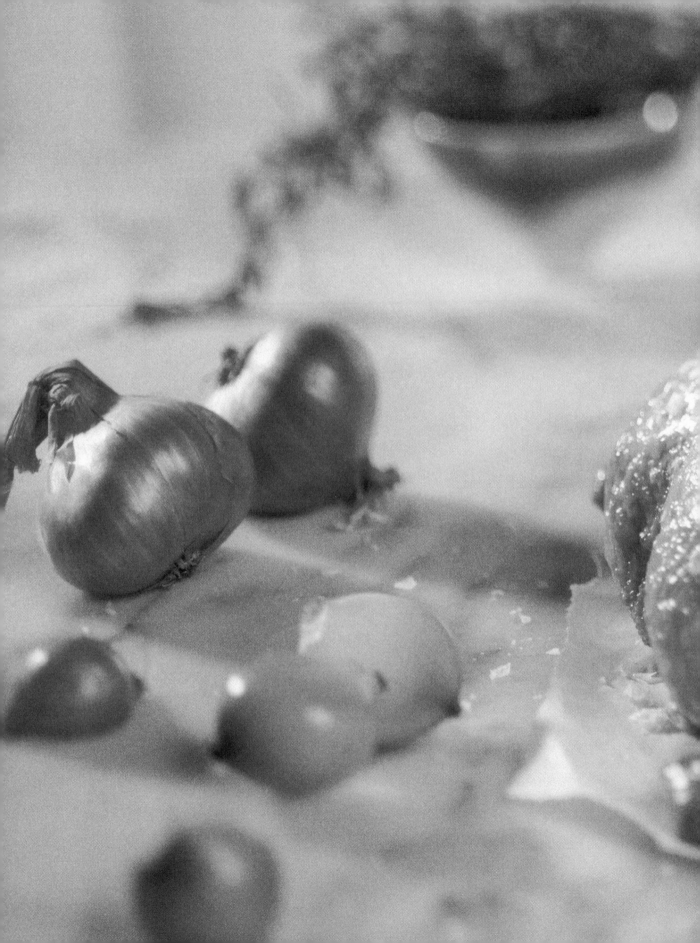

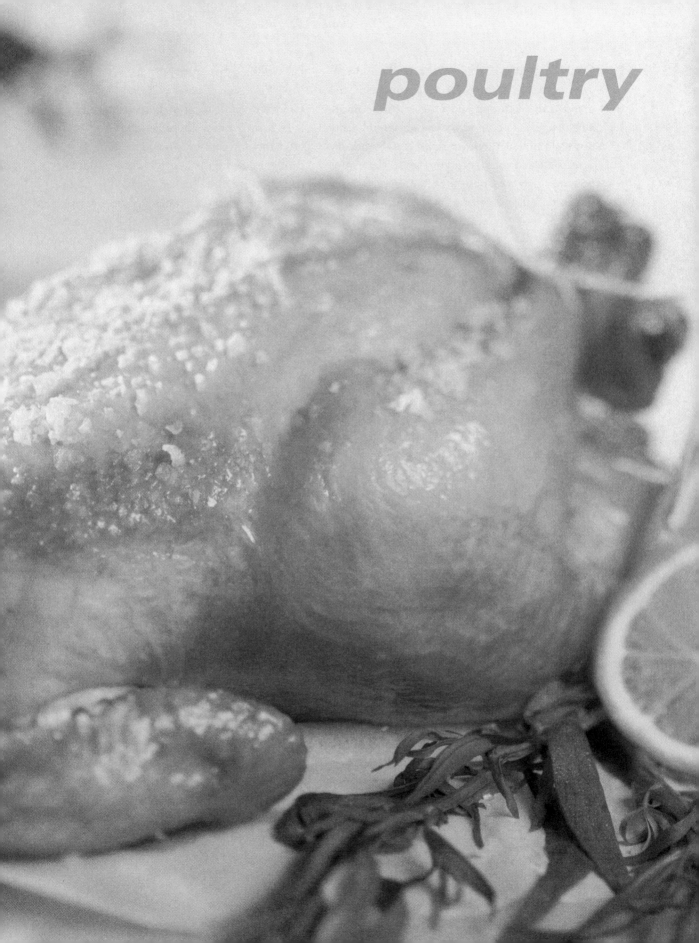

poultry

Cooking poultry for maximum flavor and tenderness, while keeping fat to a minimum, demands careful timing and temperature control. The goal is to cook poultry just until tender, but not so long that the meat turns tough and dry. The safest and most accurate way to determine doneness is to use a meat thermometer (see "How to Use a Meat Thermometer," page 107).

chicken

Chicken is cooked by either dry- or moist-heat methods. The former, which includes broiling and roasting, allows fat to melt and drain off; the latter, which encompasses braising, stewing, and poaching, tenderizes leaner cuts. When cooking cuts of chicken by themselves (i.e., not in a dish of mixed ingredients like a stew or casserole), you can leave the skin on to keep the flesh moist. The skin can then be removed before eating.

Roasting/baking Of all the cooking methods, roasting a whole bird melts away the most fat. Cooking times vary by the size of the bird (see "Chicken Cooking Chart," opposite page). Chicken parts can be roasted or baked as is, or baked with other ingredients. Baked on their own, the skin can stay on and be removed before eating; but when baked with other ingredients, or in a sauce, the chicken should be skinless, so that the rendered fat does not become part of the dish. To compensate for the moisture that could be lost with skinless chicken, you should either coat the chicken and/or cook it covered (see Chicken & Roasted Root Vegetables, page 108).

Baking in parchment One of the best ways to bake chicken so it stays moist and tender without the addition of fat is by baking it in cooking parchment or foil (see the Chicken in Parchment "Recipe Creator" on page 111).

Broiling/grilling Leaving the skin on for broiling and grilling will keep the flesh moist, but skinless cuts can also be successfully broiled (see Simple Broiled Chicken, page 108). If you do leave the skin on, you can give the chicken flavor by rubbing spices or herbs directly onto the flesh and under the skin (see Spice-Rubbed Chicken, page 110).

Frying Pan-fried chicken can be quite a healthful cooking method, especially if you use skinless chicken and a nonstick pan. And coating the skinless chicken first with flour is one way to keep the juices in (see Chicken Scallopine Provençal, page 116). Deep-frying, on the other hand, is one of the unhealthiest ways to prepare chicken, since by tradition the skin stays on, and the batter or breading absorbs a lot of the oil. A more healthful solution is to oven-fry the chicken: This method produces crisp chicken without the mess of hot oil, or the extra fat (see Spicy Oven-Fried Chicken, page 106).

Stir-frying This quick-cooking method is a good way to create dishes with lean, skinless cuts, as well as boost the ratio of vegetables to chicken. There are endless variations on the theme, and once you understand the basic con-

---

how to tell when chicken is done

In addition to the internal temperature that will tell you when chicken is done, there are certain visual clues that a cook looks for to test for doneness:

▶**Whole chicken** Hold onto a drumstick and wiggle it back and forth. The drumstick should be loose in its socket, but still firmly attached. Also, if you insert a fork or knife between the drumstick and the thigh, the juices should be clear with a tinge of yellow (and no pink).

▶**Chicken parts** Prick the chicken flesh with a knife or fork. If the juices run clear with a tinge of yellow (and no pink), the chicken is done. Chicken breasts will be white throughout, but still juicy. Bone-in thighs and drumsticks should not be pink at the bone.

chicken cooking chart

Chicken will cook faster than the times given below if you roast it in a covered pan, in a small pan, or in a small oven (more convected heat). Always check for doneness about 15 minutes before the first time listed in the range of times, and use a meat thermometer (*see "How to Use a Meat Thermometer," page 107*). Stop cooking when the internal temperature reads 165°F in the breast or 175°F in the thigh. Let the chicken stand 15 minutes; during that time, the temperature will rise another 5 degrees.

CUT	AMOUNT	METHOD
WHOLE CHICKEN	broiler/fryer, 3 to 5 lbs	**Roasting*** 350°F for 1¼ to 1½ hours, or until meat thermometer inserted in breast reads 170°F; or in thigh, 180°F
	roaster, 6 to 8 lbs	**Roasting*** 350°F for 2 to 2¼ hours, or until meat thermometer inserted in breast reads 170°F; or in thigh, 180°F
WHOLE CAPON	8 to 10 lbs	**Roasting*** 375°F for 1¾ to 2¼ hours, or until meat thermometer reads 180°F
CHICKEN BREAST	half, bone-in, 8 to 10 oz	**Roasting** 425°F for 25–30 minutes **Broiling/grilling** 4 to 6 inches from heat, 8 minutes per side
	half, boneless, 5 to 6 oz	**Baking** 350°F for 20–30 minutes **Broiling/grilling** 4 to 6 inches from heat, 6–8 minutes per side
	half, skinless, boneless, 4 to 5 oz	**Broiling/grilling** 4 to 6 inches from heat, 4 minutes per side **Pan-frying** In lightly oiled nonstick skillet, over medium heat, 4 minutes per side **Poaching** In simmering liquid to cover, 8 to 10 minutes.
	cut for stir-fry	**Stir-frying** *See Poultry Stir-Fries "Recipe Creator" on page 115*
CHICKEN THIGHS	bone-in, 5 to 7 oz	**Baking** 350°F for 30–40 minutes
	boneless, 4 to 5 oz	**Baking** 350°F for 20–30 minutes **Broiling/grilling** 4 to 6 inches from heat, 4 minutes per side
	cut for stir-fry	**Stir-frying** *See Poultry Stir-Fries "Recipe Creator" on page 115*
DRUMSTICKS	4 to 5 oz	**Baking** 350°F for 30–40 minutes
LEG (THIGH AND DRUMSTICK), BONE-IN	10 oz	**Baking** 350°F for 30–40 minutes

*roasting times are for unstuffed birds

cepts, you can make up your own recipes (*see Poultry Stir-Fries "Recipe Creator," page 115*).

Braising/stewing We tend to use dark meat in stews because it can stand up to long, slow cooking (*see Chicken Fettuccine Alfredo, page 112, Southwestern Chicken & Sweet Potato Stew, page 120, and Chicken Stew with Herbed Dumplings, page 122*). You can substitute white meat in stews, as long as you adjust the cooking times. White meat chicken will take half the cooking time of dark meat.

Poaching/steaming Steaming chicken in a vegetable steamer, or poaching in water or broth, are the best ways to prepare chicken that will later be eaten cold. You can steam or poach individual cuts (*see Cold Poached Chicken with Pepper-Caper Sauce, page 121*), or poach a whole chicken. When poaching a whole chicken, use the cooking liquid as the base for chicken soup.

Chicken broth It's easy to make your own broth to use in cooking or as the basis for soups (*see Homemade Chicken Broth, page 252*). For a good basic chicken soup, see Chicken Noodle Soup (*page 39*).

Spicy Oven-Fried Chicken

When you bake skinless chicken, you need to provide some sort of coating to keep the meat from drying out. In this oven version of fried chicken, the chicken is coated first with a sweet-spicy buttermilk mixture and then dredged in seasoned flour. Feel free to substitute skinless, boneless chicken thighs for the chicken breasts, if you prefer. **Timing alert:** If you have the time, you can let the chicken marinate in the buttermilk mixture (step 2) for several hours in the refrigerator.

> 1 cup buttermilk
> 1 tablespoon honey
> ½ teaspoon cayenne pepper
> 4 skinless, boneless chicken breast halves (5 ounces each)
> ⅔ cup flour
> 1 tablespoon chili powder
> ½ teaspoon oregano
> ½ teaspoon salt

1 In a medium bowl, stir together the buttermilk, honey, and ¼ teaspoon of the cayenne. Add the chicken and let stand 15 minutes.

2 Meanwhile, preheat the oven to 400°F. Spray a baking sheet with nonstick cooking spray.

3 On a plate, combine the remaining ¼ teaspoon cayenne, the flour, chili powder, oregano, and salt. Dredge the chicken in the flour mixture, shaking off the excess.

4 Place the chicken on the baking sheet, and spray evenly and lightly with nonstick cooking spray. Bake, without turning the chicken over, for 12 minutes, or until crisp, golden, and cooked through. *Makes 4 servings*

per serving: 279 calories, 2.9g total fat (0.9g saturated), 85mg cholesterol, 1g dietary fiber, 24g carbohydrate, 37g protein, 468mg sodium. good source of: niacin, riboflavin, selenium, vitamin B_{12}, vitamin B_6.

Apricot-Lemon Roast Chicken

Because you should not eat chicken skin, it's pointless to rub the skin of a roast chicken with any seasonings, since they will just go to waste. However, you *do* want to season the chicken flesh (as well as the pan juices). The solution is to make a seasoning mixture that gets placed underneath the skin. Here, apricots, garlic, and rosemary are pureed and used as the under-skin seasoning mixture.

⅓ cup dried apricots

¾ cup water

1 teaspoon sugar

1 teaspoon rosemary, minced

2 cloves garlic, peeled

¾ teaspoon salt

1 broiler-fryer chicken (3 to 3½ pounds)

1 large lemon

1 tablespoon flour

1 Preheat the oven to 350°F. In a food processor, combine the apricots, ¼ cup of the water, the sugar, ½ teaspoon of the rosemary, the garlic, and ¼ teaspoon of the salt. Process to a puree.

2 Rub the inside of the chicken with ¼ teaspoon of the salt and the remaining ½ teaspoon rosemary.

With a fork, prick the lemon all over. Place the lemon inside the cavity of the chicken.

3 With your fingers, carefully separate the chicken skin from the flesh of the breast and smear the apricot puree over the flesh. Pat the skin back into place so it completely covers the apricot puree.

4 Place the chicken on a rack in a roasting pan and roast for 1 hour 15 minutes, or until the internal temperature of the thigh reads 180°F.

5 When the chicken is done, transfer to a carving board and let sit 15 minutes before carving.

6 Meanwhile, make the gravy: Add the remaining ½ cup water to the roasting pan and use a whisk to scrape up any browned bits clinging to the pan. Pour the juices from the roasting pan into a gravy separator. Wait for the fat to rise to the top, then pour the degreased liquid into a small saucepan.

7 In a small bowl, combine the remaining ¼ teaspoon salt and the flour. Whisk about 3 tablespoons of the degreased cooking juices into the flour, then scrape the slurry (flour and liquid mixture) back into the saucepan. Cook, stirring, over low heat until the gravy is thickened and no raw floury taste remains, about 3 minutes. *Makes 4 servings*

per serving: 242 calories, 8.5g total fat (2.3g saturated), 101mg cholesterol, 1g dietary fiber, 7g carbohydrate, 33g protein, 389mg sodium. good source of: niacin, selenium, vitamin B_6.

how to use a meat thermometer

A meat thermometer is the surest way to judge when poultry or meat is done to the appropriate internal temperature. The temperature required will depend on how long it takes for the individual food to get tender. The cooking charts for the respective foods will give internal temperatures as a measure of doneness.

There are several styles of thermometer: There is a high-end model in which a heat sensor is inserted into the meat or poultry before it goes into the oven. The sensor is connected to a digital read-out that gives a minute-by-minute account of the internal temperature. Cheaper, and more hands-on, is what is called an instant-read thermometer. It's a metal probe about 5 inches long with a thermometer dial at one end. You insert the end of the probe into the meat or poultry and wait 5 seconds or so to read the temperature.

The trick to an accurate reading, regardless of the type of thermometer, is to be sure that the tip of the sensor is in the thickest part of the meat, and not touching any bone or surrounding metal (as in a roasting pan). If the sensor touches bone, the reading will be falsely low; if the sensor pokes all the way through and touches metal, the reading will be falsely high.

Chicken & Roasted Root Vegetables

When you bake chicken on top of vegetables, it's especially important to use skinless chicken, because the fat rendered from the skin would soak into the vegetables below. As with any other form of skinless chicken, it should be coated with something to keep it moist as it cooks. Here we use an herbed tomato paste mixture. **Serving suggestion:** This dish needs only a green salad, crusty bread, and a simple fruit dessert (*try Baked Green Apples, page 229*) to round out the meal.

¼ cup tomato paste

¾ teaspoon rosemary, minced

¾ teaspoon salt

1½ pounds skinless, boneless chicken thighs

½ cup sun-dried tomatoes

1 cup boiling water

1¼ pounds red potatoes, cut into ½-inch chunks

3 carrots, thinly sliced

3 parsnips, thinly sliced

4 garlic cloves, slivered

¼ teaspoon pepper

1 Preheat the oven to 400°F.

2 In a small bowl, stir together the tomato paste, ½ teaspoon of the rosemary, and ¼ teaspoon of the salt. Rub the chicken with the tomato paste mixture. Set aside while you prepare the vegetables.

3 In small heatproof bowl, combine the sun-dried tomatoes and boiling water. Let sit until the tomatoes have softened, about 10 minutes. Drain, reserving the soaking liquid. Coarsely chop the tomatoes.

4 In a 9 x 13-inch baking pan, stir together the remaining ¼ teaspoon rosemary, remaining ½ teaspoon salt, potatoes, carrots, parsnips, garlic, and pepper. Stir in the sun-dried tomatoes and their soaking liquid. Cover with foil and bake for 15 minutes.

5 Uncover and place the chicken on top of the vegetables. Bake for 20 minutes, or until the vegetables are tender and the chicken is cooked through. *Makes 6 servings*

per serving: 428 calories, 7.3g total fat (1.8g saturated), 141mg cholesterol, 8g dietary fiber, 52g carbohydrate, 40g protein, 772mg sodium. good source of: beta carotene, fiber, magnesium, niacin, potassium, riboflavin, selenium, thiamin, vitamin B_{12}, vitamin B_6, vitamin C, zinc.

Simple Broiled Chicken

Boneless chicken breasts come with one side thicker than the other, so you should pound them lightly (with a meat pounder or small frying pan) on the thicker side so they will cook more evenly. **Serving suggestion:** Serving broiled chicken with a chutney or salsa is a good way to get some healthful fruits and/or vegetables on your plate. It will also get you kudos for making something that seems complicated but couldn't be simpler. Try one of these: Grilled Pepper & Tomato Salsa (*page 263*), Salsa Verde (*page 258*), Spicy Cranberry Sauce (*page 259*), or Red Pepper Harissa (*page 257*).

4 skinless, boneless chicken breast halves (5 ounces each), lightly pounded

1 teaspoon grated lime zest

1 tablespoon fresh lime juice

2 teaspoons olive oil

½ teaspoon salt

⅛ teaspoon red pepper flakes

1 Preheat the broiler. Spray the broiler pan with nonstick cooking spray. Place the chicken on the broiler pan.

2 In a small bowl, combine the lime zest, lime juice, oil, salt, and red pepper flakes. Brush both sides of the chicken with the lime mixture.

3 Broil 4 to 6 inches from the heat, turning once, for 6 minutes, or until the chicken is cooked through. *Makes 4 servings*

per serving: 173 calories, 5.6g total fat (1.2g saturated), 78mg cholesterol, 0g dietary fiber, 0g carbohydrate, 29g protein, 359mg sodium. good source of: niacin, selenium, vitamin B$_6$, vitamin B$_{12}$.

Tandoori-Style Chicken with Banana Raita

Yogurt plays a double role in this Indian-inspired baked chicken. As in any tandoori dish, spiced yogurt is used as a marinade and coating mixture for food to be baked (traditionally in a hot clay oven called a tandoor). Yogurt is also used here to make an Indian condiment/accompaniment called a raita. **Timing alert:** The chicken needs to marinate for at least 2 hours.

 3 cloves garlic, minced

 2 tablespoons minced fresh ginger

 2 teaspoons paprika

 ¾ teaspoon salt

 1½ teaspoons ground coriander

 ½ teaspoon pepper

 1½ cups plain low-fat yogurt

 4 skinless, bone-in chicken breast halves
  (8 ounces each)

 ⅓ cup chopped cilantro

 2 scallions, thinly sliced

 1 small banana, coarsely chopped

1 In a shallow glass or ceramic baking dish, combine the garlic, ginger, paprika, salt, 1 teaspoon of the coriander, and ¼ teaspoon of the pepper. Stir in 1 cup of the yogurt until well blended.

2 With a sharp knife, make several slashes in the flesh of the chicken, cutting almost, but not through to the bone. Place the chicken, cut-sides down, in the yogurt mixture. Cover and refrigerate for at least 2 hours or up to overnight, turning the chicken several times.

3 Preheat the oven to 500°F. Take the dish of chicken out of the refrigerator and bring it to room temperature before placing in the oven. Bake the chicken in its marinade for about 25 minutes, or until cooked through.

4 Meanwhile, in a medium bowl, combine the remaining ½ cup yogurt, ½ teaspoon coriander, ¼ teaspoon pepper, the cilantro, scallions, and banana. Cover and chill until serving time.

5 Lift the chicken from its cooking mixture and serve hot with the chilled raita. *Makes 4 servings*

per serving: 295 calories, 4.1g total fat (1.6g saturated), 111mg cholesterol, 2g dietary fiber, 15g carbohydrate, 48g protein, 623mg sodium. good source of: niacin, potassium, riboflavin, selenium, vitamin B$_{12}$, vitamin B$_6$.

poultry safety

Never thaw frozen poultry at room temperature; the outside thaws first and becomes susceptible to bacterial growth during the time it takes for the inside to thaw. Leave it in the refrigerator to defrost on a plate to catch the drippings. Allow 3 to 4 hours of thawing time per pound; poultry parts may thaw more quickly. Use a microwave oven for thawing only if you plan to cook the poultry right away.

Keep raw poultry away from other foods, especially salad greens or any food that will be served raw or cooked only briefly. Be sure to thoroughly wash your hands, the countertop, sink, cutting board, and utensils with hot, soapy water.

Marinate poultry pieces in the refrigerator, not at room temperature. Poultry can spoil if it sits out even for three hours on a warm day. And don't use the marinade as a sauce unless you bring it to a rolling boil for several minutes before serving. Better yet, make extra marinade and store it separately until you are ready to serve it.

Spice-Rubbed Chicken

One way to protect chicken from the direct heat of broiling is to leave the skin on, and then remove it before eating. For this reason, the spice mixture is rubbed under, rather than on, the chicken skin. The chicken can be rubbed with the spice mixture several hours before cooking; if not cooking the chicken within 20 minutes, refrigerate it. **Serving suggestion:** Stay simple, with just a squeeze of fresh lemon, or be more ambitious and make a salsa to go with this broiled chicken. Try Grilled Pepper & Tomato Salsa (*page 263*) or invent your own fruit salsa using the "Recipe Creator" on page 262.

1 teaspoon paprika

1 teaspoon coriander

½ teaspoon cumin

½ teaspoon salt

4 skin-on, bone-in chicken breast halves (10 ounces each)

Lemon wedges, for serving

1 Preheat the broiler. In a small bowl, combine the paprika, coriander, cumin, and salt. With your fingers, lift the chicken skin and rub the spice mixture under the skin.

2 Broil the chicken 4 to 6 inches from the heat, turning several times, for 15 minutes, or until just cooked through.

3 Serve the chicken with lemon wedges. Remove the chicken skin before eating. *Makes 4 servings*

per serving: 228 calories, 5g total fat (1.4g saturated), 113mg cholesterol, 2g dietary fiber, 4g carbohydrate, 42g protein, 390mg sodium. good source of: niacin, selenium, vitamin B$_{12}$, vitamin B$_6$.

Chicken Fajitas for a Crowd

Any time you can shift the balance in a meal in favor of lots of colorful vegetables, the better off you'll be. Fajitas provide a perfect opportunity: Instead of loads of grilled chicken with grilled vegetables as a condiment, we've inverted the proportions to make the bell peppers, red onions, lettuce, and salsa the main focus, with grilled chicken as the "condiment." If you're not cooking for a crowd, this recipe can easily be halved.

Simple Broiled Chicken (page 108)

½ cup fresh lime juice

2 tablespoons chili powder

1 tablespoon olive oil

6 bell peppers, mixed colors, cut into thin strips

2 large red onions, thinly sliced

16 flour tortillas (6 inches)

2 cups bottled mild or medium salsa

4 cups shredded romaine lettuce

1 Prepare the Simple Broiled Chicken. Leave the broiler on. When cool enough to handle, cut the chicken across the grain into thin slices.

2 Meanwhile, in a large bowl, combine the lime juice, chili powder, oil, bell peppers, and onions.

3 Working in 2 batches, with a slotted spoon, transfer the bell peppers and onions to a broiler pan. Broil the vegetables 4 to 6 inches from the heat, turning occasionally, until tender, about 10 minutes. Repeat with the remaining vegetables.

4 Place the tortillas under the broiler for 30 seconds to warm through.

5 Place serving bowls of chicken, onion-pepper mixture, salsa, and lettuce on the table. Serve 2 tortillas per person and let each diner assemble his/her own fajitas. *Makes 8 servings*

per serving: 437 calories, 10g total fat (2.3g saturated), 72mg cholesterol, 7g dietary fiber, 52g carbohydrate, 35g protein, 676mg sodium. good source of: beta carotene, capsaicin, folate, niacin, potassium, riboflavin, selenium, thiamin, vitamin B$_6$, vitamin C.

recipe creator
chicken in parchment

Baking chicken in an enclosed packet (either of parchment paper or foil) is one of the best ways to cook skinless, boneless chicken breast and keep it moist and tender without having to use a lot of fat. The packet provides a one-pot meal with a nice balance of complex carbohydrates and vegetables to animal protein. Aside from the obvious health factors, parchment packets can be assembled in advance (and refrigerated until time to cook them) to make a super-quick meal.

Pick ingredients from each of the 4 categories and follow these basic instructions (note that the quantities given for the ingredients are *per packet*): Cut 4 pieces (12 x 18 inches) of parchment paper or foil. With a short side of the parchment (or foil) facing you, place 1 STARCH about 3 inches from the bottom edge. Place one 5-ounce skinless, boneless chicken breast on top and sprinkle with ¼ teaspoon salt, ⅛ teaspoon pepper, 1 or 2 SEASONINGS, and 1 AROMATIC. Top with 1 or 2 VEGETABLES. Fold the parchment over the ingredients and fold in the edges to seal (if using parchment, be sure to leave a bit of headroom for the steam). Bake the packets on a baking sheet for 12 to 15 minutes in a 450°F oven. The parchment packets will puff when the chicken is cooked. For foil packets (which won't puff), carefully open one packet and poke the chicken. If the juices run clear, the chicken is cooked through, if not, reseal the packet and return it to the oven for a few more minutes. *Makes 4 servings*

STARCHES

▶ Potatoes, ½ cup thinly sliced cooked

▶ White or brown rice, ½ cup cooked

▶ Sweet potatoes, ½ cup thinly sliced cooked

▶ Couscous, ½ cup cooked

▶ Bulgur, ½ cup soaked and drained

▶ Small pasta shapes, ½ cup cooked

SEASONINGS

▶ Reduced-sodium soy sauce, 1 Tbsp

▶ Fresh lemon or lime juice, 1 Tbsp

▶ Pesto sauce, 1 Tbsp

▶ Horseradish, 1 Tbsp

▶ Salsa, 2 Tbsp

▶ Hot pepper sauce, ¼ tsp

▶ Red or white wine, 2 Tbsp

▶ Balsamic vinegar, 1 Tbsp

▶ Olives, 1 Tbsp minced

▶ Capers, 1 tsp minced

AROMATICS

▶ Fresh basil, 2 Tbsp chopped

▶ Fresh dill, 2 Tbsp chopped

▶ Fresh parsley, 2 Tbsp chopped

▶ Fresh mint, 2 Tbsp chopped

▶ Cilantro, 2 Tbsp chopped

▶ Garlic, 1 clove minced

VEGETABLES

▶ Carrots, ½ cup matchsticks

▶ Leeks, ½ cup matchsticks

▶ Mushrooms, ½ cup chopped

▶ Tomatoes, ½ cup chopped

▶ Broccoli, ½ cup shredded

▶ Red bell pepper, ½ cup slivered

▶ Zucchini and/or yellow squash, ½ cup shredded

▶ Snow peas or sugar snap peas, ½ cup

Sweet & Spicy Maple-Broiled Chicken

A mixture of pineapple juice, maple syrup, and soy sauce seasoned with ginger and cayenne makes a simple basting sauce but with complex flavors. If you can find grade B maple syrup (it's often available at farmers' markets), by all means, use it here. Grade B syrup, produced from late-season sap, is dark in color and intensely flavored. **Serving suggestion:** Serve with Red Cabbage Slaw (*page 202*) and Angel Biscuits (*page 216*). For dessert, offer Strawberries with Balsamic Vinegar & Pepper (page *226*). **Timing alert:** The chicken marinates for at least 2 hours.

¼ cup pineapple juice

3 tablespoons maple syrup

2 tablespoons reduced-sodium soy sauce

3 cloves garlic, minced

½ teaspoon ground ginger

½ teaspoon salt

¼ teaspoon cayenne pepper

1 pound skinless, boneless chicken thighs

1 In a shallow nonaluminum pan, stir together the pineapple juice, maple syrup, soy sauce, garlic, ginger, salt, and cayenne. Add the chicken, cover, and marinate in the refrigerator for at least 2 hours or up to overnight.

2 Preheat the broiler. Line the broiler pan with foil for easy cleanup. Lift the chicken from the marinade and broil 4 to 6 inches from the heat for 3 minutes.

3 Brush with half the marinade remaining in the pan and broil for 3 minutes.

4 Turn the chicken over, brush with the remaining marinade, and broil until the chicken is just cooked through, about 4 minutes. When cool enough to handle, thinly slice. *Makes 4 servings*

per serving: 220 calories, 8.6g total fat (2.4g saturated), 74mg cholesterol, 0g dietary fiber, 14g carbohydrate, 21g protein, 628mg sodium. good source of: niacin, selenium, vitamin B$_6$, zinc.

did you know?

Fettuccine Alfredo is named for Alfredo DiLeo, the owner of a restaurant called Alfredo's (which still exists in Rome). According to legend, in 1914 Signor DiLeo created a simple dish of hot noodles tossed with grated cheese, cream, and butter for his wife, who was suffering from morning sickness. (The Italians are fond of treating wiggly stomachs with "white food.") The legend also includes the dramatic moment a dozen years later when Alfredo tossed together the dish at tableside for Mary Pickford and Douglas Fairbanks, an event that brought the dish to America.

Chicken Fettuccine Alfredo

Our version of fettuccine Alfredo deviates from the traditional by adding chicken and peas to make this a one-dish meal instead of an Italian pasta course. We've also greatly reduced the fat content.

10 ounces fettuccine

¾ pound skinless, boneless chicken breasts, cut into 1-inch chunks

2 tablespoons flour

2 teaspoons olive oil

1 cup low-fat (1%) milk

¾ teaspoon salt

½ teaspoon pepper

¼ teaspoon nutmeg

1 cup frozen peas

¼ cup grated Parmesan cheese

⅓ cup fat-free half-and-half

1 In a large pot of boiling water, cook the fettuccine according to package directions. Drain, reserving ⅓ cup of the cooking water.

2 Meanwhile, dredge the chicken in the flour, shaking off the excess.

3 In a large nonstick skillet, heat the oil over medium heat. Add the chicken and cook, stirring, until lightly browned, about 2 minutes.

4 Gradually add the milk, stirring until smooth. Add the reserved ⅓ cup pasta cooking water, the salt, pepper, and nutmeg. Bring to a boil, reduce to a simmer and add the peas. Cook until the sauce is slightly thickened and the chicken is cooked through, about 2 minutes.

5 Transfer to a large bowl, add the fettuccine, Parmesan, and fat-free half-and-half and toss to combine. *Makes 4 servings*

per serving: 472 calories, 6.8g total fat (2.2g saturated), 56mg cholesterol, 4g dietary fiber, 65g carbohydrate, 35g protein, 667mg sodium. good source of: niacin, selenium, vitamin B_{12}, vitamin B_6.

Sautéed Chicken with Leeks & Radicchio

A small amount of rich, flavorful chicken thigh goes a long way in this quick, vegetable-packed sauté. If you don't happen to have reduced-sodium teriyaki sauce on hand, use 2 tablespoons reduced-sodium soy sauce mixed with 1 teaspoon brown sugar.

⅓ cup dried porcini or shiitake mushrooms

1½ cups boiling water

3 teaspoons olive oil

¾ pound skinless, boneless chicken thighs, cut into ½-inch-wide strips

2 tablespoons plus 1½ teaspoons cornstarch

2 leeks, cut into matchsticks and well washed

½ pound asparagus, cut into 1-inch lengths

2 cups packed shredded radicchio (about ¼ pound)

2 cloves garlic, minced

2 shallots, minced, or 2 scallions, thinly sliced

2 tablespoons reduced-sodium teriyaki sauce

2 teaspoons grated lemon zest

1 tablespoon fresh lemon juice

½ teaspoon salt

1 In a small heatproof bowl, combine the dried mushrooms and the boiling water, and let stand for 20 minutes, or until softened. Reserving the soaking liquid, scoop out the dried mushrooms and coarsely chop. Strain the soaking liquid through a coffee filter or a paper towel-lined sieve. Set aside.

2 In a large nonstick skillet, heat 2 teaspoons of the oil over medium-high heat. Dredge the chicken in 2 tablespoons of the cornstarch, shaking off the excess. Add the chicken to the pan and sauté until crisp and golden brown, about 4 minutes. With a slotted spoon, transfer the chicken to a plate.

3 Add the remaining 1 teaspoon oil, the mushrooms, leeks, asparagus, radicchio, garlic, and shallots to the pan and stir-fry until the asparagus is crisp-tender, about 5 minutes.

4 In a small bowl, stir the reserved mushroom soaking liquid into the remaining 1½ teaspoons cornstarch. Stir in the teriyaki sauce, lemon zest, lemon juice, and salt. Add the teriyaki mixture to the pan and bring to a boil. Return the chicken to the pan, reduce to a simmer, and cook, stirring until the chicken is heated through and the sauce is slightly thickened, about 2 minutes. *Makes 4 servings*

per serving: 245 calories, 7.5g total fat (1.4g saturated), 71mg cholesterol, 4g dietary fiber, 22g carbohydrate, 23g protein, 655mg sodium. good source of: folate, niacin, vitamin B_6.

different *spins*

▶**Sautéed Chicken with Arugula** Follow the directions for *Sautéed Chicken with Leeks & Radicchio,* but substitute 1 medium red onion, sliced, for the leeks. Omit the asparagus and use ½ pound of fresh shiitakes (in addition to the dried mushrooms) instead. Use 3 cups of arugula leaves instead of the radicchio. Omit the shallots.

Pan-"Fried" Chicken Burgers

You can buy ground chicken at the supermarket, but grinding your own breast meat ensures that you won't be getting any skin ground with the meat. Mushrooms not only lend moisture to these burgers, but they give them a rich, earthy flavor. **Serving suggestion:** Keep it simple and serve these burgers on a bun, with lettuce and ketchup. Or get fancy and prepare one of these toppings: Hot & Spicy Cocktail Sauce (*page 256*), Corn Relish (*page 264*), Tomato-Orange Chutney (*page 267*), or Fresh Vidalia Onion Relish (*page 265*).

> 2 slices (1 ounce each) firm whole-wheat sandwich bread, torn into large pieces
> ¼ pound white or cremini mushrooms, quartered
> ⅓ cup packed parsley leaves
> 2 cloves garlic, peeled
> ¾ teaspoon salt
> ½ teaspoon pepper
> ½ teaspoon tarragon
> 1 pound skinless, boneless chicken breasts, cut into large chunks
> 2 scallions, thinly sliced
> ½ cup water
> 1 teaspoon reduced-sodium soy sauce

1 In a food processor, process the bread, mushrooms, parsley, garlic, salt, pepper, and tarragon until coarsely ground. Transfer to a large bowl. Do not clean the food processor bowl.

"frying" burgers

Instead of using oil to pan-fry chicken (or turkey) burgers, "fry" them in a small amount of seasoned water (or other liquid, such as broth). Here's how it works: You start the burgers off in the liquid—this keeps them from sticking to the pan. Then, as they cook, the burgers contribute their own natural juices to the pan, and the water evaporates, leaving a flavorful glaze for the burgers.

2 Add the chicken to the food processor and pulse on and off until finely ground. Add to the bowl along with the scallions and blend well. Shape the mixture into 4 patties.

3 In a large nonstick skillet, bring the water and soy sauce to a simmer over medium heat. Add the chicken patties and cook, turning the patties once, until richly browned and cooked through, about 7 minutes. *Makes 4 servings*

per serving: 177 calories, 2g total fat (0.4g saturated), 66mg cholesterol, 2g dietary fiber, 9g carbohydrate, 29g protein, 626mg sodium. good source of: niacin, riboflavin, selenium, vitamin B_{12}, vitamin B_6.

Pan-Fried Chicken with Pumpkin Seed Sauce

Pumpkin seeds develop even more flavor when briefly toasted. Look for unsalted, hulled pumpkin seeds (also called pepitas) in the nut section of the supermarket, at health-food stores, or Latin American markets. If you can only find salted pumpkin seeds, simply reduce the salt in the sauce (step 1) from ½ teaspoon to ¼ teaspoon.

> ¼ cup hulled pumpkin seeds (pepitas)
> 1 can (4½ ounces) mild green chilies, drained
> 1 plum tomato, cut into large chunks
> 1 canned or bottled jalapeño pepper
> ¼ cup cilantro sprigs
> ¾ teaspoon coriander
> ½ teaspoon salt
> 2 teaspoons olive oil
> 4 small skinless, boneless chicken breast halves (4 ounces each)
> 1 tablespoon fresh lime juice

1 In a small skillet, toast the pumpkin seeds over low heat until they begin to pop in the pan, about 5 minutes. Transfer to a blender or food processor. Add the mild green chilies, tomato, jalapeño, cilantro, coriander, and salt. Process to a smooth puree.

recipe creator
poultry stir-fries

Poultry is especially well suited to stir-frying, because it cooks quickly and pairs well with a wide range of seasonings. Pick ingredients from each of the categories and follow these basic instructions: Cut the POULTRY into strips ¼ inch wide (or buy it precut for stir-fry). In a small bowl, stir together 1 cup chicken broth, 2 teaspoons cornstarch, 1 teaspoon brown sugar, and ½ teaspoon salt to make a coating sauce; set aside. In a wok or large nonstick skillet, heat 2 teaspoons olive or canola oil over medium-high heat. Cook the POULTRY until cooked through, about 3 minutes. With a slotted spoon, transfer the poultry to a plate. Choose 2 to 5 VEGETABLES, using a total of 5 cups. Add 2 teaspoons oil and any hard vegetables (asparagus or broccoli) to the pan; stir-fry for 3 minutes. Add any soft vegetables, 1 to 3 AROMATICS, and 1 to 4 SEASONINGS. Cook until the vegetables are crisp-tender, about 3 minutes. Stir the coating sauce to recombine. Return the poultry to the pan, along with the coating sauce; cook until heated through and evenly coated, about 1 minute. *Makes 4 servings*

POULTRY	VEGETABLES	AROMATICS	SEASONINGS
▶Chicken breast, skinless, boneless, ½ pound	▶Red or green bell peppers, cut into thin strips	▶Scallions, 3 sliced	▶Red pepper flakes, ½ tsp
▶Chicken thigh, skinless, boneless, ½ pound	▶Onions or leeks, cut into matchsticks	▶Garlic, 3 cloves minced	▶Chili powder, 1 tsp
▶Turkey cutlets, ½ pound	▶Asparagus, cut into ½-inch lengths	▶Shallots, ¼ cup minced	▶Grated orange zest, 1 tsp
▶Duck breast, skinless, boneless, ½ pound	▶Sugar snaps or snow peas, strings removed	▶Grated ginger, 1 Tbsp	▶Curry powder, 1 tsp
	▶Broccoli florets		▶Dark sesame oil, 1 tsp
	▶Shredded cabbage		▶Tarragon, 1 tsp

2 In a large nonstick skillet, heat the oil over medium heat. Add the chicken and cook until browned, about 2 minutes per side.

3 Stir in the pumpkin-seed mixture, cover, and cook, turning the chicken once in the sauce, until the chicken is cooked through and the sauce is flavorful, about 7 minutes.

4 Remove the chicken from the sauce and place on 4 serving plates. Stir the lime juice into the sauce and spoon the sauce over the chicken. *Makes 4 servings*

per serving: 203 calories, 7.7g total fat (1.4g saturated), 66mg cholesterol, 2g dietary fiber, 4g carbohydrate, 29g protein, 490mg sodium. **good source of:** niacin, selenium, vitamin B_{12}, vitamin B_6.

Chicken Scallopine Provençal

Thin-sliced chicken cutlets cook in a flash. Here we cook them first (it only takes 3 minutes) and remove them from the pan while we make a quick ratatouille-like sauce to go over them. The best capers to use for the sauce are the small capers called "nonpareil," but if you can only find large capers, just chop them.

- 4 chicken cutlets (4 ounces each)
- 2 tablespoons flour
- 3 teaspoons olive oil
- 3 cloves garlic, minced
- 1 small eggplant (8 ounces), unpeeled and cut into ½-inch chunks
- 1 zucchini, halved lengthwise and cut crosswise into ½-inch slices
- ⅓ cup water
- ½ teaspoon tarragon
- 1 can (14½-ounces) stewed tomatoes, chopped with their juice
- 2 teaspoons capers, chopped if large
- ½ teaspoon salt

1 Dredge the chicken in the flour, shaking off the excess. In a large nonstick skillet, heat 2 teaspoons of the oil over medium heat. Add the chicken and cook, turning once, until golden brown, about 3 minutes. Transfer the chicken to a plate.

2 Add the remaining 1 teaspoon oil and the garlic to the pan and cook, stirring constantly, until fragrant, about 30 seconds. Add the eggplant and cook, stirring occasionally, until it begins to soften, about 3 minutes.

3 Add the zucchini, water, and tarragon, and cook, stirring frequently, until the vegetables begin to brown, about 3 minutes.

4 Add the stewed tomatoes, capers, and salt. Bring to a boil and cook until the eggplant is tender, about 3 minutes.

5 Return the chicken to the pan and spoon the sauce over it. Cook until the chicken is heated through, about 1 minute. Serve the chicken topped with the vegetable sauce. *Makes 4 servings*

per serving: 232 calories, 6.3g total fat (1.1g saturated), 66mg cholesterol, 3g dietary fiber, 15g carbohydrate, 29g protein, 637mg sodium. good source of: niacin, potassium, selenium, vitamin B$_6$.

Chicken Chow Mein

A typical chow mein includes meat, noodles, water chestnuts, and bean sprouts. We've taken some liberties with the ingredients but have preserved the spirit of the dish's textural contrasts. For example, instead of beans sprouts, we've used shredded napa cabbage; and we've replaced the water chestnuts with crunchy jícama.

- ¼ cup reduced-sodium soy sauce
- 2 tablespoons hoisin sauce or red currant jelly
- 1 tablespoon dry sherry
- ½ teaspoon hot pepper sauce
- 8 ounces linguine
- 2 tablespoons olive oil
- ½ pound skinless, boneless chicken breasts, cut into ¼-inch-wide strips
- 1 red bell pepper, diced
- 4 cloves garlic, minced
- ½ cup sliced scallions
- 2 tablespoons minced fresh ginger
- 3 cups shredded napa cabbage
- ½ cup jícama matchsticks

1 In a small bowl, combine the soy sauce, hoisin sauce, sherry, and hot pepper sauce, and stir to blend. Set aside.

2 In a large pot of boiling water, cook the fettuccine according to package directions. Drain.

---

did you know?

Most people mistake chow mein for an American invention (like chop suey), but it is in fact a perfectly respectable dish from northern China (where wheat noodles are the starch of choice instead of rice). The name chow mein comes from Mandarin and translates as "fried noodles."

3 Meanwhile, in a large nonstick skillet, heat the oil over medium heat. Add the chicken and cook, stirring frequently, until golden brown, about 4 minutes. With a slotted spoon, transfer the chicken to a plate.

4 Add the bell pepper, garlic, scallions, and ginger, and cook, stirring frequently, until the bell pepper is crisp-tender, about 4 minutes.

5 Add the cabbage and jícama, cover, and cook until the cabbage has wilted, about 4 minutes. Add the soy sauce mixture to the pan. Add the chicken and cook, stirring frequently, until the chicken is cooked through, about 1 minute.

6 Transfer the chicken mixture to a large bowl. Add the hot pasta, and toss to combine. *Makes 4 servings*

per serving: 395 calories, 8.9g total fat (1.3g saturated), 33mg cholesterol, 4g dietary fiber, 55g carbohydrate, 23g protein, 729mg sodium. **good source of:** niacin, selenium, vitamin B$_6$, vitamin C, zinc.

Warm Curried Chicken & Sweet Potato Salad

The creamy dressing for this warm salad is laced with fresh mint and cilantro. If fresh mint is not easy to come by, substitute 1 tablespoon chopped fresh basil or 1 teaspoon dried mint.

> ½ cup plain fat-free yogurt
>
> ¼ cup chopped cilantro
>
> 2 tablespoons minced red onion
>
> 1 tablespoon chopped fresh mint
>
> ¼ teaspoon cayenne pepper
>
> 2¼ teaspoons curry powder
>
> ¼ teaspoon salt
>
> 1 pound sweet potatoes, peeled and cut into 1-inch cubes
>
> ⅓ cup orange juice
>
> 2 teaspoons olive oil

different *spins*

▶**Shrimp & Vegetable Chow Mein** Follow the directions for *Chicken Chow Mein (opposite page)*, but substitute ½ pound of medium shrimp, shelled and deveined, for the chicken. In step 3, cook the shrimp for 1 minute.

▶**Pork & Vegetable Chow Mein** Follow the directions for *Chicken Chow Mein (opposite page)*, but substitute ½ pound of pork tenderloin for the chicken. Substitute 1 bunch of watercress for the napa cabbage.

> ¾ pound skinless, boneless chicken breasts
>
> 6 cups loosely packed shredded spinach leaves

1 In a small bowl, whisk together the yogurt, cilantro, red onion, mint, and cayenne. Refrigerate until serving time.

2 In a small bowl, stir together the curry powder and salt. In a vegetable steamer, cook the sweet potatoes until tender, about 8 minutes. Transfer the sweet potatoes to a bowl and add the orange juice, 1½ teaspoons of the curry powder mixture, and 1 teaspoon of the oil.

3 Rub the remaining 1 teaspoon curry powder mixture onto both sides of the chicken. In a nonstick skillet, heat the remaining 1 teaspoon oil over medium-high heat. Add the chicken and cook until golden brown and cooked through, about 3 minutes per side.

4 Line 4 dinner plates with the spinach and mound the sweet potato mixture on top.

5 Cut the chicken into strips and arrange on top. Drizzle some of the yogurt dressing over each serving and pass the remainder on the side. *Makes 4 servings*

per serving: 224 calories, 3.8g total fat (0.7g saturated), 50mg cholesterol, 4g dietary fiber, 24g carbohydrate, 24g protein, 263mg sodium. **good source of:** beta carotene, folate, lutein, niacin, potassium, riboflavin, selenium, vitamin B$_6$, vitamin C.

Chicken Cacciatore

Hunter-style chicken dishes (*cacciatore* means hunter in Italian) abound in Europe and vary widely from region to region. The version that has made it to this country as Chicken Cacciatore is a Neapolitan dish of chicken braised in a tomato sauce scented with herbs (almost always rosemary). Somewhere along the line, mushrooms got added to the American version, though this is not a standard ingredient in the Neapolitan rendition.

> 4 skinless, bone-in chicken breast halves (8 ounces each)
>
> 3 tablespoons flour
>
> 1 tablespoon olive oil
>
> 2 shallots, minced
>
> 4 cloves garlic, minced
>
> ½ pound cremini mushrooms, thinly sliced
>
> 1 can (14½ ounces) diced tomatoes
>
> ⅓ cup water
>
> ⅓ cup dry red wine
>
> ½ teaspoon salt
>
> ½ teaspoon rosemary, minced
>
> ½ teaspoon pepper

1 Dredge the chicken in the flour, shaking off the excess. In a large nonstick skillet, heat the oil over medium heat. Add the chicken and cook until golden brown, about 3 minutes per side. Transfer the chicken to a plate.

2 Reduce the heat to low, add the shallots and garlic, and cook until the shallots are soft, about 3 minutes. Add the mushrooms and cook, stirring occasionally, until they are soft, about 5 minutes.

3 Add the tomatoes, water, wine, salt, rosemary, and pepper, and bring to a boil. Return the chicken to the pan, reduce the heat to low, cover, and simmer until the chicken is cooked through, about 20 minutes. *Makes 4 servings*

per serving: 329 calories, 5.8g total fat (1.1g saturated), 105mg cholesterol, 1g dietary fiber, 19g carbohydrate, 45g protein, 825mg sodium. **good source of:** niacin, potassium, riboflavin, selenium, vitamin B_{12}, vitamin B_6.

Chicken with 40 Cloves of Garlic

This is the famous chicken dish from the Provence region of France. The chicken and vegetables (and garlic) are baked in the oven with a small amount of liquid. It's a technique caught somewhere between baking, steaming, and braising. Pernod gives a slight anise flavor to the dish, but if you don't have any on hand, increase the vermouth or white wine to ½ cup. **Serving suggestion:** The baked garlic gets meltingly soft and almost sweet in flavor. Let each diner squeeze the garlic out of its skin and mash it into the sauce.

> 1½ pounds red potatoes, cut into 1-inch chunks
>
> 1 bulb fennel, stalks discarded and bulb cut crosswise into ½-inch-thick slices
>
> 40 cloves garlic, unpeeled
>
> 1 teaspoon tarragon
>
> ¾ teaspoon salt
>
> 1 cup chicken broth, homemade (page 252) or canned
>
> ⅓ cup dry vermouth or white wine
>
> 3 tablespoons Pernod, Pastis, or Ricard
>
> 2 teaspoons olive oil
>
> 1½ teaspoons grated lemon zest
>
> 1¼ pounds skinless, boneless, chicken thighs, cut into 1-inch chunks

1 Preheat the oven to 350°F. In a Dutch oven or flameproof casserole, combine the potatoes, fennel, garlic, tarragon, and salt. Toss to combine. Add the broth, vermouth, Pernod, oil, and lemon zest, and bring to a boil over medium heat. Reduce to a simmer, cover, and cook for 10 minutes.

2 Add the chicken, cover, place in the oven, and bake for 30 minutes, or until the chicken is cooked through and the vegetables are tender.

3 Serve the chicken with the vegetables, whole garlic cloves, and pan juices spooned over the top. *Makes 4 servings*

per serving: 459 calories, 8.3g total fat (1.8g saturated), 118mg cholesterol, 6g dietary fiber, 54g carbohydrate, 35g protein, 715mg sodium. **good source of:** niacin, potassium, riboflavin, selenium, thiamin, vitamin B_6, vitamin C, zinc.

Braised Lemon Chicken

Dark-meat chicken takes longer to cook than white meat. So to keep the chicken breasts from overcooking, they are not added to the braising liquid until after the dark-meat pieces have cooked for 15 minutes. But before braising, the chicken pieces are coated with cornstarch and quickly sautéed; this helps brown the chicken as well as seal in its juices. And the cornstarch will also help thicken the lemon sauce.

1 broiler-fryer chicken (3 to 3½ pounds), cut into 8 serving pieces (see box, below)

3 tablespoons plus 1 teaspoon cornstarch

1 tablespoon olive oil

1 green bell pepper, cut into matchsticks

4 scallions, cut into 1-inch lengths

5 cloves garlic, minced

1 tablespoon slivered fresh ginger

1⅓ cups chicken broth, homemade (page 252) or canned

1½ teaspoons grated lemon zest

⅓ cup fresh lemon juice

2 tablespoons sugar

½ teaspoon salt

1 tablespoon water

1 Skin the chicken pieces. Dredge the chicken in 3 tablespoons of the cornstarch, shaking off the excess.

2 In a large nonstick skillet, heat the oil over medium heat. Add the chicken and cook until golden brown, about 4 minutes per side. With tongs, transfer the chicken to a plate.

3 Add the bell pepper, scallions, garlic, and ginger to the pan and cook until the pepper is crisp-tender, about 3 minutes.

4 Add the broth, lemon zest, lemon juice, sugar, and salt, and bring to a boil. Return just the drumsticks and thighs to the pan; reduce to a simmer, cover, and cook for 15 minutes.

5 Add the chicken breasts, cover, and cook for 10 minutes, or until all of the chicken is cooked through. Transfer the chicken to a platter and cover loosely to keep warm.

6 In a small bowl, stir together the remaining 1 teaspoon cornstarch and the water. Return the mixture in the skillet to a boil, stir in the cornstarch mixture, and cook, stirring constantly, for 1 minute or until slightly thickened. Spoon the sauce over the chicken and serve. *Makes 6 servings*

per serving: 253 calories, 8g total fat (1.9g saturated), 88mg cholesterol, 1g dietary fiber, 13g carbohydrate, 31g protein, 371mg sodium. good source of: niacin, selenium, vitamin C.

how to cut up a chicken

If you don't buy already cut-up chicken at the market, here's how you would cut a whole chicken into 8 serving pieces (2 drumsticks, 2 thighs, 4 quarter breasts):

1. Remove the legs by cutting down between the thigh and the body with a sharp chef's knife. Place the leg on a cutting board and cut through the joint between the drumstick and thigh.

2. Remove the wings by pulling them away from the body and cutting through the joint at the body. Cut off the very end of the wing (the wing tip) and discard; they are too fatty to be used. Save the meaty portion of the wings for stock.

3. Use poultry shears to cut through the ribs on one side of the backbone; repeat on the other side. Pull out the backbone and save for stock.

4. Place the breast, skin-side up, on a cutting board and cut through the breast bone to make two halves. Then cut each breast half in half crosswise.

5. To skin the chicken pieces, grab the skin with a paper towel and pull. The paper towel keeps your hand from getting greasy and slippery.

Chicken & Winter Squash Tagine

A tagine is a Moroccan stew, named for the pot it is cooked in (a round earthenware baking dish covered with a conical top). Traditional tagines were made by placing the stew ingredients in the covered baking dish, and then mounding the hot coals of a cook fire up the sides of the conical cover.

>   2 teaspoons olive oil
>
>   4 skinless, bone-in chicken thighs
>   (5 ounces each)
>
>   1 large onion, finely chopped
>
>   3 cloves garlic, minced
>
>   1 pound butternut squash, peeled,
>   seeded, and cut into ½-inch chunks
>
>   1 can (15 ounces) crushed tomatoes
>
>   ⅓ cup water
>
>   2 tablespoons honey
>
>   ¾ teaspoon salt
>
>   ¾ teaspoon coriander
>
>   ¼ teaspoon cayenne pepper
>
>   1¾ cups cooked chick-peas (page 180) or
>   canned (rinsed and drained)

1 In a nonstick Dutch oven or flameproof casserole, heat the oil over medium heat. Add the chicken and cook until golden brown, about 4 minutes per side. Transfer the chicken to a plate.

2 Add the onion and garlic to the pan and cook, stirring frequently, until the onion is soft, about 7 minutes.

3 Add the squash, tomatoes, water, honey, salt, coriander, and cayenne, and bring to a boil. Return the chicken to the pan. Reduce to a simmer, cover, and cook for 20 minutes.

4 Stir in the chick-peas. Cover and cook until the chicken is cooked through and the squash is tender, about 15 minutes. *Makes 4 servings*

per serving: 441 calories, 14g total fat (3g saturated), 72mg cholesterol, 12g dietary fiber, 53g carbohydrate, 30g protein, 799mg sodium. good source of: beta carotene, fiber, folate, magnesium, niacin, potassium, selenium, thiamin, vitamin B$_6$, vitamin C, zinc.

Southwestern Chicken & Sweet Potato Stew

Dark-meat chicken is a better choice for stews than breast meat because it stays moist and retains more of its flavor when cooked relatively slowly, and in a lot of liquid. **Serving suggestion:** If you can find blue cornmeal (a specialty of the American Southwest), use it to make cornbread to go along with this hearty chicken stew.

>   2 teaspoons olive oil
>
>   1 large onion, cut into 1-inch chunks
>
>   3 cloves garlic, minced
>
>   1½ pounds skinless, boneless chicken
>   thighs, cut into 1-inch chunks
>
>   1 tablespoon chili powder
>
>   1½ teaspoons ground coriander
>
>   ½ teaspoon salt
>
>   1 large red bell pepper, cut into 1-inch
>   chunks
>
>   2½ cups chicken broth, homemade
>   (page 252) or canned
>
>   1½ pounds sweet potatoes, peeled and
>   cut into 2-inch chunks
>
>   1½ cups cooked black beans (page 180)
>   or canned (rinsed and drained)
>
>   ½ cup chopped cilantro

1 In a nonstick Dutch oven or flameproof casserole, heat the oil over medium heat. Add the onion

---

different *spins*

▶**Chicken & Summer Squash Tagine** Follow the directions for *Chicken & Winter Squash Tagine*, but use 2 zucchini and 1 yellow squash cut into 1-inch-thick rounds instead of butternut squash, adding them after the other ingredients in step 3 have cooked for 10 minutes. Substitute 1½ cups lima beans for the chick-peas, adding them in step 4. Stir in ¼ cup chopped cilantro at the end.

and garlic, and cook, stirring occasionally, until the onion is tender, about 7 minutes.

2 Add the chicken, chili powder, coriander, and salt, stirring to combine. Stir in the bell pepper and broth. Cover and bring to a boil over high heat. Add the sweet potatoes, reduce to a simmer, cover, and cook until the sweet potatoes are tender and the chicken is cooked through, about 15 minutes.

3 With a large fork or the back of a spoon, mash about one-third of the sweet potatoes to help thicken the stew.

4 Stir in the black beans and cilantro, and cook until the beans are heated through, about 5 minutes. *Makes 6 servings*

per serving: 323 calories, 6.6g total fat (1.5g saturated), 94mg cholesterol, 6g dietary fiber, 36g carbohydrate, 29g protein, 611mg sodium. good source of: beta carotene, niacin, riboflavin, selenium, vitamin B$_6$, vitamin C, zinc.

Cold Poached Chicken with Pepper-Caper Sauce

Poaching chicken is a quick, low-fat way to cook chicken for use in other dishes, such as salads or sandwiches. Or you can serve the poached chicken as a main course, with a sauce. Here the chicken is served with a pureed roasted pepper and caper sauce, but you could also serve it with Hot & Spicy Cocktail Sauce (*page 256*), Dill-Caper Dressing (*page 253*), or Tomatillo Salsa (*page 261*). **Timing alert:** The chicken can be served at room temperature, but is good as a cold dish, making this recipe a good candidate for make-ahead. The poached chicken and the sauce can both be made a day or so before serving.

⅔ cup chicken broth, homemade (page 252) or canned

⅓ cup dry white wine

¾ teaspoon tarragon

2 cloves garlic, minced

4 skinless, boneless chicken breast halves (5 ounces each)

---

did you know?

Capers are the flower buds of an evergreen bush, which are pickled and used as an accent in dishes from salads to stews. Capers can range in size from tiny to quite large. Look for the tiny "nonpareil" capers from France. Larger (and generally cheaper) capers from Spain have a somewhat coarser flavor and texture. Capers can be found on the grocery shelf next to the olives.

---

1 cup roasted red peppers, homemade (page 190) or storebought

2 tablespoons slivered almonds, toasted

1 tablespoon tomato paste

2 teaspoons balsamic vinegar

1 teaspoon olive oil

½ teaspoon hot pepper sauce

½ teaspoon salt

1 tablespoon capers, chopped if large

1 In a large skillet, combine the broth, wine, tarragon, and garlic. Bring to a boil over medium heat. Reduce to a simmer, add the chicken, cover, and cook, turning over halfway, until the chicken is cooked through, about 10 minutes. Transfer the chicken to a plate, cover, and refrigerate. Measure out 2 tablespoons of the poaching liquid to use in the sauce (save the remainder for another use).

2 In a food processor or blender, combine the reserved 2 tablespoons chicken poaching liquid, the roasted peppers, almonds, tomato paste, vinegar, oil, hot pepper sauce, and salt, and process to a smooth puree. Stir in the capers.

3 To serve, slice the chicken across the grain on the diagonal and top with the pepper-caper sauce. *Makes 4 servings*

per serving: 228 calories, 5.2g total fat (0.8g saturated), 82mg cholesterol, 1g dietary fiber, 6g carbohydrate, 35g protein, 626mg sodium. good source of: niacin, selenium, vitamin B$_6$.

Chicken Stew with Herbed Dumplings

Skinless, boneless chicken thighs stay moist and tender under a blanket of fluffy herb-flecked dumplings. If you prefer, you can use chicken breasts instead of thighs, but reduce the initial cooking time in step 2.

1 pound skinless, boneless chicken thighs, cut into 1½-inch chunks

2 tablespoons plus 1 cup flour

1 tablespoon olive oil

1 large onion, chopped

2 carrots, diced

3 cloves garlic, minced

1½ cups water

¾ teaspoon salt

½ teaspoon rosemary, minced

1½ teaspoons baking powder

¼ teaspoon baking soda

2 scallions, thinly sliced

2 tablespoons chopped fresh dill

⅓ cup buttermilk or plain fat-free yogurt

1 Dredge the chicken in 2 tablespoons of the flour, shaking off the excess.

2 In a large nonstick skillet, heat the oil over medium heat. Add the chicken and cook, stirring frequently, until golden brown, about 5 minutes. Transfer the thighs to a plate.

different spins

▶**Chicken Stew with Pesto Dumplings**
Follow the directions for *Chicken Stew with Herbed Dumplings*, but substitute 1 diced red bell pepper for the carrots. Substitute tarragon for the rosemary. Omit the scallions. Substitute ¼ cup chopped fresh basil for the dill and add 2 tablespoons grated Parmesan to the flour mixture in step 4.

3 Add the onion, carrots, and garlic to the pan and cook, stirring frequently, until the vegetables begin to soften, about 5 minutes. Stir in the water, ½ teaspoon of the salt, and the rosemary. Return the chicken to the pan and bring to a boil.

4 Meanwhile, in a medium bowl, combine the remaining 1 cup flour, the baking powder, baking soda, and remaining ¼ teaspoon salt. Add the scallions, dill, and buttermilk, and stir to combine.

5 Drop the dough by tablespoonfuls onto the boiling chicken mixture to make 8 dumplings. Cover, reduce to a simmer, and cook until the chicken and dumplings are cooked through, about 10 minutes. ***Makes 4 servings***

per serving: 337 calories, 8.5g total fat (1.8g saturated), 95mg cholesterol, 3g dietary fiber, 36g carbohydrate, 28g protein, 736mg sodium. **good source of:** beta carotene, niacin, riboflavin, selenium, thiamin, vitamin B$_6$.

turkey

For dry-heat methods, such as roasting, broiling, or pan-frying, you can leave the turkey skin on. This will help keep the meat moist and juicy, and won't increase the fat content of the turkey as long as it is removed before eating. But for mixed-ingredient dishes, where the fat from the skin would stay in the dish (like stews or casseroles), you should use skinless turkey.

Roasting Use the information in the "Turkey Cooking Chart" (*opposite page*) for traditional turkey roasting. We give cooking times for unstuffed birds. Poultry stuffings are especially prone to bacterial contamination; the bacteria in the raw poultry can get into the stuffing and multiply, so we advise cooking the stuffing separately. Furthermore, an unstuffed bird cooks faster than a stuffed one.

Steam-roasting We use a combination of roasting and steaming to produce a particularly moist and flavorful bird. The turkey starts out in a tightly covered roasting pan with some liquid,

turkey cooking chart

Whole turkey will roast faster than the times given below if you cook it in a covered roaster, or in a small roasting pan, or in a small oven (more convected heat). Always check for doneness about 15 minutes before the first time listed in the range of times, and use a meat thermometer (*see "How to Use a Meat Thermometer," page 107*). Stop cooking when the internal temperature reads 165°F in the breast or 175°F in the thigh. Let the turkey stand 15 minutes; during that time, the temperature will rise another 5 degrees.

CUT	AMOUNT	METHOD
WHOLE TURKEY	8 to 12 lbs	**Roasting*** 325°F for 2¾ to 3 hours, or until meat thermometer inserted in breast reads 170°F; or in thigh, 180°F
	14 to 18 lbs	**Roasting*** 325°F for 3¾ to 4¼ hours, or until meat thermometer inserted in breast reads 170°F; or in thigh, 180°F
	20 to 24 lbs	**Roasting*** 325°F for 4½ to 5 hours, or until meat thermometer inserted in breast reads 170°F; or in thigh, 180°F
TURKEY BREAST	whole, 4 to 6 lbs	**Roasting*** 325°F for 1½ to 2¼ hours, or until meat thermometer reads 170°F
	whole, 6 to 8 lbs	**Roasting*** 325°F for 2¼ to 3¼ hours, or until meat thermometer reads 170°F **Poaching** In simmering liquid to cover, for 1½ hours, or until meat thermometer reads 170°F
	half, bone-in, 3 to 4 lbs	**Roasting** 325°F for 1 to 1½ hours, or until meat thermometer reads 170°F
	half, boneless, 2 to 3 lbs	**Poaching** In simmering liquid to cover, for 45 minutes, or until meat thermometer reads 170°F
	cutlets, ½ inch thick	**Broiling/grilling** 4 to 6 inches from heat, 1–2 minutes per side **Pan-frying** In a lightly oiled nonstick skillet, over medium heat, 2 minutes per side
	cut into strips for stir-fry	**Stir-frying** *See Poultry Stir-Fries "Recipe Creator" on page 115*
	ground, burgers	**Broiling/grilling** 4 to 6 inches from heat, 4 minutes per side **Pan-"frying"** In a covered skillet with a little water, 4 minutes per side
DRUMSTICKS, THIGHS	10 oz each	**Baking** 325°F for 1 to 1¼ hours **Grilling** 6 to 8 inches from heat, 45–60 minutes, turning occasionally

*roasting times are for unstuffed birds

making gravy

There are several different styles of gravy you can make to go with roast turkey (this also works for roast chicken). All of the gravies start out with the same basic technique, though:

1. Deglazing: Remove the bird from the roasting pan. Add water or broth to the pan and use a wire whisk to scrape the bottom and sides of the pan to get any browned meat juices incorporated into the liquid. This is called deglazing.

2. Degreasing: Pour the deglazed juices into a gravy separator. Wait for the fat to rise to the top, and then pour the degreased juices into a small bowl. Discard the fat.

Once you've deglazed and degreased, you have three options:

▶**For a simple "au jus":** If the degreased juices are flavorful enough, you can use them as is. If the degreased juices seem a little thin, cook them over low heat to reduce and concentrate.

▶**For a flour-thickened gravy:** In a small bowl, whisk the degreased juices into some flour (2 tablespoons flour for every 2 cups of pan juices; add broth if necessary). Cook over medium heat until thickened.

▶**For a vegetable-thickened gravy:** While the turkey is cooking, roast some vegetables in a separate pan. Try roasting carrots, turnips, parsnips, leeks, and garlic (use any combination you want) in a pan with some broth or water. You'll need about ½ cup roasted vegetables for every 2 cups of pan juices (augment with broth if necessary). Place the vegetables and the pan juices in a food processor or blender and puree. Season to taste.

which turns to steam to cook the turkey. The lid is removed for the last 20 minutes or so to brown the skin. This is really just a cosmetic issue, since for health reasons, you should not be eating the skin anyway. *(See Maple-Bourbon Roast Turkey, opposite page.)*

Broiling/grilling Turkey cutlets and burgers can be broiled or grilled, and larger turkey parts (such as thighs or drumsticks) can be grilled on a barbecue, but not in a broiler. For grilling thicker parts, such as thighs and drumsticks, be sure the grill rack is 6 to 8 inches from the heat source. Turn turkey parts occasionally as they cook; they will take 45 minutes or more, depending on size and thickness.

Pan-frying Plain turkey breast cutlets can be pan-fried in a nonstick skillet with a small amount of oil, but if you dredge them in egg whites and a coating (usually of breadcrumbs) first, it helps keep the juices in *(see Turkey Scallopine Milanese, page 130)*. Ground turkey breast, in the form of burgers, can be pan-"fried" in a nonstick skillet with a small amount of liq-

uid *(see Turkey Burgers "Recipe Creator," page 129)*.

Stir-frying Quick cooking over high heat, in a small amount of oil, is a good choice for thin strips of lean turkey breast *(see Turkey Piccata Stir-Fry, page 130, or Poultry Stir-Fries "Recipe Creator," page 115)*.

Poaching Large pieces of turkey breast can be poached in broth, or broth and wine. You can use this method to make a hot dish *(see Turkey Breast à la Ficelle, page 134)* or use it to cook turkey for later use in a cold dish *(see Turkey-Papaya Salad, page 134)*.

Braising/stewing In order to stew or braise turkey, which is very lean and will just get "raggy" if cooked too long, we use a technique that is also employed for other lean meats: First quickly pan-fry the turkey, then remove it while the other stew ingredients cook, then return the turkey to the stew at the end of the cooking *(see Hearty Turkey Stew, page 132)*. For ground turkey, you can braise it in a sauce or stew for a short amount of time *(see Spaghetti & Turkey Meatballs, page 135)*.

Maple-Bourbon Roast Turkey

The reason for tying the legs together when you roast a turkey is cosmetic: If the legs are not tied, the turkey tends to splay out and look less attractive on the carving board. Obviously, this step is completely optional. If your roasting pan doesn't have a lid (which is important to the success of this steam-roasting method), cover the pan with a couple of layers of foil, crimping it around the edges of the pan to make a tight seal. **Serving suggestion:** Make one of the following stuffings to go with the turkey, but bake it separately, not inside the bird. Try Apple & Onion Cornbread Stuffing or Sausage, Chestnut & Dried Plum Stuffing (*both on page 126*).

1 turkey (12 to 14 pounds)

4 teaspoons salt

1 teaspoon rosemary, minced

1 teaspoon rubbed sage

1 small onion, peeled

1 small apple, halved and seeded

6 cloves garlic, peeled

2 cups bourbon or dark rum

½ cup maple syrup

2 tablespoons reduced-sodium soy sauce

¼ cup flour

1 Preheat the oven to 350°F. With your fingers, carefully lift the skin of the turkey away from the flesh. Rub 2 teaspoons of the salt, ½ teaspoon of the rosemary, and ½ teaspoon of the sage under the skin.

2 Rub the cavity of the turkey with the remaining 2 teaspoons salt, ½ teaspoon rosemary, and ½ teaspoon sage. Place the onion, apple, and garlic in the turkey cavity. Tie the turkey legs together with kitchen string.

3 Place the turkey, breast-side up, in a roasting pan (not on a rack) with a tight-fitting lid. Pour the bourbon, maple syrup, and soy sauce into the pan. Cover and roast 2 hours without removing the lid.

4 Uncover and roast for 20 minutes, or until the turkey thigh registers 180°F on a meat thermometer. Transfer the turkey to a platter.

5 Pour the pan juices into a gravy separator and let stand until the fat rises to the surface of the separator. Pour the degreased juices into a medium saucepan (discard the fat). In a small bowl, whisk ½ cup of the pan juices into the flour until smooth. Whisk the flour mixture back into the saucepan of pan juices and cook over medium heat, stirring constantly, until the gravy is slightly thickened and no floury taste remains, about 7 minutes.

6 Remove the apple, onion, and garlic from the turkey cavity and discard. Carve the turkey and serve with the gravy. Remove the skin before eating. *Makes 16 servings*

per serving: 390 calories, 8.5g total fat (2.8g saturated), 128mg cholesterol, 0g dietary fiber, 9g carbohydrate, 50g protein, 477mg sodium. good source of: niacin, riboflavin, selenium, vitamin B_{12}, vitamin B_6, zinc.

how to tell when turkey is done

In addition to the internal temperature that will tell you when turkey is done (*see "How to Use a Meat Thermometer," page 107*), there are certain visual tests for doneness:

▶**Whole turkey** Hold onto a drumstick and wiggle it back and forth. The drumstick should be loose in its socket, but still firmly attached. Also, if you insert a fork or knife between the drumstick and the thigh, the juices should be clear with a tinge of yellow (but no pink).

▶**Parts** Poke the turkey with a knife or fork without touching the bones if there are any. If the juices run clear with a tinge of yellow (but no pink), the turkey is done.

▶**Burgers** Make a small cut in the center of the burger; the juices will be clear and the flesh will be a uniform color, with no pink tinge.

▶**Cutlets** Make a small cut in the center of the cutlet; the juices will run clear and the flesh will be uniformly opaque, with no hint of pink.

Apple & Onion Cornbread Stuffing

You can make the cornbread for the stuffing up to a day ahead of time. Once the cornbread has been baked, let it cool to room temperature, then tear it into ½-inch pieces and let it dry out. If you'd rather not make cornbread, you can use a whole-grain bread such as oatmeal or whole-wheat instead. You'll need 8½ cups of bread (about 12 ounces) torn into ½-inch pieces. Spread it out to let it dry for a couple of hours.

> Oniony Cornbread (page 218), crumbled
>
> 2 teaspoons olive oil
>
> 1 small onion, minced
>
> 3 cloves garlic, minced
>
> 2 Granny Smith apples, unpeeled, cut into ½-inch chunks
>
> ½ cup chopped parsley
>
> ¾ teaspoon rubbed sage
>
> ¾ teaspoon salt
>
> ½ teaspoon pepper
>
> 1½ cups chicken broth, homemade (page 252) or canned
>
> ⅓ cup chopped mixed dried fruit

1 Make the Oniony Cornbread, but bake it in a 9 x 13-inch pan for 25 minutes. Let cool to room temperature before crumbling into bite-size pieces.

2 In a large nonstick skillet, heat the oil over medium heat. Add the onion and garlic, and cook, stirring frequently, until the onion is soft, about 7 minutes. Add the apples and stir to coat.

3 Transfer to a large bowl. Add the cornbread, parsley, sage, salt, and pepper, and stir well to combine. Add the broth and the dried fruit, and stir until the cornbread is moistened.

4 Transfer to a 2½-quart shallow baking dish, cover with foil, and bake for 30 minutes, or until the stuffing is piping hot. *Makes 12 servings*

per serving: 158 calories, 4g total fat (0.7g saturated), 19mg cholesterol, 2g dietary fiber, 27g carbohydrate, 4g protein, 369mg sodium.

Sausage, Chestnut & Dried Plum Stuffing

Turkey breast and lean pork have the same amount of saturated fat (0.6 grams per ounce of cooked), but when you get into the realm of sausage, turkey is the winner: Pork sausage has more than twice the saturated fat of turkey sausage.

> 1 pound chestnuts, cooked (see below) and peeled
>
> 10 cups whole-grain bread cubes (about 15 ounces)
>
> 2 teaspoons olive oil
>
> ¼ pound Italian-style turkey sausage, casings removed
>
> 1 medium onion, finely chopped

how to cook chestnuts

▶**Roasting** With a sharp knife, cut an "X" in the flat side of each chestnut. Place in a jelly-roll pan and roast at 400°F for about 25 minutes, or until the shells pop open. When cool enough to handle, but still warm, peel the hard outer shell and inner membrane away. (Cover the remaining chestnuts while you work, as they are easier to peel while still warm.)

▶**Boiling** Cut an "X" as described above. In a large saucepan of boiling water, cook the chestnuts until their shells pop open and the chestnuts are tender, about 20 minutes. Drain and peel while still slightly warm.

▶**Reconstituting** Dried chestnuts are available at gourmet shops, and at Asian and Italian markets. Soak dried chestnuts in cold water for several hours or overnight. Drain. In a large pot of boiling water, cook the chestnuts until tender, about 20 minutes. Some dried chestnuts still have bits of membrane stuck in their crevices, but once the chestnuts are expanded and softened, it's easy to pull those pieces off.

2 stalks celery, halved lengthwise and thinly sliced crosswise

3 cups chicken broth, homemade (page 252) or canned

1 cup diced pitted dried plums (prunes)

1 teaspoon thyme

¾ teaspoon salt

½ teaspoon pepper

1 Coarsely chop the chestnuts, and set aside.

2 Preheat the oven to 350°F. Spread the bread on a baking sheet and bake for 7 to 10 minutes, stirring occasionally, or until crisp. Transfer to a large bowl. Keep the oven on.

3 Meanwhile, in a large nonstick skillet, heat the oil over medium heat. Crumble in the sausage meat and cook, stirring to break up the meat, until the sausage is lightly browned, about 5 minutes. Add the onion and cook, stirring frequently, until the onion is soft, about 7 minutes. Stir in the celery and cook until the celery is crisp-tender, about 3 minutes.

4 Add the sautéed sausage and vegetables to the bread. Then add the chestnuts, broth, prunes, thyme, salt, and pepper, and stir well to combine and evenly moisten the bread.

5 Transfer the stuffing mixture to a shallow 3-quart baking dish, cover with foil, and bake for 30 minutes, or until the stuffing is piping hot. *Makes 16 servings*

per serving: 199 calories, 3.1g total fat (0.6g saturated), 5mg cholesterol, 5g dietary fiber, 38g carbohydrate, 6g protein, 383mg sodium. good source of: fiber, riboflavin, selenium, thiamin, vitamin B$_6$.

Roast Turkey Salad with Cranberry Vinaigrette

Using frozen juice in its concentrated form makes a delicious low-fat vinaigrette for this turkey and sweet potato salad. The dressing also supplies an impressive amount of vitamin C.

1½ pounds sweet potatoes, peeled and cut into 1-inch chunks

2 navel oranges

3 cups shredded Romaine lettuce

6 ounces roasted turkey breast, torn into 1-inch pieces (about 1 cup)

½ cup thinly sliced scallions

⅓ cup frozen cranberry juice concentrate, thawed

1 tablespoon balsamic vinegar

1 tablespoon olive oil

½ teaspoon salt

½ teaspoon pepper

2 tablespoons coarsely chopped pecans, toasted (about ½ ounce)

2 tablespoons dried cranberries or raisins

1 In a vegetable steamer, cook the sweet potatoes until tender, about 8 minutes.

2 Meanwhile, remove the peel and white pith from the oranges. Cut each orange in half lengthwise, place the halves flat on a cutting board, and cut crosswise into ¼-inch-thick slices.

3 Spread the lettuce on a platter. Top with the sweet potatoes, turkey, and orange slices. Sprinkle with the scallions.

4 In a screw-top jar, combine the cranberry juice concentrate, vinegar, oil, salt, and pepper, and shake to combine. Pour the vinaigrette over the salad and sprinkle with the pecans and dried cranberries. *Makes 4 servings*

per serving: 396 calories, 6.9g total fat (0.9g saturated), 35mg cholesterol, 6g dietary fiber, 68g carbohydrate, 18g protein, 343mg sodium. good source of: beta carotene, folate, niacin, potassium, riboflavin, selenium, vitamin B$_6$, vitamin C, vitamin E.

Chili-Glazed Turkey Meatloaf

Poultry seasoning is a prepared blend of herbs—usually sage, rosemary, marjoram, and thyme—that accents the flavor of poultry. If you don't have poultry seasoning on hand, substitute ½ teaspoon sage and ¼ teaspoon rosemary.

1½ pounds skinless, boneless turkey breast, cut into large chunks

2 teaspoons olive oil

1 onion, chopped

2 cloves garlic, minced

1 large carrot, minced

2 slices (1 ounce each) whole-wheat sandwich bread, crumbled

¼ cup fat-free or low-fat (1%) milk

2 large egg whites

¾ teaspoon poultry seasoning

½ teaspoon salt

½ teaspoon pepper

⅓ cup chili sauce

1 Preheat the oven to 350°F. Spray an 8½ x 4½-inch loaf pan with nonstick cooking spray. In a food processor, grind the turkey until coarsely ground.

2 In a large nonstick skillet, heat the oil over medium heat. Add the onion and garlic, and cook until the onion is soft, about 7 minutes. Add the carrot and cook, stirring, until the carrot is crisp-tender, about 5 minutes.

3 In a large bowl, combine the bread and milk. Add the ground turkey, the sautéed vegetable mixture, the egg whites, poultry seasoning, salt, and pepper, and mix well. Transfer the meatloaf mixture to the loaf pan.

4 Spread the chili sauce evenly over the top of the meatloaf and bake for 45 minutes, or until cooked through and firm. Serve warm or chilled. *Makes 6 servings*

per serving: 205 calories, 2.8g total fat (0.6g saturated), 71mg cholesterol, 2g dietary fiber, 13g carbohydrate, 31g protein, 529mg sodium. **good source of:** niacin, selenium, vitamin B$_{12}$, vitamin B$_6$.

Turkey Enchiladas

The sauce for most enchiladas is a simple chili-based sauce. Here we've taken the opportunity to get vegetables into the mix, adding pureed roasted vegetables to the usual enchilada sauce ingredients. The reason for heating the tortillas briefly in an ungreased skillet before rolling them up is to make them pliable. Refrigerated corn tortillas (as in those you find in the supermarket) will have lost their original flexibility and will crack if you try to roll them without heating them first.

2 large carrots, very thinly sliced

1 large red onion, cut into ½-inch wedges

1 red bell pepper, cut into thick strips

5 cloves garlic, peeled

1 tablespoon olive oil

2 chipotle peppers in adobo

3 tablespoons tomato paste

1 cup water

¾ teaspoon salt

8 corn tortillas

½ pound cooked turkey breast, shredded (about 1½ cups)

½ cup cooked black beans (page 180) or canned (rinsed and drained)

1 cup shredded Mexican cheese blend or Monterey jack (4 ounces)

1 Preheat the oven to 450°F. In a roasting pan, combine the carrots, onion, bell pepper, and garlic. Add the oil and toss to coat. Roast the vegetables until very tender and brown, about 25 minutes. Reduce the oven temperature to 350°F.

different spins

▶ **Apple-Mustard Glazed Turkey Meatloaf** Follow the directions for *Chili-Glazed Turkey Meatloaf*, but substitute 1 diced red bell pepper for the carrot, and ¼ cup apple jelly blended with 1 tablespoon Dijon mustard for the chili sauce.

recipe creator
turkey burgers

Ground turkey breast is an excellent substitute for beef in a burger: Ounce for ounce, ground beef has three times the saturated fat of ground turkey breast; and even extra-lean ground beef has almost twice the saturated fat. But along with the lean turkey breast's healthful virtues comes a tendency for it to be a bit dry. To compensate for that, and to make extra-flavorful burgers, we suggest a variety of mix-ins. Choose from the categories below and follow these basic instructions: To make 4 burgers, place 1 pound lean ground turkey breast in a bowl. Add 1 EXTENDER, 1 FLAVORING, 1 or 2 SEASONINGS, and 1 FRESH HERB (optional). Shape into 4 patties. Cook in a covered nonstick skillet with ¼ cup water and 2 teaspoons reduced-sodium soy sauce for 4 to 5 minutes per side, or until cooked through. Or broil 4 inches from the heat for 4 to 5 minutes per side. *Makes 4 servings*

EXTENDERS	FLAVORINGS	SEASONINGS	FRESH HERBS
►Mushrooms, 1 cup chopped	►Mango chutney, 2 Tbsp minced	►Ground cumin, 1 tsp	►Cilantro, ½ cup finely chopped
►TVP granules, ½ cup, moistened with 2 Tbsp water	►Ketchup, 2 Tbsp	►Ground coriander, 1 tsp	►Fresh basil, ½ cup finely chopped
►Whole-wheat sandwich bread, 2 slices, crumbled and moistened with 2 Tbsp low-fat milk	►Mustard, 1 Tbsp	►Curry powder, 1 tsp	►Parsley, ¼ cup finely chopped
	►Prune butter, 2 Tbsp	►Rubbed sage, ½ tsp	►Chives, ¼ cup minced
►Bulgur, ½ cup soaked and drained	►Barbecue sauce, 2 Tbsp	►Rosemary, ½ tsp minced	►Fresh dill, ¼ cup minced

2 Transfer the vegetables to a food processor. Add the chipotle peppers, tomato paste, water, and salt, and process to a smooth puree.

3 Spoon ¾ cup of the sauce into the bottom of a 7 x 11-inch glass baking dish. In a cast-iron (or other heavy-bottomed) skillet, or on a griddle, heat 1 tortilla at a time until soft and pliable, about 10 seconds per side. Dip both sides of each tortilla briefly in the remaining sauce to coat. Dividing evenly, top the tortillas with the turkey and black beans. Sprinkle each tortilla with 1 tablespoon of the cheese. Roll the tortillas up.

4 Place the filled tortillas, seam-side down, in the baking dish. Spoon the remaining sauce over the tortillas. Sprinkle the remaining ½ cup cheese on top. Cover and bake for 25 minutes, or until piping hot and bubbling. *Makes 4 servings*

per serving: 367 calories, 9.9g total fat (3.5g saturated), 60mg cholesterol, 8g dietary fiber, 44g carbohydrate, 27g protein, 660mg sodium. **good source of:** beta carotene, calcium, fiber, folate, niacin, selenium, vitamin B_6, vitamin C, zinc.

Turkey Scallopine Milanese

Sautéed turkey cutlets, with a crisp crumb topping, are topped with a spinach salad in a takeoff on a traditional Milanese veal dish called Veal Capricciosa (in which a veal chop is served underneath a salad). The combination of chilled salad and the hot turkey scallops makes a delightful contrast.

> 1 tablespoon plus 4 teaspoons olive oil
>
> ¼ cup fresh lemon juice
>
> 2 teaspoons honey mustard
>
> ¼ teaspoon salt
>
> 3 plum tomatoes, cut into ½-inch chunks
>
> 1 Belgian endive, thinly sliced crosswise
>
> 1 small red onion, halved and thinly sliced
>
> 6 cups baby spinach or torn larger
>   spinach leaves (6 ounces)
>
> ¼ cup grated Parmesan cheese
>
> ¼ cup flour
>
> ½ cup plain dried breadcrumbs
>
> 2 large egg whites, beaten with
>   1 tablespoon water
>
> 8 thin turkey cutlets (1 pound total)

1 In a large bowl, whisk together 1 tablespoon of the oil, the lemon juice, mustard, and salt. Add the tomatoes, Belgian endive, and red onion, but do not toss. Add the spinach to the bowl, and again, do not toss the ingredients (this will happen just before you're ready to serve the salad).

2 Place the Parmesan, flour, and breadcrumbs on three separate sheets of wax paper. Place the egg whites in a shallow bowl. Dip the turkey cutlets first in the Parmesan, patting it into the turkey. Next dip the turkey into the flour, then into the egg whites, and finally into the breadcrumbs, patting the crumbs into the turkey.

3 In a large nonstick skillet, heat 2 teaspoons of the oil over medium heat. Add half the cutlets and cook until golden brown and cooked through, about 1½ minutes per side. Repeat with the remaining 2 teaspoons oil and remaining cutlets.

4 Transfer the cutlets to serving plates. Toss the salad ingredients together to coat with the dressing and spoon on top of the hot cutlets. *Makes 4 servings*

per serving: 342 calories, 12g total fat (2.5g saturated), 74mg cholesterol, 3g dietary fiber, 23g carbohydrate, 36g protein, 339mg sodium. **good source of:** niacin, potassium, riboflavin, selenium, vitamin B_{12}, vitamin B_6, vitamin C.

Turkey Piccata Stir-Fry

The technique of stir-frying is a good way to cook lean cuts of meat and poultry, such as turkey breast. Limiting the amount of time the turkey spends over high heat helps keep the meat tender and juicy. **Serving suggestion:** Serve the stir-fry over orzo pasta, pearl barley, or soft polenta.

> 1 tablespoon olive oil
>
> 2 ounces prosciutto or Canadian bacon,
>   diced (about 6 tablespoons)
>
> 1 pound turkey cutlets, cut into ½-inch-
>   wide strips
>
> 2 tablespoons flour
>
> 3 cloves garlic, finely chopped
>
> ¼ cup fresh lemon juice
>
> 1¼ cups chicken broth, homemade
>   (page 252) or canned
>
> ½ teaspoon salt
>
> 2 teaspoons cornstarch blended with
>   1 tablespoon water

1 In a large nonstick skillet, heat the oil over medium heat. Add the prosciutto and cook until it is lightly crisped, about 2 minutes. With a slotted spoon, transfer the prosciutto to a plate.

---

different spins

▶ **Shrimp with Lemon & Prosciutto** Follow the directions for *Turkey Piccata Stir-Fry*, but substitute 1 pound shelled medium shrimp for the turkey. Cook the shrimp with the prosciutto in step 1 and remove it from the pan along with the prosciutto. Omit the flour and step 2. Substitute bottled clam juice for the chicken broth.

2 Dredge the turkey in the flour, shaking off the excess. Add the turkey to the skillet and stir-fry until golden brown and just cooked through, about 2 minutes. With a slotted spoon, transfer the turkey to the plate with the prosciutto.

3 Add the garlic and cook until tender, about 1 minute. Add the lemon juice, scraping up any browned bits from the bottom of the pan. Add the broth and salt, and bring to a boil. Boil 1 minute.

4 Add the cornstarch mixture and cook, stirring, until the sauce is slightly thickened, about 1 minute. Return the prosciutto and turkey to the pan and cook just until heated through, about 1 minute. *Makes 4 servings*

per serving: 211 calories, 5.2g total fat (1g saturated), 77mg cholesterol, 0g dietary fiber, 7g carbohydrate, 32g protein, 687mg sodium. good source of: niacin, selenium, vitamin B_{12}, vitamin B_6.

Turkey-Mushroom Lasagna

This style of lasagna is called a white lasagna because it is made with a white sauce instead of a tomato sauce. Fat-free mozzarella is a good option here (it doesn't work in all recipes), because it helps to hold the lasagna together and has no saturated fat. **Timing alert:** The lasagna needs to sit for a good 20 minutes after it comes out of the oven.

½ cup dried shiitake or porcini mushrooms (½ ounce)

1 cup boiling water

9 lasagna noodles (9 ounces)

3 cups low-fat (1%) milk

¼ cup flour

¾ teaspoon salt

¼ teaspoon cayenne pepper

¼ cup plus 2 tablespoons grated Parmesan cheese

2 teaspoons olive oil

1 medium onion, finely chopped

3 cloves garlic, minced

½ pound fresh shiitake mushrooms, stems discarded and caps thinly sliced

1 pound lean ground turkey breast

¾ teaspoon fennel seeds

4 ounces fat-free mozzarella, shredded

1 In a small heatproof bowl, combine the dried mushrooms and the boiling water, and let stand for 20 minutes, or until softened. Reserving the soaking liquid, scoop out the dried mushrooms and coarsely chop. Strain the soaking liquid through a coffee filter or a paper towel-lined sieve.

2 Meanwhile, in a large pot of boiling water, cook the lasagna noodles according to package directions. Drain and transfer to a bowl of cold water to prevent the noodles from sticking together.

3 In a medium saucepan, whisk the milk into the flour. Stir in ½ teaspoon of the salt and the cayenne, and bring to a boil over medium heat, stirring constantly. Reduce to a simmer and cook until the sauce is the consistency of heavy cream, about 5 minutes. Stir in ¼ cup of the Parmesan. Set the white sauce aside.

4 Preheat the oven to 450°F. Meanwhile, in a large nonstick skillet, heat the oil over medium heat. Add the onion and garlic, and cook, stirring frequently, until tender, about 10 minutes.

5 Add the fresh shiitakes and cook until tender, about 5 minutes. Add the remaining ¼ teaspoon salt, the turkey, and fennel seeds, and cook until the turkey is no longer pink, about 5 minutes.

6 Stir in the dried mushrooms and soaking liquid, and ½ cup of the white sauce, and cook for 2 minutes. Spread ¼ cup of the white sauce over the bottom of a 9 x 13-inch baking dish and lay 3 noodles on top. Spoon on half the turkey mixture, ¾ cup of the white sauce, and half the mozzarella.

7 Top with 3 noodles, the remaining turkey, ¾ cup of the white sauce, and remaining mozzarella. Top with the last 3 noodles, the remaining white sauce, and remaining 2 tablespoons Parmesan.

8 Cover and bake for 20 minutes, or until piping hot. Uncover and bake for 10 minutes longer or until golden brown on top. Let sit for 20 minutes before cutting and serving. *Makes 8 servings*

per serving: 331 calories, 8.2g total fat (3g saturated), 50mg cholesterol, 2g dietary fiber, 38g carbohydrate, 25g protein, 510mg sodium. good source of: calcium, niacin, riboflavin, selenium, vitamin B_{12}, vitamin B_6, vitamin D.

Hearty Turkey Stew

You can use leftover or storebought roast turkey instead of the sautéed turkey breast if you'd like. Omit step 1 and add 3 cups of cooked turkey chunks in step 4, when adding the broccoli. If you are using leftover turkey from a bird you roasted yourself, then you will also have a turkey carcass you can use to make turkey broth (*see "Making Turkey Broth," opposite page*); use the turkey broth instead of the chicken broth called for.

> 2 tablespoons olive oil
>
> 1¼ pounds skinless, boneless turkey breast, cut into 1-inch chunks
>
> 1 onion, cut into ½-inch chunks
>
> 1 pound Yukon Gold potatoes, cut into 1-inch chunks
>
> 4 ounces mushrooms, halved (2 cups)
>
> 5 cloves garlic, minced
>
> 1½ cups chicken broth, homemade (page 252) or canned
>
> ½ teaspoon salt
>
> 3 cups broccoli florets and thinly sliced stems
>
> ½ cup fat-free or low-fat (1%) milk
>
> 2 tablespoons flour

1 In a nonstick Dutch oven or flameproof casserole, heat 1½ teaspoons of the oil over medium heat. Add half the turkey and sauté until browned, about 4 minutes. Transfer to a plate. Repeat with another 1½ teaspoons oil and the remaining turkey.

2 Add the remaining 1 tablespoon oil to the pan along with the onion and cook, stirring occasionally, until the onion is lightly browned and soft, about 7 minutes.

3 Stir in the potatoes, mushrooms, and garlic. Add the broth and salt, and bring to a boil. Reduce to a simmer, cover, and cook until the potatoes are firm-tender, about 10 minutes.

4 Add the broccoli, cover, and cook until the potatoes and broccoli are tender, about 5 minutes.

5 Meanwhile, in a small bowl, whisk the milk into the flour until smooth. Stir the flour mixture into the simmering stew and cook, stirring until the sauce is slightly thickened, about 2 minutes.
Makes 4 servings

per serving: 376 calories, 8.1g total fat (1.3g saturated), 89mg cholesterol, 5g dietary fiber, 33g carbohydrate, 43g protein, 565mg sodium. good source of: niacin, potassium, riboflavin, selenium, vitamin B_{12}, vitamin B_6, vitamin C.

Turkey Gumbo

Gumbo, a staple of New Orleans cuisine, is a thick soup-stew that comes from the region's Creole cuisine. Gumbo cooks divide into two camps on how the stew should be thickened: with okra (as here) or with filé powder (ground sassafras leaves). But all gumbos include a thickener called a roux, which is a cooked fat and flour mixture. A classic Creole roux is cooked slowly to a deep mahogany color and is often made with lard. In our lightened version, we toast the flour to get some of the deep flavor of a dark roux and use a bit of olive oil.

> 2 tablespoons flour
>
> 1 tablespoon olive oil
>
> 1 pound skinless, boneless turkey breast, cut into 1-inch chunks
>
> 1 large onion, finely chopped
>
> 3 cloves garlic, minced
>
> 1 red bell pepper, coarsely chopped
>
> Half of a 10-ounce package frozen sliced okra, minced
>
> 1⅔ cups chicken broth, homemade (page 252) or canned
>
> ¾ teaspoon thyme
>
> 1 teaspoon Louisiana-style hot sauce
>
> ½ teaspoon black pepper
>
> ½ teaspoon salt

1 In a small skillet, heat the flour over low heat. Cook, stirring frequently, until the flour is golden brown, about 5 minutes. Remove from the heat and transfer the flour to a small bowl to stop it from cooking any longer.

2 In a nonstick Dutch oven or flameproof casserole, heat the oil over medium heat. Add the turkey and cook until lightly browned, about 3 minutes. Transfer the turkey to a plate.

3 Add the onion and garlic to the Dutch oven and cook until the onion is golden brown and tender, about 10 minutes. Add the bell pepper and cook until soft, about 4 minutes.

4 Sprinkle the toasted flour over the vegetables and stir until evenly coated. Add the okra and stir until well combined. Gradually add the broth, stirring constantly, until the sauce is smooth.

5 Add the thyme, hot sauce, black pepper, and salt. Bring to a boil, reduce to a simmer, cover, and cook, stirring occasionally, until slightly thickened, about 15 minutes. Return the turkey to the pan and cook until the turkey is cooked through, about 5 minutes. *Makes 4 servings*

per serving: 216 calories, 4.5g total fat (0.8g saturated), 70mg cholesterol, 3g dietary fiber, 12g carbohydrate, 31g protein, 568mg sodium. **good source of:** niacin, selenium, vitamin B$_6$, vitamin C.

Three-Alarm Chili

Ordinarily, chunky Texas-style chilis are made with beef. By using lean turkey breast instead, you can substantially reduce the amount of saturated fat in this delicious, spicy stew. Cooking the turkey in two batches prevents crowding in the pan, allowing the turkey to brown rather than steam. This browning step seals in the turkey's juices, keeping it moist and juicy. **Serving suggestion:** Serve the chili over brown rice.

1 tablespoon olive oil

1 pound skinless, boneless turkey breast, cut into ½-inch chunks

1 large onion, finely chopped

5 cloves garlic, minced

2 green bell peppers, cut into ½-inch squares

2 canned or bottled jalapeño peppers, finely chopped

1 tablespoon chili powder

1½ teaspoons cumin

¼ teaspoon cayenne pepper

1 cup dark beer

1 can (15 ounces) crushed tomatoes

1¼ cups cooked pinto beans (page 180) or canned (rinsed and drained)

¾ teaspoon salt

1 In a large nonstick Dutch oven, heat the oil over medium heat. Cook the turkey in two batches, stirring frequently, until browned, about 4 minutes. With a slotted spoon, transfer the turkey to a plate.

2 Add the onion and garlic, and cook, stirring frequently, until the onion is soft, about 7 minutes.

3 Add the bell peppers and jalapeños, and cook, stirring frequently, until the bell peppers are tender, about 5 minutes. Stir in the chili powder, cumin, and cayenne, and cook 1 minute.

4 Stir in the beer and bring to a boil. Add the tomatoes, beans, and salt, and return to a boil. Return the turkey to the pan. Reduce to a simmer, cover, and cook until the turkey is tender and the sauce is richly flavored, about 35 minutes. *Makes 4 servings*

per serving: 340 calories, 5.4g total fat (0.9g saturated), 70mg cholesterol, 10g dietary fiber, 35g carbohydrate, 36g protein, 867mg sodium. **good source of:** fiber, folate, niacin, potassium, selenium, thiamin, vitamin B$_6$, vitamin C.

making turkey broth

If you've roasted a whole turkey, don't throw the carcass away—it makes wonderful broth.

With a pair of poultry shears, or a heavy knife, cut the carcass into large pieces and put them into a soup pot or stockpot. Add water to cover by 2 inches. Bring the water to a boil over high heat and skim off any foam that rises to the surface. Add 1 large unpeeled onion, quartered, 4 cloves unpeeled garlic, 2 thinly sliced carrots, 1 or 2 stalks of celery, thinly sliced (optional), 2 tablespoons tomato paste (optional), and ½ teaspoon each of rosemary and thyme. Return to a boil, then reduce to a simmer, and cook, partially covered, until the broth is very flavorful, about 2 hours. (Check the water periodically, adding a bit more water if it doesn't cover the carcass.) Strain. Use as you would chicken broth.

If you aren't using the broth right away, you should freeze it—in large or small quantities, or even in ice cube trays.

Turkey-Papaya Salad

Both papaya and kiwifruit have enzymes (papain in papaya, actinidin in kiwi) that wreak havoc with protein, so you should not assemble this salad too long before serving it, or the fruits will make the turkey mushy. Any fruit juice-blend would be good in the dressing, but use one that is not too sweet.

> 2 cups water
>
> 2 cloves garlic, minced
>
> 1 teaspoon grated lemon zest
>
> ¾ teaspoon salt
>
> 1 pound thick turkey breast cutlets
>
> ⅓ cup frozen tropical fruit juice concentrate, thawed
>
> ¼ cup rice vinegar
>
> 1 tablespoon olive oil
>
> 3 cups strawberries, quartered
>
> 1 papaya, peeled, seeded, and cut into ½-inch chunks
>
> 2 kiwifruit, peeled and diced
>
> 4 cups shredded romaine lettuce
>
> ¼ cup dry-roasted cashews or peanuts, coarsely chopped

1 In a large skillet, combine the water, garlic, lemon zest, and ¼ teaspoon of the salt, and bring to a boil over medium heat. Add the turkey cutlets and reduce to a simmer. Cover and simmer until the turkey is cooked through, about 10 minutes.

2 Transfer the turkey to a plate and let cool to room temperature; discard the poaching liquid (or save for soup). When cool enough to handle, cut the turkey into bite-size pieces.

3 In a large bowl, whisk together the remaining ½ teaspoon salt, the fruit juice concentrate, vinegar, and oil. Add the turkey, strawberries, papaya, and kiwi. Add the lettuce and toss to combine. Sprinkle with the cashews. *Makes 4 servings*

per serving: 368 calories, 8.9g total fat (1.6g saturated), 82mg cholesterol, 7g dietary fiber, 37g carbohydrate, 34g protein, 413mg sodium. **good source of:** folate, niacin, potassium, riboflavin, selenium, vitamin B$_6$, vitamin C.

Turkey Breast à la Ficelle

In French, *à la ficelle* literally means "on a string," and it's an apt description of a dish in which a large cut of meat—usually a beef roast—is tied with string and then suspended "on a string" in a large pot of broth to cook. A portion of the vegetables that cook along with the turkey get pureed into a surprisingly buttery tasting sauce.

> 1 large skinless, boneless turkey breast half (about 1½ pounds)
>
> ¾ teaspoon salt
>
> ½ teaspoon rosemary, minced
>
> ½ teaspoon pepper
>
> ½ cup parsley leaves
>
> 3 carrots, thinly sliced
>
> 2 leeks, halved lengthwise and thinly sliced crosswise
>
> 1 white turnip (6 ounces), halved and thinly sliced
>
> 1 parsnip, thinly sliced
>
> 1 large tomato, cut into chunks
>
> 1 stalk celery, thinly sliced
>
> 5 cloves garlic

1 Place the turkey breast on a cutting board with one short end facing you. With a sturdy, long, thin-bladed knife, cut the turkey breast horizontally and lengthwise, starting at the thin side and cutting toward the thick side. Do not cut all the way through. Open the turkey like a book.

2 Sprinkle the turkey with the salt, rosemary, and pepper. Scatter the parsley leaves down the center. Starting from one long end, roll the turkey breast up and tie with kitchen string (leaving an 18-inch length of string coming off the middle).

3 In a large pot, combine the carrots, leeks, turnip, parsnip, tomato, celery, and garlic, and enough water to cover the turkey by 2 inches (put the turkey in the pot to make this judgment, but remove before bringing the poaching liquid to a boil). Bring to a boil over high heat and boil for 10 minutes; then reduce to a simmer.

4 Tie the long piece of string to the handle of the pot so that the turkey is suspended in the broth, not touching the bottom. Reduce to a simmer and cook until the turkey is just cooked through, about 25 minutes. Lift the turkey out and place on a cutting board. Strain the cooking liquid through a sieve, reserving the vegetables and ½ cup of the liquid, and transfer to a food processor

5 Measure out 1 cup of the vegetables and add to the processor. Process to a smooth puree and transfer to a small saucepan. Cook over medium heat until piping hot, about 5 minutes. Thinly slice the turkey and serve with the sauce and vegetables. *Makes 4 servings*

per serving: 306 calories, 1.8g total fat (0.5g saturated), 105mg cholesterol, 6g dietary fiber, 27g carbohydrate, 45g protein, 591mg sodium. good source of: beta carotene, folate, niacin, potassium, selenium, vitamin B_{12}, vitamin B_6, vitamin C.

Spaghetti & Turkey Meatballs

Grinding turkey breast in a food processor is the best way to ensure that you are getting the leanest ground meat possible. If you don't care to do this, be sure to look for ground turkey *breast*, since packages labeled "lean ground turkey" probably include dark meat and skin and are higher in fat.

1 pound skinless, boneless turkey breast, cut into large chunks

2 teaspoons olive oil

1 medium onion, finely chopped

3 cloves garlic, minced

1 slice (1 ounce) oatmeal or whole-wheat sandwich bread, crumbled

¼ cup fat-free or low-fat (1%) milk

¼ cup grated Parmesan cheese

¾ teaspoon salt

¼ teaspoon rubbed sage

1 can (28 ounces) crushed tomatoes

½ teaspoon fennel seeds

10 ounces spaghetti

1 In a food processor, coarsely grind the turkey.

2 In a large nonstick skillet, heat the oil over medium heat. Add the onion and garlic, and cook until the onion is soft, about 7 minutes. Transfer the onion to a large bowl. (Set the skillet aside.)

3 Add the crumbled bread and milk to the onion, and stir to moisten. Add the turkey, Parmesan, ½ teaspoon of the salt, and the sage. Mix well to combine, then shape into 20 meatballs.

4 In the same skillet the onion cooked in, combine the remaining ¼ teaspoon salt, the tomatoes, and fennel seeds. Bring to a boil over medium heat. Add the meatballs, cover, and cook until the meatballs are cooked through and the sauce is flavorful, about 10 minutes.

5 Meanwhile, in a large pot of boiling water, cook the pasta according to package directions. Drain and transfer to a large bowl. Add the meatballs and sauce, tossing to combine. *Makes 4 servings*

per serving: 555 calories, 6.7g total fat (1.8g saturated), 75mg cholesterol, 7g dietary fiber, 79g carbohydrate, 45g protein, 895mg sodium. good source of: magnesium, niacin, potassium, riboflavin, selenium, thiamin, vitamin B_{12}, vitamin B_6, zinc.

different spins

▶ **Turkey Meatball & Pepper Hero** Follow the recipe for *Spaghetti & Turkey Meatballs*, but substitute rosemary for the sage in step 3. In step 4, omit the crushed tomatoes and substitute 1 can (14½ ounces) of diced tomatoes. Add 1 green bell pepper cut into matchsticks to the tomatoes and meatballs as they cook. Spoon the meatballs and peppers onto 4 whole-wheat rolls.

▶ **Turkey Meatball Soup** Follow the recipe for *Spaghetti & Turkey Meatballs*, but only through the end of step 3 (omit all of the sauce ingredients and the pasta). Shape the turkey mixture into 30 small meatballs. Drop the meatballs into 5 cups of homemade chicken or turkey broth and cook 5 minutes, or until cooked through. Serve with ¼ cup Parmesan cheese.

duck

A fat-conscious diner offered the choice between chicken breast and duck breast would undoubtedly opt for the chicken—but would be wrong. A three-ounce serving of cooked duck breast (about the size of a deck of cards), without skin, has just over 2 grams of fat. The same portion of skinless, boneless chicken breast has 3 grams of fat. The key, of course, is the skin, which is where the majority of the fat is in all poultry. And in the case of duck, the skin has a spectacular amount of fat, which is why most people assume that duck is too fatty to eat. However, once you've taken the skin off, you've leveled the playing field; and duck flesh stacks up quite favorably.

Because duck has such an enormous amount of fat in its skin, we have concentrated on cooking with just the duck breasts, which are easily skinned before cooking. Though it can be difficult to find duck breasts, if you make an effort to find them (at a butcher or some mail-order sources), you will be well rewarded. Look for the Pekin variety—the most common breed available—or the less common moulard. Both are lean and very flavorful.

Broiling/grilling Skinless duck breasts can be broiled or grilled either on a grill or stovetop grill pan (*see "The Grill Pan," opposite page*). Preheat the broiler or grill and cook 4 to 6 inches from the heat until medium-rare, 3 to 4 minutes per side.

Pan-frying Duck breasts can be treated like steak. Remove the skin and season the meat. Sauté in a small amount of oil to the desired degree of doneness.

Stir-frying Skinless duck breasts can be cut into thin strips, like chicken breast, and stir-fried for 2 minutes until done.

how to tell when duck is done

Like steaks, duck breasts cook quickly and can be eaten medium-rare (145°F on a meat thermometer). To tell whether a duck breast is cooked to your liking, check it after it has cooked for 5 minutes. A knife inserted into the breast should offer little resistance. The more resistance it offers, the more well done the duck will be. The visual clues to doneness are similar to those for beef. Cooked to medium, the duck will look slightly pink in the center and feel firm to the touch; at medium-rare, the center of the duck will be a deeper pink.

Chinese-Style Grilled Duck Breast

Five-spice powder is a blend of spices—usually cinnamon, ground cloves, fennel seed, star anise or anise seed, and Szechuan peppercorns— mainly used in Chinese cooking. Combined with brown sugar and used as a rub, it lends a wonderful sweet and spicy flavor to grilled duck.

> 2 tablespoons reduced-sodium soy sauce
> 2 teaspoons five-spice powder
> 1½ teaspoons dark brown sugar
> 1 teaspoon dark sesame oil
> 4 skinless, boneless duck breast halves
>   (5 ounces each)

1 In a shallow pan or pie plate, combine the soy sauce, five-spice powder, brown sugar, and sesame oil. Add the duck breasts and turn them to coat. Let stand for 10 minutes.

2 Spray a grill rack with nonstick cooking spray. Preheat the grill to medium. Lift the duck from the marinade, reserving any marinade.

3 Place the duck on the grill and brush with the marinade. Grill the duck 4 inches from the heat, turning over once, for 6 to 7 minutes for medium-rare, or 8 to 10 minutes for medium. When cool enough to handle, but still warm, thinly slice the duck across the grain. *Makes 4 servings* per serving: 174 calories, 4g total fat (0.8g saturated), 152mg cholesterol, 0g dietary fiber, 3g carbohydrate, 30g protein, 379mg sodium. good source of: niacin, riboflavin, selenium.

Cajun Grilled Duck

One of the few good applications for garlic powder and onion powder is in Cajun-style dry rubs such as the one used for this grilled duck. **Serving suggestion:** For a cool counterpoint to the slightly spicy duck, serve it with Tomato-Melon Salsa (*page 263*), Papaya-Corn Salsa (*page 263*), or Fresh Pineapple-Jícama Relish (*page 265*).

1 teaspoon thyme

1 teaspoon black pepper

¾ teaspoon salt

½ teaspoon sugar

½ teaspoon garlic powder

½ teaspoon onion powder

¼ teaspoon cayenne pepper

*4 skinless, boneless duck breast halves
   (5 ounces each)*

1 In a small bowl, stir together the thyme, black pepper, salt, sugar, garlic powder, onion powder, and cayenne. Rub the spice mixture over both sides of the duck.

2 Spray a grill rack with nonstick cooking spray. Preheat the grill to medium. Grill the duck 4

the grill pan

If it's cold outside, or if you don't have access to a grill, you can "grill" indoors with this special pan. Grill pans are basically skillets—usually made of cast iron or cast iron coated with a nonstick finish—that have raised ridges in them. When food is cooked on the ridges, it ends up with "grill marks." Food can be cooked in grill pans with very little or no fat. And the ridges allow any fat in the food being cooked to run off and collect in the well of the pan. For best results, get the pan very hot before placing food in it.

inches from the heat, turning it over once, for 6 to 7 minutes for medium-rare, or 8 to 10 minutes for medium. Alternatively, lightly brush a stovetop grill pan with oil and heat the pan over medium heat. Use the same cooking times as for grilling. *Makes 4 servings*

per serving: 166 calories, 2.9g total fat (0.7g saturated), 162mg cholesterol, 0g dietary fiber, 2g carbohydrate, 31g protein, 556mg sodium. good source of: niacin.

Grilled Duck Salad with Soba Noodles

Soba (buckwheat) noodles have an earthy taste and slightly firm, chewy texture. We used supermarket chili sauce (the kind you find right next to the ketchup) in our dressing.

*Chinese-Style Grilled Duck Breast
   (opposite page) or Cajun Grilled Duck
   (at left)*

*6 ounces soba (Japanese buckwheat)
   noodles*

¼ cup chili sauce

¼ cup fresh lime juice

1 tablespoon honey

½ teaspoon ground ginger

¼ teaspoon salt

1 bunch watercress, tough ends trimmed

1 red bell pepper, cut into thin matchsticks

1 Grill the duck. Meanwhile, in a large pot of boiling water, cook the soba noodles according to package directions. Drain well.

2 In a large bowl, whisk together the chili sauce, lime juice, honey, ginger, and salt. Add the noodles to the bowl, tossing to coat.

3 Add the watercress and bell pepper, and toss again. Slice the duck crosswise on the diagonal. Serve the duck on a mound of the soba noodle mixture. *Makes 4 servings*

per serving: 353 calories, 3.8g total fat (0.7g saturated), 122mg cholesterol, 3g dietary fiber, 50g carbohydrate, 33g protein, 833mg sodium. good source of: niacin, riboflavin, selenium, vitamin C.

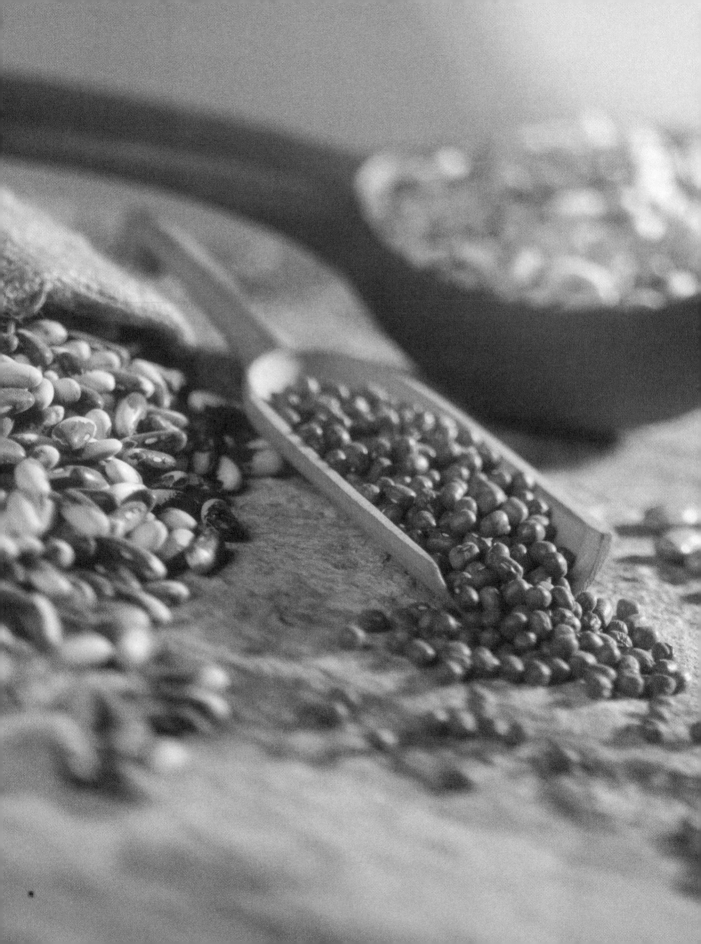

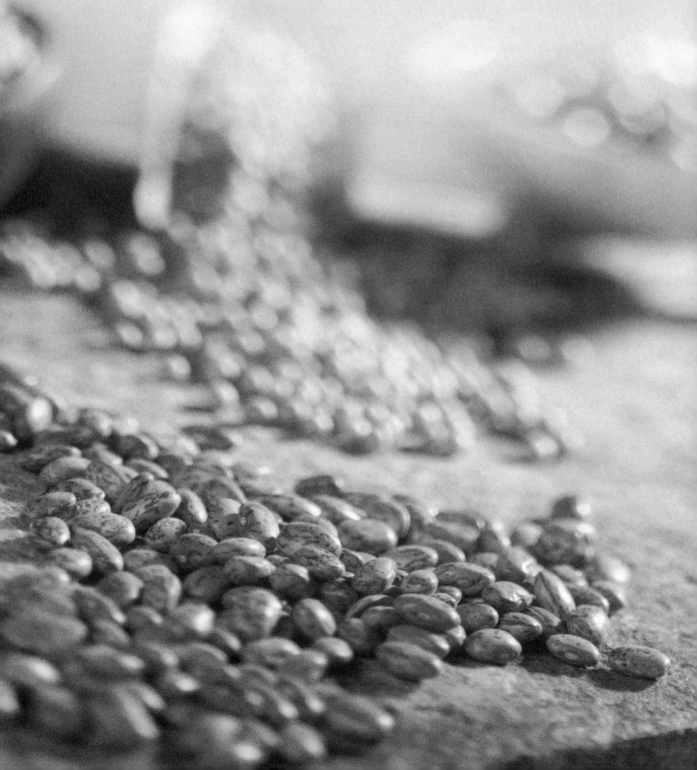

meatless
main dishes

Should you be a vegetarian? It's certainly a healthy way to eat, though strict vegetarianism is not the only option. There are all shades of vegetarianism (*see "What Type of Vegetarian Are You?" below*), ranging from the "I only eat red meat on the weekends" brand of semi-vegetarianism to the "absolutely-no-animal-product" philosophy of strict vegans. In this chapter, some of the recipes are vegan and some are not; some are lacto-ovo and some are not. But none of them is made with fish, poultry, or meat. Learning how to make delicious food that does not rely on animal protein is an important tool for healthful cooking and eating.

the health benefits

There are many clear benefits to a vegetarian diet. The clearest is that vegetarians have lower average blood cholesterol and thus a reduced risk of coronary artery disease. Vegetarians tend to weigh less than nonvegetarians and are less often afflicted with digestive-system disorders, such as constipation and diverticulosis. They have a reduced risk for type 2 (adult-onset) diabetes and gallstones. Vegetarians have a lower risk of various cancers—notably of the colon, breast, and lung—than the average American. But, of course, a vegetarian diet by itself won't cancel the effects of smoking, being sedentary, or other bad health habits.

what about protein?

Most Americans get more than enough protein. The daily Recommended Dietary Allowance (RDA) for adults is 0.8 grams of protein for each kilogram (2.2 pounds) of body weight. That adds up to 64 grams (about 2 ounces) of pure protein for a 175-pound man, and 47 grams for a 130-pound woman. (Children, teenagers, and pregnant or lactating women need a little more protein per pound of body weight.)

That isn't very much protein. Meat, chicken, and fish have 6 to 8 grams per ounce. Milk has 8 grams per cup; yogurt, 10 to 13 grams per cup; an egg, 6 grams. But plant foods also provide protein: A slice of bread or ½ cup of pasta has 3 grams. Beans have 7 grams per ½ cup cooked (soybeans are the exception, with 11 grams). Nuts and seeds average 6 grams per ounce. Grain products are often overlooked as protein sources—they supply 16% to 20% of our total protein intake. Even vegetables contain protein, though mostly in smaller amounts (½ cup of broccoli or asparagus has 2 grams).

So it's hard not to get the RDA. In fact, the average American under age 65 consumes about 50% *more* protein than the RDA. Furthermore, many Americans consume a good deal more than that. Consuming more than twice the RDA for protein is not recommended—that's the safe upper limit, according to estimates by the National Research Council. For most people, that's 100 to 120 grams of protein a day. If you eat more than that, cut back. And it's important to get as much protein as you can from plants, rather than animals.

what type of vegetarian are you?

▶**Lacto-ovo-vegetarians** eat plant-based foods, dairy products, and eggs, and exclude meat, poultry, and fish.

▶**Lacto-vegetarians** eat plant-based foods and dairy products, and exclude meat, poultry, fish, and eggs.

▶**Ovo-vegetarians** eat plant-based foods and eggs, and exclude meat, poultry, fish, and dairy products.

▶**Pesco-vegetarians** eat plant-based foods, fish, eggs, and dairy products, and exclude meat and poultry.

▶**Semi-vegetarians** eat plant-based foods, dairy products and eggs, as well as a little fish and chicken, and generally exclude meat; also called partial vegetarians.

▶**Vegans** (pronounced "VEE-guns") eat plant-based foods only, excluding all foods of animal origin; also called strict vegetarians.

plant protein

Many plant foods are good sources of protein, especially legumes, nuts, seeds, and many grains. However, the protein in most plant foods is "incomplete"—that is, it has insufficient amounts of one or more of the nine essential amino acids. (Amino acids are protein's building blocks; the essential ones are those the body can't synthesize, so you have to get them from food.) But if your diet includes a wide variety of foods each day, you will absorb a full complement of amino acids. And contrary to common belief, you do not have to eat these complementary proteins at the same meal. You can eat them hours apart or even much later in the day.

FOOD	PROTEIN (G)	FOOD	PROTEIN (G)
SOY NUTS, 2 OZ	24	FLAXSEED, ¼ CUP	6.7
TEMPEH, 4 OZ	24	PEANUTS, 1 OZ	6.7
SOYBEANS, COOKED, 1 CUP	22	WILD RICE, COOKED, 1 CUP	6.5
TOFU, BAKED, 4 OZ	20	SUNFLOWER SEEDS, 1 OZ	6.5
LENTILS, COOKED, 1 CUP	18	ALMONDS, 1 OZ	5.9
EDAMAME (GREEN SOYBEANS), ¾ CUP	17	KASHA (ROASTED BUCKWHEAT), COOKED, 1 CUP	5.7
BLACK BEANS, COOKED, 1 CUP	15	BULGUR WHEAT, COOKED, 1 CUP	5.6
CHICK-PEAS, COOKED, 1 CUP	15	TOFU, SOFT SILKEN, 4 OZ	5.4
KIDNEY BEANS, COOKED, 1 CUP	15	BARLEY, PEARL, COOKED, 1 CUP	5.0
WHITE BEANS, COOKED, 1 CUP	15	CORN, 1 CUP	5.0
TVP, DRY, ½ CUP	15	RICE, BROWN, COOKED, 1 CUP	5.0
PINTO BEANS, COOKED, 1 CUP	14	ALMOND BUTTER, 2 TBSP	4.8
BLACK-EYED PEAS, COOKED, 1 CUP	13	ASPARAGUS, COOKED, 1 CUP	4.7
BABY LIMA BEANS, COOKED, 1 CUP	12	BROCCOLI, COOKED, 1 CUP	4.7
TOFU, FIRM, REGULAR, 4 OZ	9.2	CASHEWS, 1 OZ	4.6
PEANUT BUTTER, 2 TBSP	8.1	WALNUTS, 1 OZ	4.3
WHEATBERRIES, COOKED, ¾ CUP	8.1	RICE, WHITE ENRICHED, COOKED, 1 CUP	4.3
GREEN PEAS, 1 CUP	7.5	MUSHROOMS, RAW, 4 OZ	4.1
PASTA, WHOLE-WHEAT, COOKED, 1 CUP	7.5	PASTA, COOKED, 1 CUP	3.7
BARLEY, HULLED, COOKED, 1 CUP	7.4	OATMEAL, COOKED, ⅔ CUP	3.6
QUINOA, COOKED, 1⅓ CUPS	7.4	BOK CHOY, COOKED, 1 CUP	2.7
OATS, STEEL-CUT, COOKED, 1 CUP	7.3	WHOLE-WHEAT BREAD, 1 SLICE	2.7
AMARANTH, ¼ CUP UNCOOKED	7.0	KALE, COOKED, 1 CUP	2.5
PUMPKIN SEEDS, HULLED, 1 OZ	7.0	PECANS, 1 OZ	2.2
SOY MILK, 1 CUP	6.7	GREEN BEANS, COOKED, 1 CUP	2.0

different spins

▶**Lemon-Mint Barley Salad** Follow the directions for *Chili-Lime Barley & Vegetable Salad*, but substitute 1½ cups diced fresh fennel for the corn and 1 teaspoon crushed fennel seeds for the chili powder in step 3. Substitute lemon juice for the lime juice and add ¼ cup chopped fresh mint in step 4.

▶**Linguine with Dried Plums & Feta Cheese** Follow the directions for *Linguine with Figs & Goat Cheese (opposite page)*, but substitute 1½ cups of pitted dried plums for the figs and 1 cup of crumbed feta cheese for the goat cheese.

Chili-Lime Barley & Vegetable Salad

One of the advantages of a full-fat cheese is that it melts nicely; but in cold dishes (like this salad) where meltability is not an issue, you can use a lower-fat cheese with no sacrifice—and the health benefits are obvious. If you prefer, substitute quick-cooking barley for the pearl.

- 1½ cups pearl barley
- ¾ teaspoon salt
- 4 teaspoons olive oil
- 1 red bell pepper, cut into ½-inch squares
- 1 medium red onion, coarsely diced
- 3 cloves garlic, minced
- 1½ cups frozen corn kernels
- 2 teaspoons chili powder
- ¼ cup fresh lime juice
- ½ teaspoon black pepper
- 1 cup crumbled reduced-fat feta cheese (4 ounces)

1 In a large saucepan, cook the barley according to the package directions, using ¼ teaspoon of the salt. Drain well.

2 Meanwhile, in a large nonstick skillet, heat 2 teaspoons of the oil over medium heat. Add the bell pepper, onion, and garlic. Cook, stirring frequently, until the pepper is crisp-tender, about 5 minutes.

3 Add the corn and chili powder. Increase the heat to medium-high and cook until the corn is piping hot, about 5 minutes.

4 In a large bowl, whisk together the remaining ½ teaspoon salt, lime juice, and black pepper. Add the barley, sautéed vegetables, and the remaining 2 teaspoons oil, tossing to combine. Add the cheese and toss gently. Serve at room temperature or lightly chilled. *Makes 4 servings*

per serving: 322 calories, 4.9g total fat (2.4g saturated), 10mg cholesterol, 9g dietary fiber, 63g carbohydrate, 15g protein, 828mg sodium. **good source of:** beta glucan, fiber, lutein, vitamin C.

Baked Acorn Squash with Curried Rice

The appeal of using a vegetable as an edible container for serving is obvious. Add to this the beauty of acorn squash, and the seductive flavors of a curry-scented, cheese-topped rice stuffing, and you have a winner.

- 1 cup brown rice
- ¾ teaspoon salt
- 2 large acorn squash (about 1½ pounds each)
- 2 teaspoons olive oil
- 3 garlic cloves, minced
- ¾ teaspoon ground ginger
- ¾ teaspoon curry powder
- ½ cup pitted dried plums (prunes), chopped
- ¼ cup mango chutney, chopped
- 1 tablespoon fresh lemon juice
- ¾ cup shredded reduced-fat sharp Cheddar cheese
- ½ cup plain fat-free yogurt

1 In a medium saucepan, cook the rice according to package directions, using ¼ teaspoon of salt.

2 Meanwhile, preheat the oven to 400°F. Halve the squash lengthwise and remove the seeds. Cut off a thin sliver from the bottom of each squash half so it will sit flat. Place the squash halves, cut-sides down, in a baking dish with water to come ½ inch up the sides of the squash. Bake until softened, about 20 minutes. Remove from the oven, but leave the oven on.

3 Scoop out most of the squash flesh, leaving a sturdy shell. Cut the flesh into ½-inch chunks.

4 In a large nonstick skillet, heat the oil over medium heat. Add the garlic and cook until fragrant, about 30 seconds. Add the chunks of squash and cook, stirring frequently, until lightly colored, about 5 minutes.

5 Stir in the ginger, curry powder, and remaining ½ teaspoon salt, and cook until fragrant, about 1 minute. Stir in the dried plums, chutney, and lemon juice, and cook until the squash is tender, about 10 minutes. Stir in the rice and remove from the heat.

6 Drain any liquid remaining in the baking dish and place the squash shells, cut-side up, in the dish. Spoon the stuffing mixture into the shells, sprinkle with the Cheddar, cover with foil, and bake until heated through, about 10 minutes.

7 Serve topped with the yogurt. *Makes 4 servings*

per serving: 480 calories, 9g total fat (2.9g saturated), 12mg cholesterol, 14g dietary fiber, 93g carbohydrate, 15g protein, 755mg sodium. good source of: calcium, fiber, magnesium, niacin, potassium, selenium, thiamin, vitamin B_6.

---

did you know?

If you're trying to find a cheese that won't clog your arteries, you may have heard that cheese made from goat's milk is lower in fat than cow's-milk cheese. While there are some variations, this is generally not so. All cheeses are high in fat, with from 65% to 85% of their calories coming from it, and goat cheese is no exception. One ounce of a typical soft (not aged) goat cheese has 82 calories and 6.5 g of fat (that's 71% of calories from fat), and 4.5 g of that is saturated. However, on the plus side, goat cheese has such a pronounced flavor, that you can get away with using less of it.

Linguine with Figs & Goat Cheese

Sweet, dried figs are poached in red wine to soften them, then tossed with freshly cooked pasta in a creamy goat cheese-red wine sauce.

> 1½ cups dried Calimyrna figs (4 ounces)
> ¾ cup dry red wine
> ¾ cup water
> ½ teaspoon black pepper
> ½ teaspoon tarragon
> ¼ teaspoon salt
> 1 teaspoon olive oil
> 1 red bell pepper, cut into ½-inch squares
> 10 ounces linguine
> 5 ounces soft goat cheese, crumbled
> 2 tablespoons minced chives or scallion greens

1 In a medium saucepan, combine the figs, wine, water, black pepper, tarragon, and salt. Bring to a boil, reduce to a simmer, cover, and cook until the figs are tender, about 20 minutes. When cool enough to handle, drain, reserving the cooking liquid. Remove the stems and coarsely chop the figs.

2 Meanwhile, in a large nonstick skillet, heat the oil over low heat. Add the bell pepper and sauté until crisp-tender, about 5 minutes. Add the reserved fig cooking liquid and set the skillet aside.

3 In a large pot of boiling water, cook the pasta according to package directions. Drain and transfer to a large bowl.

4 Add the goat cheese, chives, and figs to the pasta. Bring the bell pepper mixture in the skillet to a boil and pour over the pasta. Toss well. *Makes 4 servings*

per serving: 485 calories, 10g total fat (5.6g saturated), 16mg cholesterol, 6g dietary fiber, 76g carbohydrate, 17g protein, 142mg sodium. good source of: selenium, vitamin C.

Fusilli with Asparagus & Toasted Hazelnuts

Just a small amount of reduced-fat cream cheese underscored by some grated Parmesan gives the sauce for this vegetarian pasta dish a lovely creamy texture. Using some of the pasta cooking water to smooth the sauce and melt the Parmesan is an old Italian trick.

¼ cup hazelnuts

10 ounces short fusilli

1½ pounds asparagus, cut into 1½-inch lengths

1 cup frozen peas

1⅓ cups water

2 cloves garlic, minced

¾ teaspoon salt

3 tablespoons reduced-fat cream cheese (Neufchâtel)

1 teaspoon grated lemon zest

¼ cup grated Parmesan cheese

1 Preheat the oven to 375°F. Toast the hazelnuts on a baking sheet until the skins begin to flake and the nuts are fragrant, about 7 minutes. Place the nuts in a kitchen towel and rub vigorously to remove as much of the skin as possible (some skin will remain). When cool enough to handle, coarsely chop the hazelnuts and set aside.

2 In a large pot of boiling water, cook the pasta according to package directions. Drain the pasta, reserving ½ cup of the pasta cooking water.

3 Meanwhile, in a large skillet, combine the asparagus, peas, water, garlic, and salt. Cover and cook until the asparagus is crisp-tender, about 4 minutes. Uncover, increase the heat to high, bring to a boil, and stir in the cream cheese. Cook until the cream cheese has melted.

4 Transfer the pasta to a large bowl, add the reserved pasta cooking water, asparagus mixture, lemon zest, Parmesan, and hazelnuts, and toss to combine. *Makes 4 servings*

per serving: 390 calories, 11g total fat (3.4g saturated), 13mg cholesterol, 6g dietary fiber, 57g carbohydrate, 17g protein, 647mg sodium. **good source of:** folate, niacin, riboflavin, selenium, thiamin.

pasta perfect

Cooking pasta is not difficult but does require attention. The two main rules for perfect pasta are: Use plenty of water and do not overcook. Lots of water helps the pasta cook evenly and prevents clumping and sticking. Pasta is best when it is cooked to the "al dente" stage—tender but firm to the bite. Overcooked pasta will be mushy. Pasta that is to be baked, stir-fried, used in stews, or cooked further in some other way should be undercooked slightly.

▶**The pot** Choose a sufficiently large pot—one that can comfortably hold 4 quarts of water per pound of pasta. Lots of water prevents the pasta from sticking, making it unnecessary to add oil.

▶**The water** Many cooks and recipes suggest adding salt to the cooking water; about 10% of the sodium in the salt will be absorbed by the pasta. If you are sodium sensitive, you should eliminate it (try some fresh lemon juice in the water instead).

▶**The method** When the water reaches a rolling boil, uncover the pot, add the pasta, and stir to keep the pasta from clumping. Boil, uncovered, stirring occasionally with a fork to separate the pieces and keep them from sticking to the bottom of the pot.

▶**The timing** Pasta cooking time depends on the type of pasta and its shape or thickness. Package directions are generally accurate if you are cooking the whole package at once but often overestimate the time for smaller amounts. Begin checking the pasta about halfway through the recommended cooking time.

▶**The doneness test** Remove a piece from the pot, run it under cool water, and bite it. If it's still hard and white in the middle, continue cooking. If it's almost cooked through, taste another sample in 45 seconds. The pasta is done when it is translucent in the center and no longer hard, but still firm.

"Lasagna" with Fresh Dill

Broken into large pieces, lasagna noodles can be used to make a sort of unstructured lasagna. Instead of layering, these sturdy noodles are simply tossed together with the other ingredients and then baked.

> 12 ounces lasagna noodles, broken roughly into fourths
>
> 1½ cups low-fat (1%) cottage cheese
>
> 1 cup part-skim ricotta cheese
>
> 1 large egg
>
> 2 large egg whites
>
> ¼ cup grated Parmesan cheese
>
> 2 teaspoons grated orange zest
>
> 1 teaspoon cinnamon
>
> ½ teaspoon salt
>
> ½ teaspoon pepper
>
> 1 cup canned crushed tomatoes
>
> 3 tablespoons tomato paste
>
> ⅓ cup minced fresh dill

1 Preheat the oven to 350°F. Spray a 7 x 11-inch baking dish with nonstick cooking spray. In a large pot of boiling water, cook the lasagna noodles according to package directions. Drain, reserving ½ cup of pasta cooking water.

2 Meanwhile, in a food processor, combine the cottage cheese, ricotta, whole egg, egg whites, Parmesan, orange zest, cinnamon, salt, and pepper, and process to a smooth puree.

3 Transfer to a large bowl and stir in the reserved pasta cooking water, the tomatoes, tomato paste, and dill. Add the pasta, stirring to combine. Transfer the mixture to the baking dish. Bake, uncovered, until the pasta is set and the top is slightly crisp, about 30 minutes. *Makes 6 servings*

per serving: 352 calories, 6.6g total fat (3.5g saturated), 53mg cholesterol, 3g dietary fiber, 50g carbohydrate, 24g protein, 656mg sodium. good source of: folate, riboflavin, selenium, thiamin, vitamin B₁₂.

Shells with Italian Butternut Sauce

The flavors in this pasta sauce were inspired by the filling for Italian pumpkin tortellini: a mixture of naturally sweet pumpkin complemented by salty cheese and a spicy-sweet condiment (we've used chutney). Since farmers' markets now have more interesting winter squash available, you might want to substitute one of the more unusual squashes for the butternut. Try kabocha or sugar pumpkin, or buttercup or carnival squash.

> 1 butternut squash (2 pounds), halved lengthwise and seeded
>
> 10 ounces medium shells, short fusilli, or radiatore pasta
>
> 2 teaspoons olive oil
>
> 3 cloves garlic, minced
>
> ⅓ cup reduced-fat sour cream
>
> 3 tablespoons mango chutney, chopped
>
> 1 teaspoon yellow mustard
>
> ½ teaspoon rubbed sage
>
> ½ teaspoon salt
>
> ½ teaspoon pepper
>
> ⅓ cup grated Parmesan cheese

1 Preheat the oven to 425°F. Place the squash, cut-sides down, in a small baking pan. Add ½ cup water, cover, and bake for 45 minutes, or until the squash is tender. When cool enough to handle, scoop the flesh into a food processor.

2 Meanwhile, in a large pot of boiling water, cook the pasta according to package directions. Drain, reserving ½ cup of the pasta cooking water.

3 In a small nonstick skillet, heat the oil over low heat. Add the garlic and cook for 2 minutes or until softened.

4 Transfer the garlic to the food processor along with the reserved pasta cooking water, sour cream, chutney, mustard, sage, salt, and pepper, and puree. Transfer to a large bowl, add the pasta and Parmesan, and toss to combine. *Makes 4 servings*

per serving: 447 calories, 9g total fat (3.4g saturated), 13mg cholesterol, 8g dietary fiber, 81g carbohydrate, 15g protein, 273mg sodium. good source of: beta carotene, fiber, folate, magnesium, niacin, riboflavin, thiamin.

Mediterranean Orzo

Orzo is a rice-shaped pasta whose name in Italian actually means "barley" (unhulled barley has an elongated, rice-like shape). Here, orzo is tossed with feta cheese and a sauté of zucchini, tomato, and bell pepper. The Gaeta olives called for are salt-cured black olives from Italy, but Calamata olives (brine-cured Greek olives) make a fine substitute and are available in jars or at many supermarket deli counters.

1 cup orzo pasta (6 ounces)

1 tablespoon olive oil

1 red onion, finely chopped

3 cloves garlic, minced

1 red bell pepper, cut into ½-inch chunks

1 zucchini, halved lengthwise and thinly sliced crosswise

1½ cups cherry tomatoes, halved

¼ cup Gaeta or Calamata olives, pitted and coarsely chopped

2 teaspoons capers

1 teaspoon tarragon

½ teaspoon salt

¼ cup chopped fresh basil or mint

1 cup crumbled reduced-fat feta cheese (4 ounces)

1 In a large pot of boiling water, cook the pasta according to package directions. Drain well.

2 Meanwhile, in a large nonstick skillet, heat the oil over medium heat. Add the onion and garlic, and cook, stirring, until the onion is golden, about 5 minutes.

3 Add the bell pepper and zucchini, and cook until the pepper is crisp-tender, about 5 minutes.

4 Add the tomatoes, olives, capers, tarragon, and salt, and cook until the tomatoes begin to collapse, about 4 minutes. Stir in the basil.

5 Transfer the vegetables to a large bowl. Add the drained orzo and the cheese, and toss to combine. *Makes 4 servings*

per serving: 305 calories, 9.4g total fat (2.9g saturated), 10mg cholesterol, 4g dietary fiber, 44g carbohydrate, 14g protein, 837mg sodium. good source of: folate, thiamin, vitamin C.

did you know?

Many people avoid olives because they're high in fat. But the fat is mostly monounsaturated and thus heart-healthy. Six pitted Calamata olives (about ¼ cup) averages 60 calories and a little over 5 grams of fat. Olives also supply some calcium, fiber, vitamin E, and healthful phytochemicals, such as phenols and lignans. The main drawback is sodium, about 200 mg per ounce. But because olives such as Calamata are strongly flavored, you can use as few as 6 to flavor a dish to serve 4 people, meaning each person will be getting only 15 calories, a little over 1 gram of fat, and 90 mg of sodium.

Radiatore with Cauliflower, Raisins & Sun-Dried Tomatoes

Cauliflower has a shape similar to that of radiatore pasta giving you the impression that you're eating more pasta than you actually are.

⅓ cup golden raisins

⅓ cup slivered sun-dried tomatoes

1½ cups very hot water

2 slices (1 ounce each) multigrain sandwich bread, finely crumbled

8 ounces radiatore or short fusilli pasta

1 tablespoon olive oil

4 cups small cauliflower florets

5 cloves garlic, minced

2 teaspoons anchovy paste

¾ teaspoon salt

½ teaspoon red pepper flakes

⅓ cup grated Parmesan cheese

1 In a small bowl, combine the raisins, sun-dried tomatoes, and hot water. Let stand until the raisins have softened, about 10 minutes.

2 Meanwhile, in a small ungreased skillet, toast the crumbled bread over low heat until lightly crisped and golden brown, about 3 minutes. Remove from the heat.

3 In a large pot of boiling water, cook the pasta according to package directions. Drain and transfer to a large bowl.

4 Meanwhile, in a large nonstick skillet, heat the oil over low heat. Add the cauliflower and cook, stirring frequently, until golden, about 5 minutes.

5 Add the raisins, sun-dried tomatoes, their soaking liquid, the garlic, anchovy paste, salt, and red pepper flakes. Cook until the cauliflower is tender, about 4 minutes.

6 Transfer the cauliflower mixture to the bowl of pasta. Add the breadcrumbs and Parmesan, and toss to combine. *Makes 4 servings*

per serving: 381 calories, 7.3g total fat (2.2g saturated), 6mg cholesterol, 6g dietary fiber, 67g carbohydrate, 15g protein, 846mg sodium. good source of: folate, niacin, riboflavin, thiamin, vitamin C.

Couscous with Eggplant Meatballs

Eggplant meatballs (*polpettine di melanzane*) are an Italian Lenten dish. We've given our version of these meatless "meatballs" a Middle Eastern twist by flavoring them with fresh cilantro and coriander and serving them over couscous. **Timing alert:** The eggplant needs to drain for 30 minutes.

> 1 eggplant (¾ pound), peeled and cut into ½-inch cubes
>
> 2¼ teaspoons salt
>
> ½ cup plain dried breadcrumbs
>
> ¾ cup chopped cilantro
>
> 1 cup crumbled reduced-fat feta cheese (4 ounces)
>
> 1 large egg white
>
> 2 tablespoons flour
>
> 1 tablespoon olive oil
>
> 2 cans (14½ ounces each) no-salt-added diced tomatoes
>
> 2 cloves garlic, minced
>
> ¾ teaspoon ground coriander
>
> 1 cup couscous

different *spins*

▶**Italian-Style Eggplant Meatballs** Follow the directions for *Couscous with Eggplant Meatballs*, but substitute Italian-style breadcrumbs for the plain dried breadcrumbs, and use basil instead of cilantro. In step 3, omit the ¼ cup feta and use ½ cup shredded part-skim mozzarella in the meatball mixture. In step 5, omit the coriander. In step 6, omit the ¾ cup feta and substitute ¼ cup grated Parmesan instead.

1 In a colander set over a bowl, toss the eggplant with 2 teaspoons of the salt. Let the eggplant sit for 30 minutes to release liquid. Rinse the eggplant briefly under cold running water to remove the salt. Squeeze the eggplant until it's dry and has lost most of its seeds.

2 Steam the eggplant in a vegetable steamer until tender, about 15 minutes. Transfer the eggplant to a large bowl and let cool to room temperature.

3 Add the breadcrumbs, ½ cup of the cilantro, ¼ cup of the feta, and the egg white to the eggplant. Mix well to combine. Shape into 16 balls. Dredge the balls in the flour, shaking off the excess.

4 In a large nonstick skillet, heat the oil over medium heat. Add the eggplant meatballs and cook, shaking the pan occasionally, until they are lightly browned, about 7 minutes.

5 Add the tomatoes, garlic, coriander, and the remaining ¼ cup cilantro and ¼ teaspoon salt. Bring to a boil. Reduce to a simmer, cover, and cook until the meatballs are firm and hot throughout, about 10 minutes.

6 Meanwhile, prepare the couscous according to package directions, using no salt. Drain and transfer to a large bowl. Add the remaining ¾ cup feta and the meatballs and sauce, and toss to combine. *Makes 4 servings*

per serving: 367 calories, 7.6g total fat (2.7g saturated), 10mg cholesterol, 8g dietary fiber, 60g carbohydrate, 17g protein, 739mg sodium. good source of: fiber, niacin, potassium, thiamin.

Southwestern Meatless Chili

In this Southwestern-style chili, green is the color scheme (from sweet bell and jalapeño peppers, scallions, and cilantro). Also from the Southwest—and also green—is a pear-shaped squash called chayote, with a mild flavor similar to other summer squash. You can find chayotes in the produce section of large supermarkets, especially in the Southwest or in the South (where they're more likely to be called mirlitons). If you can't find a chayote, use 1 medium zucchini instead.

1 tablespoon olive oil

2 green bell peppers, diced

4 scallions, thinly sliced

3 cloves garlic, minced

1 canned or bottled jalapeño pepper, finely chopped

1 chayote, peeled, halved lengthwise, and cut crosswise into ½-inch slices

1 cup carrot juice

1¾ cups cooked chick-peas (page 180) or canned (rinsed and drained)

1 can (15 ounces) hominy, rinsed and drained

½ cup chopped cilantro

½ teaspoon salt

½ cup plain fat-free yogurt

1 In a nonstick Dutch oven, heat the oil over medium heat. Add the bell peppers, scallions, garlic, and jalapeño, and cook until the bell peppers are tender, about 7 minutes.

2 Stir in the chayote, carrot juice, chick-peas, hominy, ¼ cup of the cilantro, and the salt. Bring to a boil. Reduce the heat to a simmer, cover, and cook for 10 minutes, or until the vegetables are tender and the stew is flavorful.

3 Stir in the remaining ¼ cup cilantro. Serve the chili topped with the yogurt. *Makes 4 servings*

per serving: 311 calories, 6.7g total fat (0.9g saturated), 1mg cholesterol, 12g dietary fiber, 53g carbohydrate, 12g protein, 729mg sodium. good source of: beta carotene, fiber, folate, potassium, vitamin B$_6$, vitamin C, zinc.

Middle Eastern Veggie Loaf

Look for tahini (sesame paste) in the gourmet section of your supermarket or at Middle Eastern grocery stores. If you can't find tahini, substitute creamy peanut butter. **Serving suggestion:** You could accompany this loaf with Smashed Potatoes (*page 193*) and a green salad or make a veggie loaf sandwich and top it with some Chimichurri Sauce (*page 258*). **Timing alert:** The eggplant needs to drain for 30 minutes.

1 eggplant (1½ pounds), peeled and cut into ½-inch cubes

2½ teaspoons salt

2 cups cooked chick-peas (page 180) or canned (rinsed and drained)

1 cup plain low-fat yogurt

different spins

▶**Cincinnati Meatless Chili** Follow directions for *Southwestern Meatless Chili*, but in step 2, substitute 1½ cups canned crushed tomatoes for the carrot juice. Use kidney beans instead of chick-peas, and parsley instead of cilantro. Add 1 teaspoon cinnamon. Omit the hominy and spoon the chili over 8 ounces of pasta, cooked.

▶**Butternut & Black Bean Stew** Follow directions for *Black Bean & Yellow Squash Stew* (*opposite page*), but substitute 4 sliced scallions for the red onion in step 1. Omit the potatoes and yellow squash and substitute 1 pound of butternut squash cut into ½-inch chunks in step 2. Stir ⅓ cup of chopped cilantro into the stew just before serving.

2 tablespoons tahini (sesame paste) or creamy peanut butter

2 tablespoons tomato paste

2 teaspoons grated lemon zest

3 tablespoons fresh lemon juice

2 teaspoons paprika

1 teaspoon coriander

2 whole-wheat pita breads (7 inches), finely chopped

⅓ cup water

3 large egg whites

1 tablespoon flour

1 In a colander set over a bowl, toss the eggplant with 2 teaspoons of the salt. Let the eggplant sit for 30 minutes to release liquid. Rinse the eggplant briefly under cold running water to remove the salt. Squeeze the eggplant until it's dry and has lost most of its seeds.

2 In a vegetable steamer, steam the eggplant until tender, about 15 minutes.

3 In a large bowl, with a potato masher, mash the chick-peas with the remaining ½ teaspoon salt, ½ cup of the yogurt, the tahini, tomato paste, lemon zest, lemon juice, paprika, and coriander. Add the eggplant and lightly mash.

4 Preheat the oven to 350°F. In a small bowl, stir together the pita and water until the pita is moistened. Stir the moistened pita into the bowl with the chick-pea mixture. Stir in 2 of the egg whites.

5 In a small bowl, stir together the remaining ½ cup yogurt, remaining egg white, and the flour.

6 Spray a 9 x 5-inch loaf pan with nonstick cooking spray. Spoon the eggplant mixture into the pan. Bake for 45 minutes.

7 Spread the yogurt mixture over the top of the loaf and bake for 10 minutes, or until glazed. Cool for 20 minutes in the pan before cutting into slices and serving. *Makes 4 servings*

per serving: 369 calories, 8.4g total fat (1.6g saturated), 4mg cholesterol, 14g dietary fiber, 59g carbohydrate, 20g protein, 749mg sodium. **good source of:** fiber, folate, magnesium, potassium, riboflavin, selenium, thiamin.

Black Bean & Yellow Squash Stew

A small amount of peanut butter stirred into stews offers a lot of bang for the buck: The roasted, rich flavor permeates the entire stew and at the same time adds a satisfying thickness to the sauce.

1 tablespoon olive oil

1 large red onion, diced

1 large green bell pepper, cut into ½-inch chunks

3 cloves garlic, minced

¾ pound small red potatoes, cut into 1-inch chunks

¾ cup water

1 pound yellow squash, halved lengthwise and cut crosswise into ½-inch-thick slices

1 can (14½ ounces) stewed tomatoes, chopped with their juice

1¾ cups cooked black beans (page 180) or canned (rinsed and drained)

2 tablespoons creamy peanut butter

¾ teaspoon oregano

¾ teaspoon salt

1 cup frozen corn kernels

1 In a nonstick Dutch oven or flameproof casserole, heat the oil over medium heat. Add the onion, bell pepper, and garlic, and cook, stirring, until the onion is soft, about 7 minutes.

2 Add the potatoes and water. Cover and cook until firm-tender, about 10 minutes.

3 Add the squash, tomatoes and their juice, black beans, peanut butter, oregano, and salt. Stir to combine. Bring to a boil, reduce to a simmer, cover, and cook until the squash and potatoes are tender, about 10 minutes.

4 Stir in the corn and cook until the corn is heated through, about 2 minutes. *Makes 4 servings*

per serving: 313 calories, 8.6g total fat (1.5g saturated), 0mg cholesterol, 15g dietary fiber, 51g carbohydrate, 15g protein, 712mg sodium. **good source of:** fiber, folate, magnesium, niacin, potassium, thiamin, vitamin B$_6$, vitamin C.

Summer Squash Parmesan

The problem with most baked dishes called "Parmesan" or "alla Parmigiana" is that the breaded ingredients are invariably pan-fried in a good deal of oil (or butter) before being layered with cheese and baked. The more healthful solution is to bake rather than fry the breaded ingredients. **Serving suggestion:** Serve this with a green salad.

1 cup plain dried breadcrumbs

⅓ cup grated Parmesan cheese

1 teaspoon grated lemon zest

¼ teaspoon pepper

4 large egg whites

¼ cup water

¾ pound yellow summer squash, cut lengthwise into ½-inch-thick slabs

¾ pound zucchini, cut lengthwise into ½-inch-thick slabs

1 can (14½ ounces) stewed tomatoes, chopped with their juice

1 can (8 ounces) tomato sauce

3 tablespoons tomato paste

½ cup shredded part-skim mozzarella

1 Preheat the oven to 400°F. Spray a large baking sheet with nonstick cooking spray.

2 In a shallow bowl, combine the breadcrumbs, Parmesan, lemon zest, and pepper. In another shallow bowl, beat the egg whites with the water. Dip the yellow squash and zucchini first in the egg white mixture, then in the breadcrumb mixture, patting on the crumb mixture.

3 Place the yellow squash and zucchini on the prepared baking sheet and bake for about 20 minutes, turning them over after 10 minutes, until crispy and golden brown.

4 Meanwhile, in a small bowl, combine the stewed tomatoes and their juice, tomato sauce, and tomato paste. Spray a 7 x 11-inch baking dish with nonstick cooking spray. Place half of the baked squash in a single layer in the dish. Spoon half of the tomato mixture over the squash. Top with the remaining squash and remaining tomato mixture.

5 Bake, covered, for 10 minutes. Uncover and sprinkle the mozzarella over the top. Bake for 10 minutes, or until piping hot and bubbling. *Makes 4 servings*

per serving: 277 calories, 6.1g total fat (3.1g saturated), 13mg cholesterol, 7g dietary fiber, 40g carbohydrate, 17g protein, 589mg sodium. good source of: calcium, potassium, riboflavin, selenium, thiamin, vitamin C.

Tex-Mex Butternut Stew

The texture of the bulgur gives the impression that there's meat in this hearty stew. **Serving suggestion:** Serve the stew topped with plain fat-free yogurt and a sprinkling of cilantro and scallions, if you like.

½ cup bulgur

1 cup boiling water

1 tablespoon olive oil

1 large onion, cut into ½-inch chunks

3 cloves garlic, minced

2 red bell peppers, cut into ½-inch squares

1 pound butternut squash or sweet potato, peeled and cut into ½-inch cubes

1 tablespoon chili powder

1 teaspoon cumin

1 teaspoon cinnamon

½ teaspoon salt

1¾ cups cooked chick-peas (page 180) or canned (rinsed and drained)

1 can (14½ ounces) no-salt-added diced tomatoes

1 In a small heatproof bowl, combine the bulgur and boiling water. Set aside to soak while you prepare the rest of the stew.

2 In a nonstick Dutch oven or large saucepan, heat the oil over medium heat. Add the onion and garlic, and cook, stirring, until the onion is soft, about 7 minutes.

3 Add the bell peppers and cook, stirring, until the peppers are crisp-tender, about 5 minutes.

4 Add the butternut squash and cook, stirring, until the squash begins to soften, about 4 minutes.

5 Add the chili powder, cumin, cinnamon, and salt, stirring to combine. Add the chick-peas and the tomatoes and their juice, and bring to a boil.

6 Drain the bulgur and add to the pan. Reduce to a simmer, cover, and cook until the squash is tender, the chili is slightly thickened, and the flavors are blended, about 7 minutes. *Makes 4 servings*

per serving: 485 calories, 9g total fat (1.1g saturated), 0mg cholesterol, 25g dietary fiber, 88g carbohydrate, 20g protein, 526mg sodium. **good source of:** beta carotene, fiber, folate, magnesium, niacin, potassium, thiamin, vitamin B$_6$, vitamin C, vitamin E, zinc.

Multigrain Pilaf with Beans & Greens

This grain-based meatless main course could also serve 8 as a side dish.

> 3¾ cups water
> 1½ teaspoons grated lemon zest
> ¾ teaspoon salt
> 1 cup brown basmati rice
> ½ cup pearl barley
> 1 tablespoon olive oil
> 1 small red onion, finely chopped
> 4 cloves garlic, minced
> 1¾ cups cooked black beans (page 180) or canned (rinsed and drained)
> 12 cups shredded Swiss chard or kale
> ¼ cup dried currants

1 In a large saucepan, bring the water, lemon zest, and salt to a boil over medium heat. Add the brown rice and barley, reduce to a simmer, cover, and cook until tender, 35 to 40 minutes. Drain any remaining liquid.

2 Meanwhile, in a large nonstick skillet, heat the oil over medium heat. Add the onion and garlic and cook, stirring frequently, until the onion is soft, about 7 minutes.

3 Stir in the beans and Swiss chard, cover, and cook until the chard is tender, about 7 minutes.

4 Stir the black beans and Swiss chard into the rice-barley mixture along with the currants. *Makes 4 servings*

per serving: 421 calories, 5.8g total fat (0.6g saturated), 0mg cholesterol, 13g dietary fiber, 81g carbohydrate, 14g protein, 615mg sodium. **good source of:** fiber, folate, magnesium, potassium.

Jasmine Rice Salad

Jasmine rice is a traditional Thai rice variety and one of the so-called aromatic rices, which have a distinctive nutty flavor. If you can't find jasmine, substitute basmati, Texmati, or pecan rice.

> 1⅓ cups jasmine rice
> ¾ teaspoon salt
> 1 cup plain fat-free yogurt
> 3 tablespoons fresh lemon juice
> 1 tablespoon light mayonnaise
> ¾ cup crumbled feta cheese (3 ounces)
> 3 tablespoons minced fresh dill
> 2 tablespoons chopped fresh mint
> 1 cup cherry tomatoes, halved
> 2 Granny Smith apples, cut into ½-inch cubes
> ⅓ cup hulled pumpkin seeds (pepitas)
> ⅓ cup raisins

1 In a medium saucepan, cook the rice according to package directions, using ½ teaspoon of the salt.

2 In a large bowl, whisk together the yogurt, lemon juice, mayonnaise, feta cheese, dill, mint, and the remaining ¼ teaspoon salt.

3 Add the rice and fluff with a fork. Add the tomatoes, apples, pumpkin seeds, and raisins, and toss to combine. Serve warm or at room temperature. *Makes 4 servings*

per serving: 473 calories, 11g total fat (4.4g saturated), 21mg cholesterol, 4g dietary fiber, 81g carbohydrate, 14g protein, 756mg sodium. **good source of:** riboflavin, vitamin B$_{12}$.

Lentil, Goat Cheese & Beet Salad

You can either use homemade roast beets (*start with ¾ pound uncooked beets and see cooking times in "Vegetable Cooking Chart," page 174*) or canned beets.

> 3 cups water
>
> 3 cloves garlic, minced
>
> 1½ teaspoons grated lemon zest
>
> 1 teaspoon tarragon
>
> ¾ teaspoon salt
>
> 1½ cups lentils
>
> ⅓ cup fresh lemon juice
>
> 4 teaspoons olive oil
>
> 4 teaspoons Dijon mustard
>
> 1 red bell pepper, diced
>
> 1½ cups diced cooked beets
>
> 6 cups mixed greens or watercress
>
> ½ cup crumbled goat cheese or feta cheese (2 ounces)
>
> 2 tablespoons coarsely chopped pecans

1 In a medium saucepan, combine the water, garlic, lemon zest, tarragon, and salt, and bring to a boil over high heat. Add the lentils. Reduce to a simmer, cover, and cook until firm-tender, about 25 minutes. Drain off any liquid remaining.

2 In a medium bowl, combine the lemon juice, oil, and mustard. Add the lentils, bell pepper, and beets, tossing until well coated.

3 Mound the lentil salad on a bed of greens and sprinkle with the goat cheese and pecans. *Makes 4 servings*

different spins

▶**Spinach & Lentil Salad** Follow the directions for *Lentil, Goat Cheese & Beet Salad*, but substitute ½ teaspoon of thyme for the tarragon. Omit the beets and add 1½ cups halved seedless red grapes. Substitute small spinach leaves for the mixed greens. Add the spinach to the bowl and toss with the warm lentils.

per serving: 403 calories, 12g total fat (3g saturated), 7mg cholesterol, 26g dietary fiber, 54g carbohydrate, 26g protein, 758mg sodium. good source of: fiber, folate, magnesium, potassium, riboflavin, thiamin, vitamin B$_6$, vitamin C, zinc.

Panzanella

Panzanella is a Tuscan salad designed to make good use of stale bread (we re-create the dryness of the bread by toasting it). If you like, add a seeded and sliced cucumber or replace the plum tomatoes with halved grape or cherry tomatoes. **Timing alert:** The salad needs to be refrigerated for at least 1 hour to chill before serving.

> 8 ounces whole-wheat Italian bread, halved lengthwise
>
> 3 bell peppers, mixed colors, roasted (page 190)
>
> ⅓ cup balsamic vinegar
>
> 1 tablespoon olive oil
>
> 1 clove garlic, minced
>
> ¾ teaspoon salt
>
> ½ teaspoon black pepper
>
> 1 pound plum tomatoes, cut into ½-inch chunks
>
> 3 tablespoons chopped fresh basil
>
> 4 ounces part-skim mozzarella, cut into ½-inch cubes

1 Preheat the broiler. Broil the bread 4 to 6 inches from the heat until lightly toasted, about 1 minute. Cut into 1-inch cubes. Transfer the bread to a large bowl and sprinkle with enough cold water to thoroughly moisten. Let stand 10 minutes, then gently squeeze to get rid of any excess water.

2 Roast the peppers as directed on page 190, and when cool enough to handle, peel them and cut into ½-inch pieces.

3 In a large bowl, whisk together the vinegar, oil, garlic, salt, and black pepper. Add the bread cubes, roasted peppers, tomatoes, basil, and mozzarella, and toss well.

4 Refrigerate for at least 1 hour or up to 4 hours before serving. *Makes 4 servings*

per serving: 323 calories, 10g total fat (3.7g saturated), 16mg cholesterol, 5g dietary fiber, 45g carbohydrate, 14g protein, 917mg sodium. good source of: beta carotene, selenium, thiamin, vitamin C.

Strawberry, Mango & Lentil Salad with Balsamic Dressing

The combination of fragrant mango, silky avocado, sweet-tart strawberries and tomatoes, and peppery-savory lentils in a balsamic dressing makes this a multidimensional salad.

- 1 cup lentils
- 1/3 cup balsamic vinegar
- 4 teaspoons olive oil
- 3/4 teaspoon salt
- 1/2 teaspoon pepper
- 1 pint strawberries, quartered
- 2 cups grape tomatoes or small cherry tomatoes, halved
- 2 medium mangoes, pitted, peeled, and cut into 1/2-inch chunks (2 cups)
- 1 small Hass avocado, pitted, peeled, and cut into 1/2-inch chunks (3/4 cup)

1 In a large pot of boiling water, cook the lentils until tender but not mushy, about 25 minutes. Drain.

2 Meanwhile, in a large bowl, whisk together the vinegar, oil, salt, and pepper. Add the warm lentils and toss to combine.

3 Add the strawberries, tomatoes, mangoes, and avocado, and toss again. Serve at room temperature or chilled. *Makes 4 servings*

per serving: 355 calories, 10g total fat (1.5g saturated), 0mg cholesterol, 21g dietary fiber, 56g carbohydrate, 16g protein, 458mg sodium. good source of: beta carotene, fiber, folate, potassium, thiamin, vitamin B$_6$, vitamin C.

Quinoa & Corn Salad

Rinsing quinoa before cooking removes some of its slightly bitter, green taste. The enoki mushrooms—found at many supermarkets—contribute a satisfying chewy texture to the salad.

- 4 teaspoons olive oil
- 4 scallions, thinly sliced
- 5 cloves garlic, minced
- 1 3/4 cups quinoa
- 3 1/2 cups boiling water
- 1 teaspoon salt
- 1/2 teaspoon pepper
- 1/3 cup fresh lime juice
- 2 packages (3 1/2 ounces each) enoki mushrooms, tough ends removed
- 1 package (10 ounces) frozen corn kernels, thawed
- 2 tablespoons hulled pumpkin seeds (pepitas)
- 1/4 cup chopped fresh basil

1 In a nonstick Dutch oven, heat 2 teaspoons of the oil over medium-low heat. Add the scallions and garlic, and cook, stirring occasionally, until the scallions are tender, about 2 minutes.

2 Rinse the quinoa under cold water and drain. Add the quinoa to the pan and cook, stirring occasionally, for 2 minutes.

3 Add the boiling water, salt, and pepper, and return to a boil. Reduce to a simmer, cover, and cook until no liquid remains and the quinoa is tender, about 12 minutes.

4 Transfer the quinoa to a large bowl and add the remaining 2 teaspoons oil and the lime juice. Stir to combine. Add the enoki mushrooms, corn, pumpkin seeds, and basil, and stir to combine. Serve at room temperature or chilled. *Makes 4 servings*

per serving: 434 calories, 12g total fat (1.5g saturated), 0mg cholesterol, 8g dietary fiber, 74g carbohydrate, 15g protein, 604mg sodium. good source of: fiber, magnesium, niacin, potassium, riboflavin, saponins, vitamin E, zinc.

Black-Eyed Pea & Shiitake Salad

For a chewier texture, you could make this with brown rice instead of white rice: In step 1, cook the brown rice about 25 minutes before adding the black-eyed peas.

4 cups water

1 cup rice

1 teaspoon salt

1 package (10 ounces) frozen black-eyed peas

2 tablespoons olive oil

¾ cup fresh lemon juice

1 tablespoon Dijon mustard

¾ teaspoon pepper

1 pound shiitake mushrooms, stems discarded and caps thinly sliced

1 teaspoon tarragon

½ pound sugar snap peas, strings removed

4 scallions, thinly sliced

1 In a medium saucepan, bring the water to a boil. Add the rice and ¼ teaspoon of the salt. Reduce to a simmer, cover, and cook for 5 minutes. Add the black-eyed peas, cover, and simmer until the rice and black-eyed peas are tender, about 15 minutes. Drain any liquid remaining in the pan.

2 Meanwhile, in a large bowl, whisk together 1 tablespoon of the olive oil, the remaining ¾ teaspoon salt, the lemon juice, mustard, and pepper. When the rice and peas have finished cooking, add them to the bowl and toss to combine.

3 In a large nonstick skillet, heat the remaining 1 tablespoon oil over medium heat. Add the mushrooms and tarragon, cover, and cook until the mushrooms are tender, about 5 minutes.

4 Add the sugar snaps and cook, uncovered, until tender, about 3 minutes. Add to the bowl. Add the scallions to the bowl and toss again. Serve at room temperature or chilled. *Makes 4 servings*

per serving: 402 calories, 8g total fat (1.2g saturated), 0mg cholesterol, 8g dietary fiber, 69g carbohydrate, 14g protein, 707mg sodium. good source of: beta glucan, fiber, thiamin, vitamin C.

Sweet & Spicy Broiled Tofu

Here's a recipe for those who still insist that tofu dishes are flavorless. **Timing alert:** The tofu needs to marinate for at least 6 hours.

15 ounces extra-firm tofu

⅓ cup reduced-sodium soy sauce

2 tablespoons fresh lemon juice

4 teaspoons dark brown sugar

1 teaspoon dark sesame oil

1 tablespoon grated fresh ginger

2 cloves garlic, peeled and smashed

2 teaspoons Dijon mustard

4 scallions, thinly sliced

1 Slice the block of tofu horizontally in half, then cut each piece in half crosswise. Place on paper towels to drain while you prepare the marinade.

2 In a shallow container large enough to hold the tofu in a single layer, stir together the soy sauce, lemon juice, brown sugar, sesame oil, ginger, garlic, and mustard.

3 Add the tofu, cover, and refrigerate for at least 6 hours, turning the tofu over midway.

4 Line a broiler pan with foil. Preheat the broiler. Lift the tofu from the marinade, reserving any leftover. Place the tofu on the broiler pan and spoon any leftover marinade over the tofu. Broil 4 to 6 inches from the heat for 5 minutes per side, or until richly browned.

5 Serve topped with the sliced scallions. *Makes 4 servings*

per serving: 205 calories, 11g total fat (1.5g saturated), 0mg cholesterol, 3g dietary fiber, 13g carbohydrate, 18g protein, 786mg sodium. good source of: calcium, isoflavones, selenium.

Crispy Pan-Fried Tofu

The chili sauce used here is the mildly hot, tomato-based type that you can find right next to the ketchup on the supermarket shelf. Don't confuse it with Asian chili sauces, which can be searingly hot. **Serving suggestion:** To round out the meal, serve the tofu with a bowl of Sushi Rice Salad (*page 207*) and Cucumber Salad (*page 202*). For dessert, Mexican Chocolate Angel Food Cake (*page 242*).

15 ounces extra-firm tofu

1 large egg white

2 tablespoons chili sauce

1 tablespoon water

½ cup plain dried breadcrumbs

1 tablespoon sesame seeds

½ teaspoon salt

3 tablespoons cornstarch

4 teaspoons olive oil

1 Slice the block of tofu horizontally in half. Cut each half into 4 squares. Place on paper towels to drain.

2 In a shallow bowl, whisk together the egg white, chili sauce, and water. In a separate bowl, stir together the breadcrumbs, sesame seeds, and salt. Place the cornstarch on a sheet of wax paper or on a small plate.

3 Dip the tofu first in the cornstarch, then in the chili sauce mixture, and finally in the breadcrumb mixture, patting it on.

4 In a large nonstick skillet, heat the oil over medium heat. Add the tofu and cook until golden brown, crisp, and heated through, about 3 minutes per side. *Makes 4 servings*

per serving: 297 calories, 16g total fat (2.3g saturated), 0mg cholesterol, 3g dietary fiber, 22g carbohydrate, 20g protein, 551mg sodium. **good source of:** calcium, isoflavones, selenium, thiamin.

Cuban-Style Tofu Stew

Ropa vieja—a Cuban shredded beef dish whose name translates as "old clothes"—was the inspiration for this stew. Here, we've taken the liberty of making it with storebought baked tofu, which absorbs the wonderful flavors of the sauce. It's best to use an unflavored baked tofu; but failing that, try to find one with Tex-Mex or mesquite flavors.

2 teaspoons olive oil

1 medium onion, finely chopped

5 cloves garlic, minced

1 red bell pepper, cut into 1-inch chunks

1 green bell pepper, cut into 1-inch chunks

12 ounces baked tofu, cut into ½-inch cubes

½ cup dry red wine

1 can (14½ ounces) diced tomatoes

½ cup chopped cilantro

2 canned or bottled jalapeño peppers, minced

1 tablespoon semisweet chocolate chips

2 tablespoons prune butter (lekvar)

½ teaspoon salt

1 In a nonstick Dutch oven or flameproof casserole, heat the oil over medium heat. Add the onion and garlic, and cook, stirring frequently, until the onion is soft, about 7 minutes.

2 Stir in the bell peppers, and cook, stirring frequently, until the peppers are crisp-tender, about 5 minutes.

3 Add the tofu and stir to combine. Add the wine and cook until evaporated, about 3 minutes.

4 Stir in the tomatoes, ¼ cup of the cilantro, the jalapeños, chocolate, prune butter, and salt, and bring to a boil. Reduce to a simmer. Cover and cook until the sauce is richly flavored and slightly thickened, about 20 minutes. Stir in the remaining ¼ cup cilantro. *Makes 4 servings*

per serving: 282 calories, 11g total fat (2g saturated), 0mg cholesterol, 5g dietary fiber, 27g carbohydrate, 18g protein, 727mg sodium. **good source of:** isoflavones, vitamin C.

Shiitake, Tofu & Bok Choy Stir-Fry

If you find get bok choy, you can approximate the combination of textures and flavors of this Asian vegetable by using 8 ounces of napa cabbage and 4 ounces of Swiss chard instead. **Serving suggestion:** Serve this satisfying stir-fry over a bowl of brown rice.

>   15 ounces extra-firm tofu
>
>   ½ cup apple cider or juice
>
>   2 tablespoons plus 1 teaspoon reduced-sodium soy sauce
>
>   2 tablespoons cider vinegar
>
>   1½ teaspoons cornstarch
>
>   2 teaspoons olive oil
>
>   ¾ pound shiitake mushrooms, stems discarded and caps quartered
>
>   1 carrot, halved lengthwise and thinly sliced crosswise
>
>   ¼ teaspoon salt
>
>   ½ cup water
>
>   1 head bok choy (¾ pound), sliced crosswise into 1-inch-wide strips
>
>   5 scallions, thinly sliced
>
>   4 cloves garlic, minced

1 Slice the block of tofu horizontally in half, then cut each piece into 12 cubes. Place the tofu on paper towels to drain while you continue with the preparation.

2 In a small bowl, stir together the apple cider, soy sauce, vinegar, and cornstarch. Set aside.

3 In a large nonstick skillet, heat the oil over medium heat. Add the shiitakes, carrot, and salt, and stir until well combined. Add the water and cook until the carrot and mushrooms are firm-tender, about 5 minutes.

4 Add the bok choy, and cook, stirring frequently, until tender, about 5 minutes. Add the scallions and garlic, and cook until the scallions are tender, about 1 minute.

5 Add the tofu. Stir the cider mixture to recombine and add it to the pan. Cook until the tofu is heated through and the sauce is slightly thickened, about 2 minutes. *Makes 4 servings*

per serving: 188 calories, 9g total fat (1.3g saturated), 0mg cholesterol, 4g dietary fiber, 16g carbohydrate, 15g protein, 196mg sodium. **good source of:** beta carotene, beta glucan, calcium, indoles, isoflavones, vitamin C.

different spins

▶ **"Spaghetti" Picadillo** Make the *Vegetarian Picadillo (opposite page)* and use it as a "pasta" sauce to serve over spaghetti squash. To cook spaghetti squash, preheat the oven to 400°F. With a fork or a small paring knife, prick the skin of a 2½- to 3-pound spaghetti squash all over. Wrap the squash in foil and place it on a baking sheet. Bake for 1 hour 15 minutes, or until the squash is soft to the touch. Remove from the oven and let cool in the foil. When cool enough to handle, halve the squash, scoop out and discard the seeds. With a fork, pull out the spaghetti-like strands. Mound the spaghetti squash on a plate and top with the picadillo.

▶ **Mushroom, Tofu & Broccoli Rabe Stir-Fry** Follow the directions for *Shiitake, Tofu & Bok Choy Stir-Fry*, but substitute ¾ pound of cremini, portobello, or fresh porcini mushrooms for the shiitake. Substitute 1 large bunch of broccoli rabe for the bok choy. Trim off the ends of the broccoli rabe and cut the remainder into small pieces. Add ¼ teaspoon red pepper flakes when adding the broccoli rabe in step 4, and cook for about 10 minutes, or until the broccoli rabe is tender.

meat substitutes

For those who miss the chewy texture of meat (or who don't miss meat at all but like chewy texture), there are a number of plant-based ingredients that are designed to be like meat. Although some of these products are seasoned and formed to make meat look-alikes ("not-dogs" and mock chicken nuggets, for example), you can also buy these meat substitutes in their "natural" state and incorporate them into recipes for their texture. The most commonly available are tempeh and TVP.

Tempeh (pronounced "TEHM-pay") is a flat, fermented soybean cake, which is rich in protein and is commonly found at health-food stores. To make tempeh, whole soybeans are mixed with grains, usually rice or millet, and then incubated with a starter, which begins the process of fermentation. Tempeh has a nutty, yeasty flavor.

TVP, which stands for Texturized Vegetable Protein, is technically called TSP (Texturized Soy Protein), though most stores sell it under its more familiar name of TVP. Derived from isolated protein extracted from soybeans, TVP is a nutritious substance, low in fat and rich in protein. It is a highly versatile ingredient that absorbs flavors well and is available in powder form, chunks, slices, and granules.

Vegetarian Picadillo

Found in a number of Spanish-speaking countries, *picadillo* is a chopped meat stew that often includes olives and raisins. In this vegetarian version, TVP granules stand in for the meat. Like most stews, it's even better reheated and served the next day. **Serving suggestion:** Serve the stew over a mound of brown rice or pasta.

1¼ cups water
1 cup TVP granules
2 teaspoons olive oil
1 small red onion, finely chopped
3 cloves garlic, minced
2 cups cubes (1-inch) butternut squash (12 ounces)
½ pound green beans, halved crosswise
2 cans (14½ ounces) no-salt-added stewed tomatoes, chopped with their juice
⅓ cup raisins
¼ cup pitted green olives, coarsely chopped
¾ teaspoon salt
½ teaspoon oregano
⅛ teaspoon cayenne pepper

1 In a large bowl, stir together ¾ cup of the water and the TVP until well combined. Let stand for 10 minutes to soften.

2 Meanwhile, in a nonstick Dutch oven or flame-proof casserole, heat the oil over medium heat. Add the onion and garlic, and cook, stirring frequently, until the onion is soft, about 7 minutes. Stir in the TVP until well coated.

3 Add the remaining ½ cup water, the butternut squash, green beans, stewed tomatoes and their juice, raisins, olives, salt, oregano, and cayenne, and bring to a boil. Reduce to a simmer, cover, and cook until the butternut squash and green beans are tender, about 20 minutes. *Makes 4 servings*

per serving: 253 calories, 4.5g total fat (0.6g saturated), 0mg cholesterol, 13g dietary fiber, 44g carbohydrate, 16g protein, 812mg sodium. good source of: beta carotene, fiber, folate, magnesium, potassium, vitamin C.

Meatless Burgers

These burgers combine mushrooms, pinto beans, and tempeh to make a satisfying burger with no meat. Tempeh, like other soyfoods, readily absorbs the flavors of the ingredients with which it's cooked.

2 teaspoons olive oil

2 tablespoons water

½ pound portobello mushrooms, finely chopped

1 cup cooked pinto beans (page 180) or canned (rinsed and drained)

3 tablespoons reduced-sodium soy sauce

2 teaspoons Worcestershire sauce

12 ounces tempeh

¼ cup chili sauce

1 In a large nonstick skillet, heat the oil and water over medium heat. Add the mushrooms and cook, stirring frequently, until the mushrooms are very tender, about 5 minutes.

2 In a large bowl, combine the pinto beans, soy sauce, and Worcestershire sauce, and mash with a potato masher. Stir in the mushrooms.

3 Grate the tempeh on the large holes of a box grater. (Or, finely chop it with a knife.) Stir the tempeh into the mushroom mixture until well combined. Shape the mixture into 4 patties.

4 Spray the broiler pan with nonstick cooking spray. Preheat the broiler. Broil the burgers 4 to 6 inches from the heat for 5 minutes. Turn the burgers over and brush the tops with the chili sauce. Broil for 3 to 5 minutes, or until the burgers are heated through. *Makes 4 servings*

per serving: 255 calories, 7.1g total fat (1.9g saturated), 0mg cholesterol, 10g dietary fiber, 26g carbohydrate, 24g protein, 669mg sodium. good source of: fiber, isoflavones, riboflavin.

Tempeh & Sweet Potatoes in Barbecue Sauce

Tempeh's sturdy, chewy texture makes it well suited to slow cooking. **Serving suggestion:** Serve with squares of Oniony Cornbread (*page 218*) and a tossed salad of red onion and shredded romaine with Orange-Balsamic Dressing (*page 254*).

2 teaspoons olive oil

1 small onion, finely chopped

3 cloves garlic, minced

1 can (28 ounces) tomatoes, chopped with their juice

1 tablespoon balsamic vinegar

1 tablespoon molasses

1 tablespoon light brown sugar

½ teaspoon ground ginger

½ teaspoon salt

8 ounces tempeh, cut into ½-inch chunks

¾ pound sweet potatoes, peeled and cut into 1-inch chunks

1 In a nonstick Dutch oven, heat the oil over medium heat. Add the onion and garlic, and cook, stirring frequently, until the onion is soft, about 7 minutes.

2 Add the tomatoes and their juice, the vinegar, molasses, brown sugar, ginger, and salt, and bring to a boil.

3 Add the tempeh, reduce to a simmer, cover, and cook for 20 minutes.

4 Add the sweet potatoes, cover, and cook until tender, about 20 minutes. *Makes 4 servings*

per serving: 277 calories, 8.9g total fat (1.7g saturated), 0mg cholesterol, 7g dietary fiber, 40g carbohydrate, 14g protein, 603mg sodium. good source of: beta carotene, potassium, riboflavin, vitamin B$_6$, vitamin C.

Creamy Polenta with Meatless Ragù

Polenta (cornmeal) can be cooked until quite firm—you may have seen logs of precooked, firm polenta in the refrigerated section of Italian markets—or it can be cooked until soft and creamy, as here. Creamy-style polenta makes a good base for toppings. In place of the meatless sauce used here, you could also try spooning chili on top.

¾ cup TVP granules

4½ cups water

2 teaspoons olive oil

1 small red onion, finely chopped

3 cloves garlic, minced

2 cans (14½ ounces each) no-salt-added diced tomatoes

1 teaspoon salt

1 cup yellow cornmeal

¼ teaspoon cayenne pepper

⅔ cup grated Parmesan cheese

½ cup plain fat-free yogurt

1 In a medium bowl, combine the TVP with 1 cup of the water. Let stand 10 minutes to soften.

2 In a large nonstick skillet, heat the oil over medium heat. Add the onion and garlic, and cook, stirring frequently, until the onion is soft, about 7 minutes.

3 Add the TVP, stirring to combine. Add the tomatoes and ½ teaspoon of the salt, and bring to a boil. Reduce to a simmer and cook until slightly thickened and richly flavored, about 20 minutes.

4 Meanwhile, in a small bowl, stir the cornmeal and 1 cup of the cold water until blended and smooth.

5 In a medium saucepan, bring the remaining 2½ cups of water, remaining ½ teaspoon salt, and the cayenne to a simmer over low heat. Stirring constantly, pour in the cornmeal-water mixture. Cook the cornmeal over low heat, stirring constantly, until thick and creamy, about 10 minutes.

6 Remove from the heat. Stir in the Parmesan cheese and yogurt. Serve the polenta in a mound, with the sauce spooned into the center. *Makes 4 servings*

per serving: 290 calories, 7g total fat (3g saturated), 11mg cholesterol, 7g dietary fiber, 44g carbohydrate, 15g protein, 935mg sodium. good source of: calcium.

Bow-Ties with Mushroom Sauce

The earthy flavor of mushrooms and the chewy texture of TVP are used to create a pasta dish that even diehard carnivores will find satisfying.

½ cup dried porcini mushrooms (½ ounce)

3 cups boiling water

10 ounces bow-tie pasta

1 tablespoon olive oil

1 medium onion, finely chopped

3 cloves garlic, minced

¾ pound fresh shiitake mushrooms, stems discarded and caps thinly sliced

¾ cup TVP granules

3 tablespoons tomato paste

1 teaspoon salt

¾ teaspoon pepper

½ teaspoon rosemary, minced

⅓ cup grated Parmesan cheese

1 In a small heatproof bowl, combine the dried mushrooms and the boiling water, and let stand for 20 minutes, or until softened. Reserving the soaking liquid, scoop out the dried mushrooms and coarsely chop. Strain the soaking liquid through a coffee filter or a paper towel-lined sieve.

2 In a large pot of boiling water, cook the pasta according to package directions. Drain and place in a large bowl.

3 Meanwhile, in a large nonstick skillet, heat the oil over medium heat. Add the onion and garlic, and cook, stirring frequently, until the onion is soft, about 7 minutes.

4 Add the softened porcini mushrooms, ½ cup of their soaking liquid, and the shiitake mushrooms, and cook, stirring frequently, until the mushrooms are tender, about 5 minutes.

5 Add the remaining mushroom soaking liquid, the TVP, tomato paste, salt, pepper, and rosemary, and bring to a boil. Reduce to a simmer and cook, uncovered, stirring occasionally, until the sauce is slightly thickened and richly flavored, about 10 minutes.

6 Add the sauce and Parmesan to the drained pasta and toss to combine. *Makes 4 servings*

per serving: 356 calories, 7.2g total fat (2.2g saturated), 7mg cholesterol, 5g dietary fiber, 57g carbohydrate, 17g protein, 836mg sodium. good source of: beta glucan, folate, selenium, thiamin.

eggs

Eggs can be part of a sensible "meatless" diet. They are a good source of protein, as well as vitamin B_{12}, iron and good amounts of the mineral selenium. On the downside, eggs have huge amounts of dietary cholesterol. The American Heart Association recommends that healthy people consume less than 300 mg of cholesterol a day from all sources. Eggs average 215 mg each. If you're healthy and know that your cholesterol is at a desirable level, you can eat an egg a day. But be sure to have your cholesterol level tested to make sure it doesn't shoot up (the response to dietary cholesterol varies from person to person, depending largely on genetic factors).

There are a couple of good tricks for making egg dishes that don't tip the cholesterol scales. One is to use eggs as a binder for other healthful ingredients, rather than as the centerpiece of a dish. A good example of that is a frittata (*see the "Recipe Creator," opposite page*).

The other trick is to use a combination of whole eggs and egg whites. A small amount of egg yolk (where all of the cholesterol resides) is all it takes to give egg flavor to an egg mixture such as that in scrambled eggs, frittatas, and even omelets. For example, in Scrambled Eggs with Asparagus & Potatoes (*below*), 2 whole eggs and 5 egg whites combine to provide only a little more than 100 mg of cholesterol per serving.

Scrambled Eggs with Asparagus & Potatoes

Stirring eggs over low heat produces creamy scrambled eggs. To keep saturated fat and cholesterol levels reasonable, a combination of whole eggs and egg whites is used here.

> 1 pound asparagus, cut into 1-inch lengths
>
> ¾ pound red potatoes, cut into ¼-inch cubes
>
> 2 teaspoons olive oil
>
> 2 scallions, thinly sliced
>
> 2 large eggs
>
> 5 large egg whites
>
> ½ cup low-fat (1%) cottage cheese
>
> 3 tablespoons grated Parmesan cheese
>
> 2 teaspoons flour
>
> ½ teaspoon salt
>
> ½ teaspoon tarragon
>
> ¼ teaspoon pepper

1 In a vegetable steamer, cook the asparagus until crisp-tender, about 3 minutes. Remove. Add the potatoes to the steamer and cook until firm-tender, about 4 minutes. Drain well.

recipe creator
meatless frittatas

A frittata is an Italian egg pancake, somewhat like an omelet, but with the balance of ingredients shifted significantly toward the filling and away from the egg. Pick ingredients from the categories below and follow these basic instructions. Beat 5 whole eggs, 7 egg whites, and ½ teaspoon salt. Mix in 1 HERB. In a large nonstick broilerproof skillet, heat 1 tablespoon of olive or canola oil over medium heat. Add 2½ cups of VEGETABLES (all one type or a combination) and 1½ cups of CARBO-HYDRATE (choose just one). Pour the egg mixture over the filling; sprinkle with 1 CHEESE (if desired). Reduce the heat to low. Cook, without stirring, until the sides are set but the center is still slightly wet, about 15 minutes. Once the frittata is mostly set, preheat the broiler. Run the skillet under the broiler for 2 minutes to cook the center and puff the frittata. Cut into wedges to serve. *Makes 6 servings*

HERBS	VEGETABLES	CARBOHYDRATE	CHEESE*
▶Fresh basil, 2 Tbsp minced	▶Asparagus, diced cooked	▶White beans, cooked	▶Parmesan cheese, ⅓ cup grated
▶Fresh dill, 2 Tbsp minced	▶Green beans, diced cooked	▶Lentils, cooked	▶Reduced-fat Cheddar cheese, ½ cup shredded
▶Fresh mint, 2 Tbsp minced	▶Broccoli, chopped cooked	▶Pasta, cooked	▶Feta cheese, ⅓ cup crumbled
▶Dried oregano, ¼ tsp	▶Spinach, chopped cooked	▶Brown or white rice, cooked	▶Soft goat cheese, ⅓ cup crumbled
▶Dried rosemary, ¼ tsp minced	▶Red or green bell peppers, diced cooked	▶Sweet or white potatoes, diced cooked	
▶Dried thyme, ¼ tsp		▶Peas, thawed	*optional

2 In a large nonstick skillet, heat the oil over medium heat. Add the cooked potatoes and scallions and cook until the scallions are tender, about 2 minutes.

3 Meanwhile, in a food processor, blender, or with an electric mixer, combine the whole eggs, egg whites, cottage cheese, Parmesan, flour, salt, tarragon, and pepper, and process until smooth.

4 Add the asparagus to the skillet, stirring to coat. Add the egg mixture, reduce the heat to low, and cook, stirring, until the eggs are just set, about 7 minutes. *Makes 4 servings*

per serving: 204 calories, 6.7g total fat (2.2g saturated), 111mg cholesterol, 3g dietary fiber, 20g carbohydrate, 16g protein, 603mg sodium. good source of: folate, riboflavin, selenium, vitamin B_{12}.

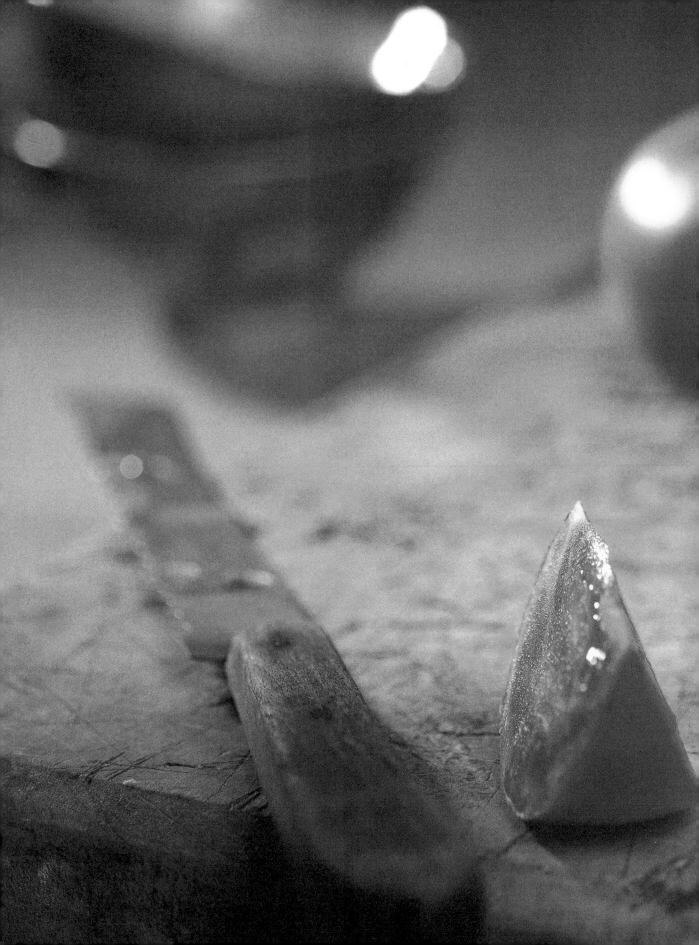

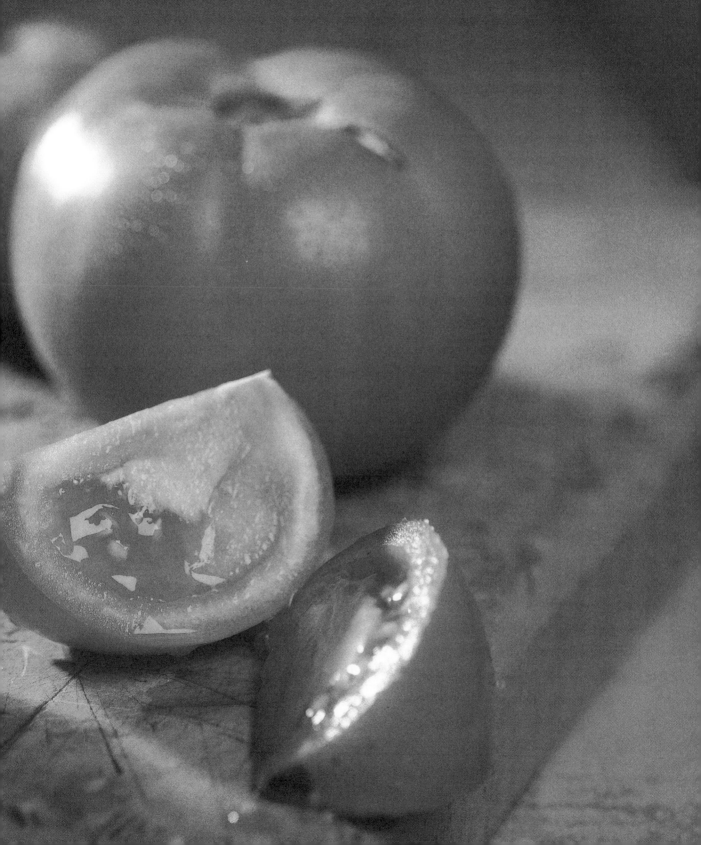

side dishes

grains

In most countries of the world, grains and grain products—flour, bread, cereal, and pasta—are the chief forms of sustenance. They provide about 50% of the world's calories and indirectly contribute much of the other half, since grains are also fed to the animals from which we get meat, eggs, and dairy products.

Between 65% and 90% of the calories in grains come from carbohydrates (mostly complex). Grains are also rich in both soluble fiber (the kind that lowers blood-cholesterol levels) and insoluble (the kind that helps to prevent constipation and help protect against some forms of cancer). Moreover, grains—especially whole grains—and grain products offer significant amounts of B vitamins (riboflavin, thiamin, and niacin), vitamin E, iron, zinc, calcium, selenium, and magnesium.

All grains need to be cooked in a liquid to make them edible. Unlike pasta, which is cooked in large quantities of water, grains are cooked in just the amount of liquid necessary to soften and plump them. This also preserves the grains' considerable B vitamin content, which would be lost to any excess cooking liquid.

what's in a grain?

Not all grains are botanically related—true grains, such as wheat, rice, oats, rye, millet, corn, triticale, and barley, are members of the grass family, Gramineae; other so-called grains, such as amaranth, quinoa, and buckwheat, belong to different botanical families. But the kernels of the different grains all have a similar composition:

▶**Kernel** A kernel is an edible seed composed of three parts—the bran, the endosperm, and the germ, or embryo. Some grains, notably rice, oats, and some varieties of barley, are also covered by an inedible papery sheath called the hull, which must be removed before the grain can be processed or consumed. Within each kernel are the nutrients needed for the embryo to grow until the plant can take root and get nourishment from outside sources.

▶**Bran** The bran is the outer covering of the kernel. It makes up only a small portion of the grain but consists of several layers—including the nutrient-rich aleurone—and contains a disproportionate share of nutrients. The bran layers supply 86% of the niacin, 43% of the riboflavin, and 66% of all the minerals in the grain, as well as practically all of the grain's dietary fiber. In some grains—wheat and corn, for example—the fiber is primarily insoluble, while in other grains, such as oats and barley, it is mainly soluble. Whole grains almost always contain the bran, but it is usually stripped away during milling and so is missing from most refined grain products.

▶**Endosperm** The starchy endosperm accounts for about 83% of the grain's weight. Most of the protein and carbohydrates are stored in the endosperm, as are some minerals and B vitamins (though less than are in the bran). This layer also has some dietary fiber; for example, about 25% of the fiber in wheat is found in the endosperm. In wheat, the endosperm is the part of the grain used to make white flour.

▶**Germ** The smallest part of the grain is the germ; it constitutes about 2% of the kernel's weight. Located at the base of the kernel, the germ is the part of the seed that if planted would sprout to form a new plant. It contains a good amount of polyunsaturated fat, and, as a consequence, is often removed during milling to prevent grain products from turning rancid. The germ is also relatively rich in vitamin E and the B vitamins—though it has fewer of the latter than are found in the bran or endosperm—and some minerals.

grains cooking chart

Here are some general guidelines for cooking grains: Place the appropriate amount (see chart) of water and/or broth in a saucepan; cover and bring to a boil over high heat. Add the grain (and ¼ teaspoon of salt, if desired) and return to a boil. Reduce to a simmer and cook, stirring occasionally, according to the method/times listed below. Toward the end of the cooking time, you may need to stir more frequently. This is especially true of the finer granulations, such as cornmeal, grits, oatmeal, teff, and bulgur. Note: The cooking methods, times, and yields for the grains in this chart are all based on **½ cup of uncooked grain**.

GRAIN	LIQUID	METHOD/TIME	YIELD
AMARANTH	1½ cups	Simmer, covered, for 30 minutes	1⅓ cups
BARLEY, HULLED	2 cups	Simmer, covered, for 1 hour 40 minutes	1¼ cups
BARLEY, PEARL	1½ cups	Simmer, covered, for 35–45 minutes	2 cups
BARLEY, QUICK-COOKING	1 cup	Simmer, covered, for 10–12 minutes. Let stand 5 minutes	1½ cups
BARLEY, GRITS	2 cups	Simmer, covered, for 20 minutes	1¾ cups
BUCKWHEAT, WHOLE GROATS, UNROASTED	1 cup	Simmer, covered, for 15 minutes	1¾ cups
BUCKWHEAT, WHOLE GROATS, ROASTED	1 cup	Simmer, covered, for 13 minutes	1½ cups
KASHA	1 cup	Simmer, covered, for 12 minutes	2 cups
CORNMEAL	(2 cups total; see method)	Whisk ½ cup cold water into cornmeal. Stir mixture into 1½ cups boiling water. Cook, stirring, for 10 minutes	2 cups
HOMINY, WHOLE DRIED	Soak for 8 hours	Drain and simmer, covered, in 3 cups water for 2½ to 3 hours	1½ cups
HOMINY GRITS, COARSE	2½ cups	Simmer, uncovered, for 30 minutes	1½ cups
FARRO/SPELT	2 cups	Simmer, covered, for 1 hour	1¾ cups
KAMUT	1½ cups	Simmer, covered, for 1 hour 10 minutes	1¼ cups

continued on page 166

grains cooking chart

Note: The cooking methods, times, and yields for the grains in this chart are all based on **½ cup of uncooked grain**.

GRAIN	LIQUID	METHOD/TIME	YIELD
continued from page 165			
MILLET	1½ cups	Simmer, covered, for 25 minutes. Let stand 10 minutes.	2½ cups
OATS, STEEL-CUT	2 cups	Simmer, uncovered, for 40–45 minutes	1½ cups
OATS, ROLLED	1 cup	Simmer, uncovered, for 5 minutes	1 cup
OATS, QUICK-COOKING	1 cup	Simmer, uncovered, for 1 minute. Let stand 3–5 minutes	1 cup
QUINOA	1 cup	Rinse the quinoa well. Simmer, uncovered, for 15 minutes	2 cups
RICE, BROWN, LONG-GRAIN	1 cup	Simmer, covered, for 25–30 minutes	1½ cups
RICE, BROWN, SHORT-GRAIN	1 cup	Simmer, covered, for 40 minutes	1½ cups
RICE, WHITE, LONG-GRAIN	1 cup	Simmer, covered, for 20 minutes	1¾ cups
RICE, WHITE, SHORT-GRAIN	1½ cups	Simmer, covered, for 20 minutes	1¾ cups
RICE, WHITE, BASMATI	1 cup	Simmer, covered, for 15–18 minutes	2 cups
RICE, WHITE, JASMINE	1 cup	Simmer, covered, for 18 minutes	1¾ cups
RYE BERRIES	1½ cups	Simmer, covered, for 2 hours	1½ cups
TEFF	1½ cups	Simmer, covered, for 15 minutes	1½ cups
TRITICALE BERRIES	1½ cups	Simmer, covered, for 1 hour 10 minutes	1¼ cups
WHEAT BERRIES	1½ cups	Simmer, covered, for 1 hour 10 minutes	1¼ cups
CRACKED WHEAT	1 cup	Simmer, covered, for 15 minutes	1 cup
BULGUR	1 cup	Simmer, covered, for 15 minutes	1½ cups
WILD RICE	2 cups	Simmer, covered, for 45–50 minutes	2 cups

Green & Gold Risotto

Arborio, a high-starch white rice with an almost round grain, is traditionally used to make the Italian rice dish risotto. Arborio absorbs up to five times its weight in liquid as it cooks, resulting in an extremely creamy dish. This risotto gets its gold color from the carrot juice used in the cooking liquid, a nice backdrop for the bright green peas.

> 2 teaspoons olive oil
>
> 1 small onion, finely chopped
>
> 2 carrots, cut into ¼-inch dice
>
> 1 cup Arborio rice
>
> 1½ cups chicken broth, homemade (page 252) or canned
>
> 1½ cups carrot juice
>
> ½ cup dry white wine
>
> ½ teaspoon salt
>
> 1 cup frozen peas
>
> ¼ cup grated Parmesan cheese
>
> 2 teaspoons butter
>
> ¼ teaspoon pepper

1 In a medium nonstick saucepan, heat the oil over medium heat. Add the onion and carrots, and cook, stirring, until the onion is soft, about 7 minutes. Add the rice, stirring to coat. Reduce the heat to low.

2 Meanwhile, in a medium saucepan, combine the broth and carrot juice, and bring to a simmer over low heat.

3 Add the wine to the rice, and cook, stirring occasionally, until evaporated by half, about 2 minutes. Add 1½ cups of the broth mixture and the salt, and cook, stirring, until the liquid has been absorbed, about 10 minutes.

4 Add ¾ cup of the warm broth mixture and cook, stirring, until absorbed, about 10 minutes. Then add the remaining ¾ cup broth mixture and cook, stirring, until absorbed, about 10 minutes. Stir in the peas and cook about 2 minutes to heat through.

5 Remove from the heat. Stir in the Parmesan, butter, and pepper. *Makes 6 servings*

per serving: 260 calories, 4.3g total fat (1.8g saturated), 7mg cholesterol, 3g dietary fiber, 43g carbohydrate, 7g protein, 438mg sodium. good source of: beta carotene.

Barley with Cilantro & Garlic

A puree of scallions, cilantro, garlic, and fresh ginger gives this creamy barley dish its exotic flavor. If you'd like to make this dish vegetarian, substitute carrot juice for the chicken broth. **Serving suggestion:** Serve this mildly spiced barley alongside a curried poultry or meat dish instead of rice.

> 4 scallions, sliced
>
> ½ cup packed cilantro sprigs
>
> 4 cloves garlic, peeled
>
> 1 tablespoon minced fresh ginger
>
> 1¼ cups water
>
> 1 tablespoon olive oil
>
> 1 green bell pepper, diced
>
> ¾ cup pearl barley
>
> 1¾ cups chicken broth, homemade (page 252) or canned
>
> ½ teaspoon salt

1 In a blender or food processor, combine the scallions, cilantro, garlic, ginger, and ¼ cup of the water. Process to a smooth puree.

2 In a large saucepan, heat the oil over medium heat. Add the bell pepper and cook for 2 minutes.

3 Add the scallion puree and cook, stirring, until the liquid in the puree has evaporated, about 2 minutes.

4 Add the barley, stirring to coat. Add the remaining 1 cup water, the broth, and salt, and bring to a boil. Reduce to a simmer, cover, and cook until the barley is tender, about 55 minutes. *Makes 4 servings*

per serving: 189 calories, 4g total fat (0.6g saturated), 0mg cholesterol, 7g dietary fiber, 34g carbohydrate, 6g protein, 496mg sodium. good source of: beta glucan, fiber, selenium, vitamin C.

Basmati Rice, Chick-Peas & Toasted Almonds

The age-old combination of rice and beans takes on a bit of an Indian flavor here with the use of basmati rice (an aromatic rice grown primarily in India) and chick-peas, another ingredient common to Indian cuisine. If you can't find basmati rice, substitute Texmati, jasmine, or any long-grain rice.

2 teaspoons olive oil

1 large onion, finely chopped

3 cloves garlic, finely chopped

1 large red bell pepper, cut into ½-inch pieces

1 cup basmati rice

2 cups water

1½ teaspoons grated lemon zest

¾ teaspoon salt

1 can (19 ounces) chick-peas, rinsed and drained

⅓ cup chopped cilantro

¼ cup sliced almonds, toasted

1 In a medium nonstick saucepan, heat the oil over medium heat. Add the onion and garlic, and cook, stirring frequently, until the onion is soft, about 7 minutes.

2 Add the bell pepper and rice, stirring to coat. Stir in the water, lemon zest, and salt, and bring to a boil. Reduce to a simmer, cover, and cook until the rice is tender, about 15 minutes.

3 Stir in the chick-peas and cook until heated through, about 3 minutes. Stir in the cilantro and toasted almonds at serving time. *Makes 6 servings*

per serving: 242 calories, 5g total fat (0.6g saturated), 0mg cholesterol, 5g dietary fiber, 42g carbohydrate, 8g protein, 395mg sodium. good source of: fiber, folate, thiamin, vitamin C.

Wild Rice Pilaf with Pumpkin Seeds

Wild rice and brown rice are good companions in a pilaf: first, because they have similar chewy textures, but second because they both take about the same amount of time to cook. A third benefit is that using a mixture stretches the expensive wild rice with a less expensive grain.

1 tablespoon olive oil

1 large onion, finely chopped

1 carrot, quartered lengthwise and thinly sliced crosswise

¾ cup wild rice (4 ounces)

toasting nuts & seeds

You can enhance the flavor of both nuts and seeds by toasting them before adding them to dishes. There are several ways to do this:

▶**Skillet** Toast the nuts or seeds in an ungreased skillet over medium to medium-low heat. Stir them and keep an eye on them, because they can turn from golden to burned very quickly. Depending on how many you are toasting at once, this can take from 1 or 2 minutes to 5 minutes. Once they are lightly toasted, immediately transfer them to a plate so the heat from the skillet will not keep cooking them. Pumpkin seeds have a very specific visual test for doneness: They will begin to pop and jump in the pan.

▶**Oven** Place the nuts or seeds in a baking pan, in a single layer, and toast them in a 350°F oven for about 7 minutes. Keep an eye on them, checking them at 5 minutes and stirring them around. Remove them from the hot pan immediately to keep them from burning.

▶**Toaster oven** This method is good for a small amount of nuts or seeds. Place them in the toaster oven tray and toast at 350°F. Because a toaster oven is small, nuts or seeds will toast much more quickly than in a standard oven, so keep an eye on them. It may take only 1 or 2 minutes. Remove them from the oven as soon as they are done and transfer them to a plate to stop the cooking.

did you know?

Whole grains reduce the risk of type 2 diabetes, according to a study of nearly 43,000 male health professionals. Men who ate three or more servings a day were 40% less likely to develop diabetes over the next 12 years than those who rarely ate whole grains. These foods include whole-grain cereals and breads, oats, and brown rice. Even obese men, who are at greatest risk for diabetes, benefited from whole grains. Refined grain products, such as white bread and pasta, did not reduce the risk (nor did they increase it).

½ cup brown rice

2 cups water

1½ cups chicken broth, homemade (page 252) or canned

½ teaspoon thyme

½ teaspoon salt

¼ cup hulled pumpkin seeds (pepitas)

¼ cup dried currants

1 In a medium nonstick saucepan, heat the oil over medium heat. Add the onion and carrot, and cook, stirring frequently, until the onion is soft, about 7 minutes.

2 Add the wild rice and brown rice, stirring to combine. Stir in the water, broth, thyme, and salt. Bring to a boil, reduce to a simmer, cover, and cook until the rices are tender, about 45 minutes.

3 Meanwhile, in a small ungreased skillet, toast the pumpkin seeds over low heat until fragrant and they begin to pop in the pan, about 5 minutes. Remove from the heat and transfer the seeds onto a plate to prevent them from burning.

4 Stir the toasted pumpkin seeds and currants into the pilaf before serving. *Makes 6 servings*

per serving: 231 calories, 6.7g total fat (1.2g saturated), 1mg cholesterol, 3g dietary fiber, 38g carbohydrate, 7g protein, 454mg sodium. good source of: beta carotene, magnesium, vitamin B$_6$, zinc.

Onion, Mushroom & Bulgur Pilaf

Bulgur is wheat kernels that have been steam-cooked, dried, and then cracked. It's available in three different granulations: coarse, medium, and fine. Coarse bulgur is the best for pilafs. For a vegetarian pilaf, use Mushroom-Onion Broth (*page 252*) instead of chicken broth.

1 tablespoon olive oil

2 medium onions, thinly sliced

3 cloves garlic, minced

¾ pound cremini mushrooms, thinly sliced

1 cup coarse bulgur

1½ cups chicken broth, homemade (page 252) or canned

1 cup water

¾ teaspoon tarragon

½ teaspoon salt

½ teaspoon pepper

⅓ cup chopped parsley

2 tablespoons coarsely chopped walnuts

1 Preheat the oven to 350°F. In a Dutch oven or flameproof casserole, heat the oil over medium heat. Add the onions and garlic, and cook, stirring frequently, until the onions are golden brown and slightly caramelized, about 15 minutes.

2 Add the mushrooms and cook until the mushrooms have softened, about 5 minutes.

3 Stir in the bulgur, broth, water, tarragon, salt, and pepper, and bring to a boil. Cover, place in the oven, and bake for 20 minutes or until the bulgur is tender and the liquid has been absorbed.

4 Stir in the parsley and walnuts before serving. *Makes 4 servings*

per serving: 235 calories, 6g total fat (0.7g saturated), 0mg cholesterol, 10g dietary fiber, 37g carbohydrate, 11g protein, 504mg sodium. good source of: beta glucan, fiber.

recipe creator
grain pilafs

A pilaf (which comes from an Indo-European word that means "rice porridge") is a rice side dish that is cooked in a seasoned broth, and often with sautéed onion. By extension, a pilaf can be any grain dish cooked in this manner. Choose the grain and other components from the categories below and follow these basic instructions: In a 3-quart saucepan, heat 1 tablespoon of olive or canola oil over medium heat. Add 1 AROMATIC, 2 cloves minced garlic, and 1 VEGETABLE, and cook until the aromatic is tender, about 7 minutes. Stir in 1 cup of GRAIN and cook 1 minute. Stir in boiling liquid (this can be water and/or broth; use the quantity specified for the particular grain being cooked), ¾ teaspoon salt, and 1 or 2 SEASONINGS, and return to a boil. Reduce to a simmer, cover tightly, and cook until tender (use the cooking time listed for the particular grain being cooked). Stir in 1 or 2 ADD-INS, cover, and let stand 5 minutes. Fluff with a fork before serving. *Makes 4 servings*

AROMATICS

▶ Onion, 1 medium, chopped

▶ Scallions, 6, sliced

▶ Leeks, 2, diced

VEGETABLES

▶ Red or green bell pepper, 1, chopped

▶ Mushrooms, ½ pound, sliced

▶ Celery, 1 stalk, sliced

▶ Carrot, 1, sliced

▶ Butternut squash, 1 cup diced

GRAINS

▶ White rice + 2¼ cups liquid (*cooking time: 15–18 mins*)

▶ Basmati or jasmine rice + 2 cups liquid (*cooking time: 18–20 mins*)

▶ Brown rice + 2½ cups liquid (*cooking time: 30–45 mins*)

▶ Quinoa, rinsed and drained + 1¾ cups liquid (*cooking time: 17–20 mins*)

▶ Pearl barley + 3½ cups liquid (*cooking time: 35–45 mins*)

▶ Millet + 3 cups liquid (*cooking time: 25–30 mins; let stand 10 minutes*)

▶ Whole-grain kasha + 2 cups liquid (*cooking time: 10–12 mins*)

SEASONINGS

▶ Rosemary, ½ tsp minced

▶ Rubbed sage, ½ tsp

▶ Bay leaf, 1 (remove after cooking)

▶ Marjoram, ½ tsp

▶ Lemon zest, 2 tsp grated

▶ Thyme, ½ tsp

ADD-INS

▶ Dried currants or raisins, ⅓ cup

▶ Dried cherries or cranberries, ½ cup

▶ Dried apricots or plums (prunes), ½ cup chopped

▶ Walnuts or pecans, ¼ cup chopped, toasted

▶ Green peas, ½ cup

▶ Grated Parmesan cheese, 3 Tbsp

▶ Pumpkin or sunflower seeds, 2 Tbsp

▶ Corn kernels, ½ cup

Farro with Wild Mushrooms

Farro is an ancient grain with a texture similar to that of barley. Farro's slightly nutty flavor is underscored by the earthiness of dried wild mushrooms and sage.

> ½ cup dried shiitake or porcini
>   mushrooms (½ ounce)
> 2½ cups boiling water
> 1 tablespoon olive oil
> 1 small onion, finely chopped
> 2 cloves garlic, minced
> 1 cup farro
> 2 cups carrot juice
> ¾ teaspoon salt
> ½ teaspoon rubbed sage

1 In a small heatproof bowl, combine the dried mushrooms and the boiling water, and let stand for 20 minutes or until softened. Reserving the soaking liquid, scoop out the dried mushrooms and coarsely chop. Strain the soaking liquid through a coffee filter or a paper towel–lined sieve.

2 In a large nonstick saucepan, heat the oil over medium heat. Add the onion and garlic, and cook, stirring frequently, until the onion is golden brown, about 10 minutes.

3 Add the farro and stir to coat. Add the mushrooms and their soaking liquid, the carrot juice, salt, and sage, and bring to a boil. Reduce to a simmer, cover, and cook until the farro is tender and most of the liquid has been absorbed, about 1 hour and 15 minutes. *Makes 4 servings*

per serving: 232 calories, 4.8g total fat (0.5g saturated), 0mg cholesterol, 2g dietary fiber, 47g carbohydrate, 6g protein, 473mg sodium. good source of: beta carotene, magnesium, potassium, vitamin B_6.

Kasha Varnishkes

Kasha varnishkes is a Middle European dish of roasted buckwheat groats (kasha) and bow-tie noodles (varnishkes). Traditionally, a whole egg (in this recipe, just an egg white) is stirred into the kasha to coat the grains so they remain separate instead of cooking into a mush. Our version ups the flavor ante with lots of caramelized onions.

> 1 tablespoon olive oil
> 2 medium onions, thinly sliced
> 1 cup kasha (roasted buckwheat groats)
> 1 large egg white
> 2 cups chicken broth, homemade
>   (page 252) or canned
> ½ teaspoon salt
> ½ teaspoon pepper
> ¼ teaspoon rosemary, minced
> 10 ounces bow-tie pasta

1 In a large nonstick skillet, heat the oil over medium-low heat. Add the onions and cook, stirring frequently, until the onions are golden brown and caramelized, about 25 minutes. Transfer the onions to a plate.

2 Meanwhile, in a medium bowl, stir together the kasha and egg white until the kasha is well coated. Add the kasha to the same skillet the onions were cooked in, and stir over medium-high heat until the grains look dry and separate, about 5 minutes.

3 Add the broth to the kasha along with the salt, pepper, and rosemary, and bring to a boil. Stir in the onions. Reduce to a simmer, cover, and cook for 10 minutes. Uncover and stir the kasha. Cover and cook until the liquid has been absorbed and the kasha is tender but not mushy, 3 to 5 minutes.

4 Meanwhile, in a large pot of boiling water, cook the pasta according to package directions. Drain. Transfer to a large bowl, add the kasha and toss to combine. *Makes 6 servings*

per serving: 224 calories, 3.2g total fat (0.5g saturated), 0mg cholesterol, 3g dietary fiber, 40g carbohydrate, 8g protein, 356mg sodium. good source of: folate, selenium, thiamin.

Baked Ratatouille & Grits

Grits are coarsely ground grains, and though they can be any type of grain, the word is most commonly used to refer to a processed white corn called hominy. Although the more typical way to serve grits in this country is as a breakfast dish, here they have a savory ratatouille-like topping and would make a good accompaniment to grilled poultry or fish.

3⅓ cups water

⅔ cup hominy grits

¾ teaspoon salt

2 teaspoons olive oil

1 large red onion, diced

3 cloves garlic, minced

1 large red bell pepper, diced

1 small eggplant (8 ounces), unpeeled and cut into ½-inch cubes

1 medium zucchini, halved lengthwise and thinly sliced crosswise

1 can (8 ounces) no-salt-added tomato sauce

1 tablespoon red wine vinegar

¾ teaspoon tarragon

1 In a medium saucepan, bring 3 cups of the water to a boil. Slowly stir in the grits and ½ teaspoon of the salt, stirring until the grits are thick and creamy, about 20 minutes. Spoon into a 9-inch square baking dish and set aside.

2 In a large nonstick skillet, heat the oil over medium heat. Add the onion and garlic, and cook, stirring occasionally, until the onion is soft, about 7 minutes.

3 Preheat the oven to 400°F.

4 Add the bell pepper to the skillet and cook, stirring frequently, until almost tender, about 4 minutes. Stir in the eggplant, toss to coat, and add the remaining ⅓ cup water and ¼ teaspoon salt. Cover and cook, stirring occasionally, until the eggplant is tender, about 7 minutes.

5 Stir in the zucchini, tomato sauce, vinegar, and tarragon. Cook, stirring occasionally, until the sauce is lightly thickened and the zucchini is tender, about 5 minutes.

6 Spoon the sauce over the grits, cover with foil, and bake until the grits are piping hot, about 10 minutes. *Makes 4 servings*

per serving: 181 calories, 3g total fat (0.4g saturated), 0mg cholesterol, 5g dietary fiber, 36g carbohydrate, 5g protein, 448mg sodium. good source of: beta carotene, fiber, folate, niacin, potassium, thiamin, vitamin B$_6$, vitamin C.

Quinoa Pilaf with Cherries & Pecans

Quinoa, in addition to being a good source of plant protein (it contains all eight essential amino acids), is rich in vitamin E, iron, and magnesium.

¾ cup quinoa

2 teaspoons olive oil

3 scallions, thinly sliced

3 cloves garlic, minced

1½ cups boiling water

¾ teaspoon salt

¼ teaspoon pepper

¼ cup dried cherries

2 tablespoons chopped pecans or walnuts

1 Place the quinoa in a colander and rinse under cold running water. Drain well.

2 In a large skillet, heat the oil over medium heat. Add the scallions and garlic, and cook, stirring frequently, until the scallions are tender, about 2 minutes. Stir in the quinoa and cook until lightly toasted, 2 to 3 minutes.

3 Add the boiling water, salt, and pepper. Reduce to a simmer, cover, and cook until the quinoa is tender, 15 to 20 minutes.

4 Stir in the dried cherries and chopped pecans. *Makes 4 servings*

per serving: 211 calories, 7.1g total fat (0.7g saturated), 0mg cholesterol, 3g dietary fiber, 34g carbohydrate, 6g protein, 446mg sodium. good source of: magnesium, saponins, vitamin E.

vegetables

The nutritional content of vegetables, as well as their taste and texture, is affected by how you handle them, and especially by how you cook them. Here are some general rules to keep in mind:

Nutrient loss occurs when vegetables are exposed to light and air; therefore, don't wash, chop, or slice vegetables until you are ready to use them. While vegetables should always be washed before you cook or serve them raw, long soaking is not recommended, as it can leach out water-soluble vitamins. You can quickly but thoroughly rinse vegetables under cold running water, or dunk them in several changes of water in a basin. Use a soft brush to remove dirt that clings; lukewarm water also helps to release sand and grit from leafy vegetables.

When peeling and chopping vegetables, remember that many nutrients are concentrated just beneath the skin. If possible, do not peel vegetables such as potatoes and beets; or, cook them in their skins and peel them after cooking, when their thin skins will slip off. (Even if you don't eat the skin, leaving it intact during cooking helps preserve nutrients.)

In general, most vegetables should be cooked until they are barely tender or crisp-tender. Only then will they retain most of their nutrients, bright colors, and fresh flavors. Of course, this rule does not apply to every vegetable: Potatoes, for instance, need to be cooked until tender, or they will be inedible.

Roasting/baking Because roasting and baking are dry-heat methods, they can be used successfully for vegetables with a thick skin that will retain the vegetable's internal moisture. Examples of this are baked potatoes or winter squash. Other vegetables need oil, moisture, or a combination to keep them from drying out as they cook (*see "Roasting Root Vegetables," below*). Very wet vegetables, such as tomatoes, are sometimes roasted in order to partially dehydrate them, thus concentrating their flavors (*see Roasted Tomatoes with Garlic, page 196*).

Grilling/broiling This high-temperature, dry-heat method cooks vegetables quickly and preserves their flavor and texture; but it also requires oil to prevent them from burning. Use a pastry brush or an oil spray for a light and even coating of oil.

Sautéing/stir-frying Although traditional sautéing and stir-frying require a good deal of oil, you can adapt these techniques to make them more healthful: Cook the vegetables in a nonstick skillet with a bit of oil and some water or broth. The broth and the natural moisture from the vegetables will pan-steam the food.

continued on page 178

roasting root vegetables

Roots and tubers (turnips, parsnips, carrots, rutabagas, sweet potatoes, potatoes, beets) take exceptionally well to roasting. The trick is to do this without a lot of fat, as tradition would dictate.

The general concept is this: Toss the vegetables in a mixture of liquid (broth, water, or wine) and olive oil. The liquid helps disperse the oil so that you get more coverage. As a general rule, you would make this mixture about 6 parts liquid to 1 part oil. The total amount required will depend on how much you're cooking. You can also throw in herbs, salt, pepper, and other seasonings (whole garlic cloves are good).

Then, place the vegetables in a roasting pan large enough to hold them in a single layer. For harder vegetables (such as carrots, turnips, or beets), you should cover the roasting pan for all or part of the cooking time. This will help them oven-steam. For softer, more porous vegetables (such as potatoes), you can roast them uncovered.

Roast the vegetables at 400°F and stir them around occasionally as they cook.

vegetable cooking chart

For all the cooking methods below, the cooking times are based on the vegetables not being crowded in the pan (or steamer). Crowding, at the very least, will increase the amount of time it takes to cook the vegetables. But in the case of roasting, baking, or grilling, it will also keep the vegetables from browning. Microwaving, which is one of the more healthful ways to cook vegetables, is not included here because oven strength and size, and the quantity of vegetables being cooked makes it impossible to give useful cooking times. It's best to consult the manual that came with your microwave oven for details.

VEGETABLE	PREP	METHOD
ACORN SQUASH	halved and seeded	**Baking** 350°F for 45–50 minutes
ARTICHOKES	whole	**Steaming** 25–40 minutes, depending on size
	hearts, sliced	**Stir-frying** 3–5 minutes with a bit of olive oil or broth
ASPARAGUS	whole spears	**Roasting** 450°F, tossed with a bit of olive oil, 10 minutes **Steaming** 4–7 minutes
	1- to 2-inch pieces	**Stir-frying** 3–5 minutes with a bit of olive oil or broth
BEANS, SHELL: LIMA/FAVA	removed from pod	**Steaming** 3–5 minutes
BEANS, SNAP: GREEN, WAX, OR ITALIAN	whole, trimmed	**Steaming** 3–5 minutes
BEET GREENS		*See Sautéed Greens "Recipe Creator" on page 183*
BEETS	whole, unpeeled	**Baking** 350°F, in roasting pan covered with foil, 1½ to 2 hours. Peel when cool
	peeled and shredded	**Stir-frying** 3–5 minutes with a bit of olive oil or broth
BOK CHOY	1-inch pieces	**Stir-frying** 5–7 minutes with a bit of olive oil or broth
BROCCOLI	small florets	**Steaming** 3–5 minutes
	whole spears	**Steaming** 5–7 minutes
BROCCOLI RABE	tough ends trimmed, thinly sliced	**Stir-frying** 7–10 minutes with a bit of olive oil or broth
BRUSSELS SPROUTS	whole	**Steaming** 6–12 minutes, depending on size
	quarters	**Stir-frying** 5–7 minutes with a bit of olive oil or broth
BURDOCK	matchsticks	**Steaming** 3–5 minutes **Stir-frying** 5–7 minutes with a bit of olive oil or broth

vegetable cooking chart

VEGETABLE	PREP	METHOD
BUTTERNUT SQUASH	halved and seeded	**Baking** 350°F for 45–50 minutes
	peeled, seeded, and cut into 1-inch cubes	**Baking** 350°F, in roasting pan with a little water and olive oil, 20–25 minutes **Steaming** 5–7 minutes
CABBAGE	whole head, cored and quartered	**Steaming** 10–15 minutes
	shredded	**Stir-frying** 5–7 minutes with a bit of olive oil or broth
CARROTS	baby carrots, whole	**Steaming** 5–7 minutes
	thinly sliced	**Steaming** 5–7 minutes
	shredded	**Stir-frying** 3–5 minutes with a bit of olive oil or broth
CAULIFLOWER	small florets	**Steaming** 4–5 minutes **Roasting** 375°F, tossed with a bit of olive oil and broth, 40 minutes
CELERIAC (CELERY ROOT)	matchsticks	**Steaming** 5–7 minutes
CELERY	whole head, halved lengthwise	**Oven-braising** 350°F, in covered baking pan with boiling broth to come halfway up the depth of the celery, 15–20 minutes
	2-inch lengths	**Stir-frying** 5 minutes with a bit of olive oil or broth
CHAYOTE	peeled and cut into 1-inch chunks	**Steaming** 5–7 minutes
CORN	whole ears, husked and wrapped individually in foil	**Roasting/grilling** 15–20 minutes
	whole ears, husked	**Boiling** Add to rapidly boiling water and remove 1 minute after water returns to a boil
EGGPLANT	whole, pierced	**Baking** 400°F for 30–40 minutes
	halved lengthwise	**Baking** 400°F, cut-sides down, for 20–30 minutes
	thick lengthwise slices lightly brushed with oil	**Grilling** 4–6 minutes per side over medium heat
	1-inch cubes	**Steaming** 8–10 minutes

continued on page 176

vegetable cooking chart

VEGETABLE	PREP	METHOD
ENDIVE, BELGIAN	whole heads, core end removed	**Braising** In covered skillet, with boiling broth to come halfway up the depth of the endives, 10 minutes
ESCAROLE		*See Sautéed Greens "Recipe Creator" on page 183*
FENNEL	quartered	**Oven-braising** 350°F, in covered baking pan with boiling broth to come halfway up the depth of the fennel, 30–40 minutes
	½-inch slices	**Stir-frying** 3–5 minutes with a bit of olive oil or broth
HUBBARD SQUASH	peeled, seeded, and cut into 1-inch cubes	**Baking** 350°F, in baking pan with a little water and olive oil, 20–25 minutes
JERUSALEM ARTICHOKES	whole, scrubbed	**Baking** 350°F, in baking pan, with a little oil, 45–50 minutes
KALE		*See Sautéed Greens "Recipe Creator" on page 183*
KOHLRABI	peeled and thinly sliced	**Steaming** 5–10 minutes
LEEKS	halved lengthwise and thoroughly rinsed	**Oven-braising** 350°F, in covered baking pan with boiling broth to come halfway up the depth of the leeks, 45 minutes **Steaming** 5–7 minutes
MUSHROOMS	portobello caps	**Grilling** Brush with olive oil. Grill 5 minutes per side over medium heat
	large mushroom caps, such as portobello	**Oven-braising** 350°F, in covered baking pan with boiling broth to come halfway up the depth of the mushrooms, 15 minutes
	button mushrooms, quartered	**Stir-frying** 3–5 minutes with a bit of olive oil or broth
MUSTARD GREENS		*See Sautéed Greens "Recipe Creator" on page 183*
NAPA CABBAGE	1-inch slices	**Stir-frying** 5–7 minutes with a bit of olive oil or broth
OKRA	whole	**Steaming** 5–6 minutes
ONIONS	whole, peeled	**Oven-braising** 350°F, in covered baking pan with boiling broth to come halfway up the depth of the onions, 40–50 minutes
PARSNIPS	peeled and thickly sliced	**Steaming** 5–7 minutes

vegetable cooking chart

VEGETABLE	PREP	METHOD
PEAS	shelled	**Steaming** 3 minutes
PEAS, SUGAR SNAP	whole, strings removed	**Steaming** 2–3 minutes **Stir-frying** 3–4 minutes with a bit of olive oil or broth
PEPPERS, BELL	cut into thin slivers	**Stir-frying** 3–5 minutes with a bit of olive oil or broth
	whole	**Broiling** *see "Roasted Peppers" on page 190*
POTATOES	whole, scrubbed, unpeeled, and pierced with a fork	**Baking** 375°F for 50–60 minutes
	1-inch chunks	**Steaming** 7–10 minutes
	whole small boiling potatoes, unpeeled	**Steaming** 15–20 minutes
RADICCHIO	halved	**Braising** In covered skillet, with boiling broth to come halfway up the depth of the radicchio, 10 minutes
RUTABAGA	peeled and cut into 1-inch chunks	**Steaming** 8–10 minutes
SNOW PEAS	whole, strings removed	**Steaming** 2–3 minutes **Stir-frying** 3–4 minutes with a bit of olive oil or broth
SPAGHETTI SQUASH	halved lengthwise and seeded	**Baking** 350°F, cut-sides down, for 50–60 minutes
SPINACH	thoroughly rinsed, tough stems removed	**Steaming** In skillet, with water clinging to leaves, 2–3 minutes
SWEET POTATOES	whole, scrubbed, unpeeled, and pierced with a fork	**Baking** 400°F for 35–45 minutes
	thickly cut	**Steaming** 10–15 minutes
SWISS CHARD		*See Sautéed Greens "Recipe Creator" on page 183*
TURNIPS	peeled, cut into 1-inch chunks	**Steaming** 5–7 minutes
ZUCCHINI/SUMMER SQUASH	cut crosswise into thin slices	**Steaming** 3–4 minutes **Stir-frying** 3–5 minutes with a bit of olive oil or broth
	thickly sliced lengthwise, and brushed lightly with oil	**Grilling** 5 minutes per side over medium heat

continued from page 173

Then, as the moisture evaporates, the small amount of oil that's left (and is now coating the vegetables), will help the vegetables brown a bit.

Boiling Of the various cooking methods, boiling takes the severest toll on vegetable nutrients, causing most of the vitamin C and other water-soluble vitamins to leach into the cooking liquid. The heat can also destroy vitamin C, and if thiamin is present, it converts this B vitamin into a form that the body cannot utilize. So except where boiling is unavoidable (huge quantities of corn on the cob, for example), boiling is not recommended.

Steaming For simple vegetable side dishes, steaming is one of the best methods available. It is quick and keeps nutrient loss to a minimum. If you eat a lot of vegetables, it would be wise to buy a Chinese-style bamboo steamer. It is larger than most steamer inserts and will fit over most large saucepans or skillets (as well as woks).

Pan-steaming This is a method very similar to healthful sautéing or stir-frying. If you cook vegetables in just a small amount of water or broth (not necessarily with oil) in a tightly closed pot, the added liquid will come to a boil and start to cook the vegetables. The vegetables will then give up their own liquid. The two liquids together will turn into steam and cook the vegetables. This works best for relatively soft vegetables (such as onions) or harder vegetables that have been thinly sliced or shredded (see Orange-Mint Carrots, page 186). For leafy vegetables, such as spinach and other greens, the only additional moisture needed to cook them is the water clinging to their leaves after they have been washed.

Microwaving Microwaving, like steaming, is a good, nutrient-preserving cooking method. Consult your microwave oven manual for vegetable-specific information.

Braising/stewing In these wet-heat methods, vegetables are cooked in a flavorful liquid with little to no fat. In the case of stews and soups, the cooking liquid gets eaten as part of the dish, thus preserving a maximum amount of the vegetable's nutrients. For braised vegetables, the cooking liquid can be flavorful enough to serve along with the vegetable, as a sauce (*see Braised Leeks with Tomato & Coriander, page 190*).

Roasted Asparagus Parmesan

These roasted asparagus spears could be served as a side dish, as part of a buffet, or as an appetizer.

> 2 pounds thick asparagus, tough ends trimmed
> ¼ cup water
> 2½ teaspoons olive oil
> ¼ teaspoon salt
> ¼ cup grated Parmesan cheese
> ⅓ cup balsamic vinegar
> 1 tablespoon dark brown sugar

1 Preheat the oven to 450°F. Place the asparagus in a baking pan large enough to hold them in a single layer. Add the water and oil and toss to coat. Arrange them in a single layer. Sprinkle the salt over the asparagus.

2 Bake until the asparagus are crisp-tender, about 10 minutes. Sprinkle the Parmesan over the asparagus and bake until the asparagus are tender and the cheese has melted and is crisp, about 5 minutes.

3 Meanwhile, in a small skillet, heat the vinegar and brown sugar until reduced to 3 tablespoons, about 3 minutes.

4 Serve the asparagus drizzled with the balsamic glaze. *Makes 4 servings*

per serving: 100 calories, 4.7g total fat (1.4g saturated), 4mg cholesterol, 2g dietary fiber, 11g carbohydrate, 5g protein, 257mg sodium. good source of: folate, riboflavin, thiamin, vitamin C.

Artichoke Hearts & Baby Limas

If you prefer, substitute two 9-ounce packages of frozen artichoke hearts for the fresh artichokes. Skip step 1 and reduce the lemon juice to 1 tablespoon (to be used in step 3). The cooking time should be about the same.

> 3 tablespoons fresh lemon juice
>
> 4 artichokes (about 10 ounces each)
>
> 2 teaspoons olive oil
>
> 1 small onion, finely chopped
>
> 3 cloves garlic, minced
>
> 1 carrot, finely chopped
>
> ½ teaspoon salt
>
> ½ teaspoon thyme
>
> 1½ cups frozen baby lima beans

1 In a large bowl, combine 4 cups of cold water and 2 tablespoons of the lemon juice. Pull off the tough outer leaves of the artichokes until you get to the paler leaves with pale tips. With a sharp knife, cut off and discard the top 1 inch of the artichokes. Cut off the tough bottoms of the stems, then peel the stems. Halve the artichokes lengthwise and remove the fuzzy chokes from the center. Cut each artichoke half in half again. Place the artichoke quarters in the lemon-water.

2 In a large nonstick skillet, heat the oil over low heat. Add the onion and garlic, and cook, stirring frequently, until the onion is tender, about 7 minutes. Add the carrot and cook 5 minutes.

3 Lift the artichokes from the water and add to the pan along with the salt, thyme, remaining 1 tablespoon lemon juice, and 2 cups of water. Bring to a boil, reduce to a simmer, and cook for 10 minutes.

4 Add the lima beans to the skillet and cook until the artichokes are tender enough to pierce with a knife, about 15 minutes. *Makes 4 servings*

per serving: 176 calories, 2.8g total fat (0.4g saturated), 0mg cholesterol, 11g dietary fiber, 33g carbohydrate, 9g protein, 450mg sodium. **good source of:** beta carotene, fiber, folate, magnesium, potassium, thiamin, vitamin B$_6$, vitamin C.

Braised Shiitakes & Artichokes

Mushrooms, potatoes, and artichokes seem to have a natural affinity for one another. Their earthy flavors complement each other while the sprightly taste of lemon gives the dish a boost.

> ½ cup dried shiitake mushrooms
> (½ ounce)
>
> 1¼ cups boiling water
>
> 1 tablespoon olive oil
>
> 5 cloves garlic, minced
>
> 1 pound fresh shiitake mushrooms, stems discarded and caps quartered
>
> 1 pound small red potatoes, quartered
>
> 1 package (9 ounces) frozen artichoke hearts
>
> 1½ teaspoons grated lemon zest
>
> 2 tablespoons fresh lemon juice
>
> ¾ teaspoon salt
>
> ½ teaspoon tarragon

1 In a small heatproof bowl, combine the dried mushrooms and the boiling water, and let stand for 20 minutes, or until softened. Reserving the soaking liquid, scoop out the dried mushrooms and coarsely chop. Strain the soaking liquid through a coffee filter or a paper towel-lined sieve.

2 In a large skillet, heat the oil over low heat. Add the garlic and cook, stirring frequently, until soft, about 2 minutes. Add the fresh and dried mushrooms, and cook until the fresh mushrooms begin to soften, about 5 minutes.

3 Stir in the potatoes, artichokes, lemon zest, lemon juice, salt, tarragon, and reserved mushroom soaking liquid, and bring to a boil. Reduce to a simmer, cover, and cook until the potatoes and artichokes are tender, about 25 minutes. *Makes 4 servings*

per serving: 273 calories, 3.9g total fat (0.6g saturated), 0mg cholesterol, 10g dietary fiber, 48g carbohydrate, 7g protein, 676mg sodium. **good source of:** fiber, folate, magnesium, niacin, potassium, riboflavin, selenium, thiamin, vitamin B$_6$, vitamin C, vitamin D, zinc.

Boston Baked Beans

Massachusetts settlers adopted the Indian custom of slow-cooking beans with bits of meat (venison) and maple syrup, but changed the meat to salt pork and the sweetener to molasses. This dish eventually came to be called Boston Baked Beans, earning Boston the name "Bean Town." Our version uses lean turkey bacon in place of the salt pork, and supplements the molasses with maple syrup. **Timing alert:** The beans bake for 2 hours. And cooking beans from scratch will add several more hours (plus soaking).

1 can (14½ ounces) crushed tomatoes
¾ cup water
3 tablespoons molasses
3 tablespoons maple syrup
2 tablespoons cider vinegar
2 teaspoons dry mustard
½ teaspoon salt
½ teaspoon pepper
1 bay leaf
3 cups cooked white beans (see below), such as Great Northern, navy, or cannellini, or 2 cans (19 ounces each) cannellini beans, rinsed and drained
4 slices turkey bacon, chopped (2 ounces)
1 small onion, finely chopped

1 Preheat the oven to 250°F. In a small Dutch oven (1½ quarts), stir together the tomatoes, water, molasses, maple syrup, vinegar, dry mustard, salt, pepper, and bay leaf. Bring to a boil and boil for 1 minute.

2 Stir in the beans, bacon, and onion. Cover and bake for 2 hours or until the beans are richly flavored and well coated. Remove the bay leaf before serving. *Makes 6 servings*

how to cook beans

Beans are cooked in water until tender, but you should adjust the cooking time to the final use you have planned. For instance, for salads, cook the beans until just done (firm but not mushy). For purees, cook them until they are very soft. And for recipes where the beans will continue to cook, such as soups or casseroles (*see Boston Baked Beans, above*), slightly undercook the beans.

▶ **To soak or not soak** There are several schools of thought on presoaking beans before you cook them. Most people will tell you that the reason for soaking them first is that it cuts down on the cooking time. The fact of the matter is that it saves only about 45 minutes (not much when you're already committed to 1 to 2 hours anyway). The other reason put forth for presoaking beans is their oligosaccharides, carbohydrates responsible for causing unwanted gas in the bean consumer. Some research suggests that presoaking beans, and then discarding the soaking water before cooking them, will get rid of some of the oligosaccharides.

▶ **Soaking methods** You can quick-soak beans in an hour, or soak them for 8 hours or overnight (in the refrigerator). For either method, place the beans in a large pot (they will double in size during soaking) and add enough water to cover: about 10 cups of water per pound of beans, or two to three times the beans' volume in water. For quick-soaking, bring the water to a boil and cook at a boil for 2 minutes. Remove the pot from the heat and let stand, covered, for 1 hour. For long soaking, let the beans stand in cold water at room temperature for no longer than 8 hours. For longer than 8 hours, or in warm weather, soak the beans in the refrigerator; otherwise they will begin to ferment.

▶ **How to cook** With either soaking method, pour off the soaking water. Then add fresh water (or broth) to cover the beans by about 2 inches. Bring the liquid slowly to a boil, skimming off the scum that rises to the surface. When the liquid boils, reduce the heat, partially cover the pot, and simmer until the beans are tender. Stir occasionally, and add more water, if necessary. The beans are done when they can be easily pierced with the tip of a knife.

▶ **Cooking times** The amount of time it takes to cook beans varies with the size, density, and age of the bean. Small beans, such as adzuki, take 30 to 40 minutes to cook (after soaking). Medium-size beans (the bulk of the bean family), such as black beans and kidney beans, take 1½ to 2 hours. Older beans (of any size) will take longer.

per serving: 235 calories, 2.8g total fat (0.6g saturated), 8mg cholesterol, 7g dietary fiber, 43g carbohydrate, 12g protein, 419mg sodium. good source of: fiber, folate, magnesium, potassium, vitamin B$_6$.

Green Beans with Fresh Tomatoes & Basil

While these beans are delicious hot, they are equally good at room temperature or chilled. The vibrant green color of the beans may become somewhat duller, but the flavor will not suffer.

> 1½ pounds green beans, halved crosswise on the diagonal
>
> 2 teaspoons olive oil
>
> 1 small red onion, halved and thinly sliced
>
> 3 cloves garlic, slivered
>
> ¾ pound plum tomatoes, coarsely chopped
>
> ¼ cup chopped fresh basil
>
> ½ teaspoon salt
>
> 1 tablespoon red wine vinegar

1 In a vegetable steamer, steam the green beans until crisp-tender, 3 to 5 minutes.

2 Meanwhile, in a large nonstick skillet, heat the oil over medium heat. Add the onion and garlic, and cook until the onion is soft, about 5 minutes.

3 Add the tomatoes, basil, and salt, and bring to a boil. Add the beans and cook, stirring frequently, until the sauce is slightly reduced and the beans are tender, about 3 minutes. Stir in the vinegar. *Makes 4 servings*

per serving: 108 calories, 3.1g total fat (0.5g saturated), 0mg cholesterol, 7g dietary fiber, 20g carbohydrate, 4g protein, 305mg sodium. good source of: fiber, folate, magnesium, niacin, potassium, riboflavin, thiamin, vitamin B$_6$, vitamin C.

Lemon-Dill Beans & Peas

A very small amount of butter added to the dish at the end softens the lemon sauce and gives the beans a very rich flavor. However you can omit the butter for a tarter, more lemony sauce.

> ¾ pound yellow wax beans or green beans, halved crosswise
>
> ¾ pound sugar snap peas, strings removed
>
> 3 cloves garlic, minced
>
> 2 tablespoons plus ¼ cup water
>
> ½ teaspoon cornstarch
>
> 1 teaspoon grated lemon zest
>
> ¼ cup fresh lemon juice
>
> ½ teaspoon salt
>
> ⅓ cup minced fresh dill
>
> 1½ teaspoons butter
>
> 1 teaspoon sesame seeds, toasted

1 In a vegetable steamer, steam the wax beans and sugar snaps until crisp-tender, about 5 minutes.

2 Meanwhile, in a large nonstick skillet, heat the garlic and 2 tablespoons of the water over low heat until the garlic is soft, about 2 minutes.

3 In a small bowl, whisk together the cornstarch and the remaining ¼ cup of water. Add to the pan along with the lemon zest, lemon juice, and salt, and bring to a boil. Cook, stirring constantly, until the sauce has thickened slightly, about 1 minute.

4 Add the beans and sugar snap peas, and toss to coat. Add the dill, and stir to combine. Remove from the heat and swirl in the butter until melted. Serve sprinkled with toasted sesame seeds. *Makes 4 servings*

per serving: 85 calories, 2.3g total fat (1.1g saturated), 4mg cholesterol, 6g dietary fiber, 16g carbohydrate, 4g protein, 297mg sodium. good source of: fiber, folate, magnesium, potassium, riboflavin, thiamin, vitamin C.

Roasted Beets with Their Greens

Anyone who likes beets will love beet greens. They taste vaguely of beets, but have the soft, rich flavors of spinach or Swiss chard.

> *4 pounds beets, preferably small, with tops (about 2½ pounds of beets weighed without the tops)*
>
> *½ cup water*
>
> *¾ cup orange juice*
>
> *½ teaspoon cornstarch*
>
> *¼ cup red wine vinegar*
>
> *2 tablespoons light brown sugar*
>
> *¾ teaspoon salt*
>
> *¼ teaspoon caraway seeds*
>
> *2 teaspoons olive oil*

1 Preheat the oven to 350°F.

2 Twist the tops (leaves and stems) off the beets. Remove and discard the tough stems. Coarsely shred the leaves with their tender stems. Wash well.

3 Place the beets in a baking dish large enough to hold them in a single layer. Add the water to the baking dish and cover tightly with foil. Bake for 1½ to 2 hours (depending on the size of the beets), or until they are fork-tender. Remove from the oven and let cool. Discard any remaining water.

4 Meanwhile, in a small nonreactive saucepan, whisk the orange juice into the cornstarch. Add the vinegar, brown sugar, ½ teaspoon of the salt, and the caraway seeds. Bring to a boil over medium-high heat. Cook, stirring, until the mixture is slightly thickened, about 1 minute. Remove from the heat and let cool to room temperature.

5 When the beets are cool enough to handle, peel, halve, and thinly slice. Place in a large bowl and toss with the orange dressing.

6 In a large nonstick skillet, heat the oil over medium-high heat. Add the beet greens and the remaining ¼ teaspoon salt, and cook, stirring frequently, until tender, about 5 minutes. Serve the baked beets on a bed of the wilted greens. *Makes 4 servings*

per serving: 168 calories, 2.8g total fat (0.4g saturated), 0mg cholesterol, 9g dietary fiber, 34g carbohydrate, 5g protein, 344mg sodium. **good source of:** betacyanins, beta carotene, fiber, folate, magnesium, potassium, riboflavin, thiamin, vitamin B_6, vitamin C, vitamin E.

Sicilian-Style Broccoli Rabe

The slight bitterness of broccoli rabe is tempered here by the sweetness of raisins. If you prefer, substitute milder broccolini for the broccoli rabe. All of the broccoli rabe is edible, though it's best to trim off the very ends, which may be tough.

> *¼ cup sun-dried tomatoes*
>
> *½ cup boiling water*
>
> *1 tablespoon olive oil*
>
> *3 cloves garlic, peeled*
>
> *1 medium onion, finely chopped*
>
> *1 bunch broccoli rabe (1 pound), thinly sliced*
>
> *⅓ cup raisins*
>
> *½ teaspoon red pepper flakes*
>
> *½ teaspoon salt*

1 In a small heatproof bowl, combine the sun-dried tomatoes and boiling water. Let stand until the tomatoes have softened, 15 to 20 minutes (depending on the dryness of the tomatoes). Drain, reserving the soaking liquid, and coarsely chop the tomatoes.

2 In a large nonstick skillet, heat the oil over medium-low heat. Add the garlic and cook until the garlic is golden brown, about 5 minutes. Remove the garlic, and when cool enough to handle, mince.

recipe creator
sautéed greens

Cooking greens couldn't be simpler. Simply wash them well, and then cook them in a skillet with just the water still clinging to the leaves (this is how you cook spinach, too). You could leave it at that, but these healthful vegetables also provide an opportunity to get creative; greens have a special affinity for salty-sour tastes. Choose from the categories below and follow these basic instructions: In a non-stick Dutch oven, heat 1 tablespoon of olive oil over low heat. Add 3 minced garlic cloves and ½ cup chopped onion, and sauté until tender. Add 1 VEGETABLE and cook until tender, 5 to 10 minutes. Stir in 12 cups of GREENS (with any water still clinging to them), 1 or 2 ADD-INS, and ¼ teaspoon salt. Cover and cook over medium-low heat, stirring occasionally, until the greens are soft and tender, from 5 to 15 minutes. The timing will vary with the sturdiness of the greens; soft Swiss chard will be done first, and hardier greens, such as kale and collards, will take longer. Once the greens are cooked, stir in 1 FINAL TOUCH. *Makes 4 servings*

VEGETABLES	GREENS	ADD-INS	FINAL TOUCH
▶Red bell peppers, 1 cup diced	▶Mustard greens, chopped	▶Sun-dried tomatoes, ¼ cup chopped	▶Cider vinegar, 1 Tbsp
▶Green bell peppers, 1 cup diced	▶Turnip greens, chopped	▶Raisins or currants, ¼ cup	▶Red wine vinegar, 1 Tbsp
▶Carrots, 1 cup sliced	▶Swiss chard, stems and leaves, chopped	▶Anchovy paste, 2 tsp	▶Rice vinegar, 1 Tbsp
▶Butternut squash, 1 cup diced	▶Escarole, chopped	▶Canadian bacon, 3 Tbsp chopped	▶Malt vinegar, 1 Tbsp
▶Mushrooms, 2 cups sliced	▶Kale, chopped	▶Canned or bottled jalapeño, 1, minced	▶Lemon juice, 1 Tbsp
	▶Collard greens, chopped	▶Lemon zest, 2 tsp grated	
	▶Beet greens, chopped	▶Mango chutney, 2 Tbsp chopped	
	▶Watercress, tough stems trimmed, chopped	▶Calamata olives, 6, pitted and chopped	

3 Add the onion to the skillet and cook, stirring frequently, until the onion is soft, about 7 minutes.

4 Add the sun-dried tomatoes, broccoli rabe, raisins, red pepper flakes, and salt to the pan and cook, stirring frequently, until the broccoli rabe starts to wilt, about 5 minutes.

5 Add the reserved soaking liquid and the minced garlic, cover, and cook until the broccoli rabe is very tender, about 10 minutes. *Makes 4 servings*

per serving: 118 calories, 3.6g total fat (0.5g saturated), 0mg cholesterol, 2g dietary fiber, 21g carbohydrate, 4g protein, 385mg sodium. good source of: beta carotene, indoles, potassium, vitamin C.

Baby Bok Choy with Shiitake Mushrooms

Small heads of tender baby bok choy are often available at Asian markets. If you can't find baby bok choy, look for the smallest heads of regular bok choy and cook the stems a minute or two longer.

2 pounds baby bok choy

2 teaspoons olive oil

¾ cup water

2 tablespoons minced fresh ginger

4 cloves garlic, minced

*½ pound fresh shiitake mushrooms,
  stems discarded and caps sliced into
  ¼-inch-wide strips*

1 teaspoon cornstarch

¾ teaspoon salt

½ teaspoon pepper

1 Trim ¼ inch off the root ends of the bok choy. Cut into 2-inch sections.

2 In a large nonstick skillet, heat the oil and ¼ cup of the water over medium-high heat. Add the ginger and garlic, and cook until the garlic is soft, about 2 minutes.

3 Add the bok choy and mushrooms, and cook, stirring, until the mushrooms are tender and the bok choy is crisp-tender.

4 Meanwhile, in a small bowl, combine the cornstarch, salt, pepper, and the remaining ½ cup water, stirring until the cornstarch is dissolved. Add the cornstarch mixture to the pan and cook, stirring constantly, for 1 minute or until the sauce is slightly thickened and the vegetables are well coated. *Makes 4 servings*

per serving: 83 calories, 2.8g total fat (0.4g saturated), 0mg cholesterol, 3g dietary fiber, 13g carbohydrate, 4g protein, 586mg sodium. **good source of:** beta carotene, calcium, folate, indoles, potassium, riboflavin, selenium, vitamin B$_6$, vitamin C, vitamin D.

Chopped Broccoli Piccata

Many people (grown-ups included) will eat the florets off a broccoli spear, leaving the nutritious stems behind. Here's a recipe that should encourage diners to eat the whole thing (well, they won't actually have a choice). If the pungent flavors of arugula are not to your liking, you can use ⅓ cup of chopped fresh basil or parsley instead.

*1 large bunch broccoli (about 1¾ pounds),
  separated into spears*

½ cup water

1 tablespoon plus 1 teaspoon olive oil

5 cloves garlic, minced

¼ teaspoon red pepper flakes

1½ teaspoons grated lemon zest

¾ teaspoon salt

2 cups arugula, shredded

2 tablespoons fresh lemon juice

1 Trim off just the tough bottoms of each spear. Peel the stalks. Very coarsely chop both the stalks and the florets.

2 In a large nonstick skillet, heat the water and oil over low heat. Add the garlic and red pepper flakes, and cook, stirring occasionally, until the garlic is tender, about 2 minutes.

3 Add the broccoli, lemon zest, and salt, and cook, stirring frequently, until the broccoli is tender but not mushy, about 5 minutes.

4 Stir in the arugula and lemon juice, and cook until the arugula has wilted, about 1 minute. *Makes 4 servings*

per serving: 99 calories, 5.2g total fat (0.7g saturated), 0mg cholesterol, 6g dietary fiber, 12g carbohydrate, 6g protein, 341mg sodium. **good source of:** beta carotene, fiber, folate, indoles, potassium, riboflavin, sulforaphane, thiamin, vitamin B$_6$, vitamin C, vitamin E.

Brussels Sprouts with Chestnuts

Brussels sprouts, in addition to looking like mini heads of cabbage, are in the cabbage family, making them cruciferous vegetables. The earthy, cabbage-y flavor of sprouts is nicely complemented by chestnuts. If you're not up for cooking and peeling chestnuts, look for cans of whole cooked chestnuts. Thyme is a sweet yet savory herbal underscore for the dish.

6 cups Brussels sprouts

2 teaspoons olive oil

¼ cup minced onion

1 clove garlic, minced

½ cup cooked chestnuts (page 126) or canned

½ teaspoon salt

½ teaspoon thyme

¼ teaspoon pepper

1 Remove the very bottom of the stem ends of the Brussels sprouts. Cut each sprout in half through the core. In a vegetable steamer, steam the Brussels sprouts for 3 minutes.

2 Meanwhile, in a large nonstick skillet, heat the oil over medium heat. Add the onion and garlic, and cook, stirring, until the onion is soft, about 5 minutes.

3 Add the Brussels sprouts, chestnuts, salt, thyme, and pepper, and cook, stirring frequently, until the Brussels sprouts are fork-tender and golden, 5 to 7 minutes; add a couple of tablespoons of water if the pan seems too dry. *Makes 4 servings*

per serving: 122 calories, 3.4g total fat (0.5g saturated), 0mg cholesterol, 5g dietary fiber, 22g carbohydrate, 4g protein, 322mg sodium. good source of: fiber, folate, indoles, potassium, riboflavin, thiamin, vitamin B_6, vitamin C, vitamin E.

the brassica bunch

The *Brassica* genus, we admit, is not as well loved as it ought to be. It's the cabbage family of vegetables, also known as cruciferous, because their flowers are shaped like a cross. These vegetables are definitely in the very-good-for-you category. They are loaded with vitamin C, beta carotene and other carotenoids, plus lots of fiber; some (the dark greens) contain calcium, too. In addition, they offer anticancer compounds such as indoles.

Here's a roster of family members, including some recipe suggestions to inspire you:

►**Bok choy** Baby Bok Choy with Shiitake Mushrooms (*opposite page*)

►**Broccoli & Broccolini** (a cross between broccoli and kale) Chopped Broccoli Piccata (*at left*)

►**Broccoli rabe** Sicilian-Style Broccoli Rabe (*page 182*)

►**Brussels sprouts** Brussels Sprouts with Chestnuts (*above*)

►**Cabbage** Colcannon (*page 186*) or Red Cabbage Slaw (*page 202*)

►**Cauliflower** Cauliflower with Cheese Sauce (*page 187*)

►**Greens (kale, collards, mustard, turnip, Swiss chard)** Sautéed Greens "Recipe Creator" (*page 183*)

►**Kohlrabi** Kohlrabi Gratin (*page 189*)

►**Turnip & Rutabaga** Roasted White & Yellow Turnips (*page 197*)

Colcannon

This traditional Irish dish (the name means "white cabbage" in Gaelic) was originally created to use up vegetable leftovers from the previous evening's meal. In Ireland colcannon would commonly have included potatoes (naturally) and cabbage.

1½ pounds baking potatoes, quartered

2 teaspoons olive oil

3 slices (1½ ounces) turkey bacon, coarsely chopped

1 large onion, finely chopped

¾ teaspoon salt

6 cups shredded green and/or red cabbage

¼ teaspoon caraway seeds

⅓ cup low-fat (1%) milk

1 In a vegetable steamer, steam the potatoes until tender, about 10 minutes. Transfer to a large bowl.

2 Meanwhile, in a large skillet, heat the oil over medium heat. Add the bacon and cook for 2 minutes. Add the onion and cook, stirring frequently, until the onion is golden brown and tender, about 10 minutes.

3 Add ¼ teaspoon of the salt, the cabbage, and caraway seeds, and cook, stirring frequently, until the cabbage is wilted and tender, about 7 minutes.

4 Drain the potatoes and return them to the pot. Shake the pot over low heat for 2 minutes to dry the potatoes. Off the heat, with a potato masher or electric mixer, beat the milk and remaining ½ teaspoon salt into the potatoes.

5 Add the mashed potatoes to the skillet and cook, stirring frequently, until the potatoes are heated through, about 5 minutes. *Makes 6 servings*

per serving: 281 calories, 5.1g total fat (1.1g saturated), 10mg cholesterol, 7g dietary fiber, 53g carbohydrate, 8g protein, 618mg sodium. good source of: fiber, folate, indoles, magnesium, niacin, potassium, sulforaphane, thiamin, vitamin B$_6$, vitamin C.

Orange-Mint Carrots

These can be made early in the day and gently reheated at serving time. If the liquid has evaporated before the carrots are tender, add a little water.

1½ pounds carrots, halved lengthwise and thinly sliced crosswise

¾ teaspoon finely slivered orange zest

1 cup orange juice

1 tablespoon honey

2 teaspoons butter

½ teaspoon salt

¼ cup chopped fresh mint

1 In a large skillet, combine the carrots, orange zest, orange juice, honey, butter, and salt. Cover and bring to a gentle boil over medium heat. Cook, stirring occasionally, for 10 minutes.

2 Uncover and cook until the carrots are tender and glazed, about 5 minutes. Stir in the mint. *Makes 4 servings*

per serving: 133 calories, 2.3g total fat (1.3g saturated), 5mg cholesterol, 5g dietary fiber, 28g carbohydrate, 2g protein, 396mg sodium. good source of: beta carotene, fiber, folate, potassium, vitamin B$_6$, vitamin C.

different spins

▶ **Glazed Carrots & Turnips** Follow the directions for *Orange-Mint Carrots*, but reduce the carrots to ¾ pound and add ¾ pound white turnips, quartered and thinly sliced. Substitute 1 tablespoon brown sugar for the honey. In step 1, add ¼ teaspoon pepper when adding the salt.

▶ **Orange-Cilantro Root Vegetables** Follow the directions for *Orange-Mint Carrots*, but reduce the carrots to ½ pound and add ½ pound parsnips, thinly sliced, and ½ pound rutabaga, peeled and thinly sliced. In step 1, add 2 cloves minced garlic, 1 teaspoon coriander, and ⅛ teaspoon cayenne pepper when adding the other ingredients. Use chopped cilantro instead of mint.

Cauliflower with Cheese Sauce

To give the milk in the cheese sauce a little heft, we've boosted it with nonfat dry milk powder, which adds milk solids (and calcium) but no fat.

> *¼ cup nonfat dry milk powder*
>
> *3 tablespoons flour*
>
> *½ teaspoon salt*
>
> *½ teaspoon thyme*
>
> *¼ teaspoon cayenne pepper*
>
> *1½ cups fat-free milk*
>
> *1 cup finely diced red bell pepper*
>
> *¼ cup shredded reduced-fat sharp Cheddar cheese*
>
> *¼ cup grated Parmesan cheese*
>
> *2 scallions, minced*
>
> *2 teaspoons Dijon mustard*
>
> *1 head cauliflower, cut into small florets*

1 In a medium saucepan, whisk together the dry milk powder, flour, salt, thyme, and cayenne. Gradually whisk in the liquid milk until no lumps remain. Cook, stirring constantly, over medium heat until the sauce is slightly thickened, about 5 minutes. Stir in the bell pepper and cook until crisp-tender, about 2 minutes.

2 Stir in the Cheddar and Parmesan, and cook until the cheeses have melted, about 1 minute. Remove from the heat and stir in the scallions and mustard.

3 Meanwhile, in a vegetable steamer, steam the cauliflower until tender, about 4 minutes. Transfer to a medium bowl. Add the cheese sauce, tossing until the cauliflower florets are well coated. *Makes 4 servings*

per serving: 145 calories, 3.7g total fat (2.1g saturated), 11mg cholesterol, 3g dietary fiber, 18g carbohydrate, 12g protein, 611mg sodium. good source of: calcium, fiber, folate, potassium, riboflavin, selenium, thiamin, vitamin B₁₂, vitamin B₆, vitamin C, vitamin D.

Celeriac Puree

The flavor of celeriac (celery root) is difficult to describe: It's decidedly celerylike, but also is slightly nutty, with very faint licorice undertones. Cooking celeriac in milk helps preserve its color—in fact, as you peel the celeriac, dropping it into the milk will keep it from discoloring. The small amount of rice cooked with the root makes a very light, creamy puree.

> *2 cups low-fat (1%) milk*
>
> *1½ pounds celeriac (celery root), peeled, halved, and thinly sliced*
>
> *2 tablespoons uncooked long-grain rice*
>
> *3 cloves garlic, peeled and smashed*
>
> *1 teaspoon salt*

1 In a medium saucepan, combine the milk, celeriac, rice, garlic, and salt. Bring to a boil over medium heat.

2 Reduce to a simmer, cover, and cook until the celeriac is very tender, about 20 minutes. (The milk will look curdled, but don't worry, it will smooth out again once the mixture is pureed.)

3 Strain the celeriac, garlic, and rice, reserving the cooking liquid. Add the solids to a food processor. With the processor running, gradually add the cooking liquid until the mixture is the consistency of creamy mashed potatoes. You may not need all of the cooking liquid (discard any you don't need). *Makes 4 servings*

per serving: 137 calories, 1.8g total fat (0.9g saturated), 5mg cholesterol, 3g dietary fiber, 25g carbohydrate, 7g protein, 790mg sodium. good source of: calcium, magnesium, potassium, riboflavin, thiamin, vitamin B₁₂, vitamin B₆, vitamin D, zinc.

different *spins*

▶**Succotash & Chicken Salad** Follow the directions for *Succotash*, but omit the butter. Let the succotash cool to room temperature, then stir in 2 teaspoons olive oil, 1 tablespoon red wine vinegar, 3 diced plum tomatoes, and 2 cups shredded cooked chicken. Serve at room temperature or chilled.

Succotash

If fresh sweet corn is in season, strip the kernels from 4 or 5 ears of corn and use them in place of the frozen kernels.

> 2 teaspoons olive oil
>
> 4 shallots, minced
>
> 1 package (10 ounces) frozen baby lima beans
>
> ¼ cup water
>
> ¾ teaspoon thyme
>
> ½ teaspoon salt
>
> 3 cups frozen corn kernels
>
> ¼ cup chopped parsley
>
> 2 teaspoons butter

1 In a medium saucepan, heat the oil over medium heat. Add the shallots and cook, stirring frequently, until softened, about 4 minutes.

2 Add the lima beans, water, thyme, and salt, and bring to a boil. Reduce to a simmer, cover, and cook until the lima beans are almost tender, about 10 minutes.

3 Stir in the corn and cook, covered, until the corn and lima beans are tender, about 4 minutes.

4 Remove from the heat, stir in the parsley and butter, and stir until the butter has melted. *Makes 4 servings*

per serving: 233 calories, 5.4g total fat (1.7g saturated), 5mg cholesterol, 8g dietary fiber, 42g carbohydrate, 9g protein, 320mg sodium. good source of: fiber, folate, magnesium, niacin, potassium, vitamin B$_6$.

Baked Fennel with Garlic & Herbs

Raw fennel is a wonderful addition to salads, but when you bake it, it becomes a meltingly tender side dish. The celerylike stalks attached to most fennel bulbs are too woody to be edible, but occasionally you'll find some tender enough to eat. Test the stalks to see, and any that aren't too tough can be baked along with the bulbs.

> 2 bulbs fennel (about 1 pound each)
>
> ¼ cup water
>
> 4 teaspoons olive oil
>
> ½ teaspoon grated lemon zest
>
> 2 tablespoons fresh lemon juice
>
> ½ teaspoon oregano
>
> ½ teaspoon salt
>
> 3 cloves garlic, slivered

1 Preheat the oven to 400°F.

2 Cut off and discard the fennel stalks. Reserve the fennel fronds and coarsely chop. Finely chop enough of the fronds to make ¼ cup and set aside. Cut the bulbs lengthwise into ¼-inch-thick slices.

3 In a large bowl, whisk together the water, oil, lemon zest, lemon juice, oregano, and salt. Add the sliced fennel and garlic, and toss until coated. Transfer to a glass or ceramic baking dish. Cover with foil.

4 Bake for 25 minutes, or until the fennel is tender. Sprinkle the reserved fennel fronds over the fennel and serve with any pan juices that have collected. *Makes 4 servings*

per serving: 96 calories, 4.9g total fat (0.6g saturated), 0mg cholesterol, 5g dietary fiber, 13g carbohydrate, 2g protein, 376mg sodium. good source of: fiber, folate, potassium, vitamin C.

Kohlrabi Gratin

Kohlrabi, a member of the turnip family, has a mild, sweet taste and a crisp, crunchy texture.

1 pound kohlrabi, peeled, halved, and thinly sliced

1 cup low-fat (1%) milk

4 teaspoons flour

1 tablespoon minced chives or 1 scallion, thinly sliced

½ teaspoon salt

¼ teaspoon pepper

¼ cup plain dried breadcrumbs

2 tablespoons grated Parmesan cheese

1 Preheat the oven to 375°F. Spray an 8-inch square baking pan with nonstick cooking spray. In a vegetable steamer, steam the kohlrabi until tender, about 7 minutes.

2 Meanwhile, in a small bowl, stir the milk into the flour. Add the chives, salt, and pepper.

3 Arrange a layer of overlapping kohlrabi slices in the bottom of the pan. Spoon ⅓ cup of the milk mixture over the kohlrabi. Repeat with 2 more layers, ending with the milk mixture.

4 In a small bowl, stir together the breadcrumbs and Parmesan. Scatter the mixture over the kohlrabi. Cover and bake for 20 minutes, or until piping hot.

5 Preheat the broiler. Place the pan under the broiler and broil 4 to 6 inches from the heat for about 1 minute, or until the crumbs are crisp and golden brown. *Makes 4 servings*

per serving: 87 calories, 1.8g total fat (1g saturated), 4mg cholesterol, 2g dietary fiber, 13g carbohydrate, 5g protein, 434mg sodium. **good source of:** calcium, potassium, riboflavin, selenium, thiamin, vitamin B_{12}, vitamin C.

---

making your own breadcrumbs

It's easy to make your own breadcrumbs. Not only is it a good solution for what to do with bread that's gone stale, but it's a good ingredient to have on hand for recipes. And if you make the crumbs from whole-grain bread, you'll also have a more healthful ingredient, since most commercial brands are not made from whole-grain bread. To make the crumbs, either toast the bread until dried and crisp, or tear it into small pieces and spread it out to air-dry. Then transfer the dried bread to a food processor and pulse on and off until you've got the desired consistency—fine or coarse. Store the breadcrumbs in the freezer (especially if you've made them with whole-grain bread).

Cipolline Agrodolce

Cipolline, small flat onions, take very well to this *agrodolce* (sweet-sour) preparation. If you can't find cipolline, use small white or red onions.

2 pounds yellow or red cipolline

⅓ cup red wine vinegar

⅓ cup chicken broth or water

2 tablespoons sugar

½ teaspoon salt

¼ teaspoon pepper

¼ teaspoon rubbed sage

⅛ teaspoon allspice

1 In a large pot of boiling water, cook the onions for 3 minutes. Drain and peel, leaving the stem end intact (this will keep the onions from falling apart).

2 In a large skillet, combine the vinegar, broth, sugar, salt, pepper, sage, and allspice. Bring to a boil over medium heat. Add the onions and reduce to a simmer. Cover and cook, shaking the pan occasionally to coat the onions evenly, until the onions are tender, about 25 minutes.

3 Increase the heat to high, uncover the skillet, and cook, stirring constantly, until the onions are glazed, about 3 minutes. *Makes 4 servings*

per serving: 112 calories, 0.4g total fat (0.1g saturated), 0mg cholesterol, 3g dietary fiber, 26g carbohydrate, 3g protein, 336mg sodium. **good source of:** potassium, vitamin B_6.

Braised Leeks with Tomato & Coriander

Leeks, the aristocrat of the onion family, have a sweet, mellow onion flavor and when gently cooked, a very tender, delicate texture. Serve these as a side dish, part of a buffet, or as an appetizer.

6 medium leeks (2 pounds total), roots removed and dark green ends trimmed

1 can (14½ ounces) diced tomatoes

1 teaspoon grated orange zest

⅓ cup orange juice

2 teaspoons olive oil

2 cloves garlic, minced

¼ teaspoon ground coriander

¼ teaspoon salt

6 Gaeta or Calamata olives, pitted and coarsely chopped

2 tablespoons chopped cilantro

1 Halve the leeks lengthwise. Soak the leeks in a bowl of warm water, gently pulling back the top several inches of the layers to get the dirt that usually lodges right where the leek starts to turn green. Use several changes of warm water until there is no grit remaining in the bottom of the bowl. Lift the leeks out of the water and pat dry.

2 In a large nonstick skillet, combine the tomatoes, orange zest, orange juice, oil, garlic, coriander, and salt, and bring to a boil over medium heat.

Add the leeks, cover, and cook until fork-tender, turning them occasionally, about 15 minutes.

3 Stir in the olives and cilantro. Serve warm, at room temperature, or chilled. *Makes 4 servings*

per serving: 150 calories, 4.2g total fat (0.5g saturated), 0mg cholesterol, 4g dietary fiber, 27g carbohydrate, 3g protein, 396mg sodium. **good source of:** fiber, folate, magnesium, potassium, vitamin B$_6$, vitamin C.

Lentils with Fennel & Tomato

Small green-black French lentils have a slight chewiness and a nutty flavor, but they are not as readily available as green lentils (the type most commonly found in supermarkets), which can easily be substituted here.

2 teaspoons olive oil

1 small red onion, finely chopped

3 cloves garlic, minced

¾ cup French lentils

3 tablespoons tomato paste

¾ teaspoon salt

¾ teaspoon fennel seeds

2½ cups water

½ cup small pasta shapes, such as farfalline, alphabets, or stelline

roasted peppers

Roasting bell peppers is a good way to cook them with absolutely no fat. You also add a slight roasted flavor to the vegetables, because you char the peppers' skin in the process.

The standard pepper-roasting method that you will find in most cookbooks is to roast the pepper whole, turning it over an open flame, and then steaming it in a paper bag. Our method streamlines this process and makes it more user-friendly:

1. Choose meaty peppers with thick walls.

2. Cut the peppers lengthwise into flat panels. Follow the natural shape of the pepper; you will end up with 4 or 5 panels, depending on the pepper. The

object here is to have surfaces flat enough that will broil at the same rate, making removal of the skin easier.

3. Preheat the broiler. Place the pepper pieces, skin-side up, on a broiler pan (you can also do this on a grill, skin-side down). Broil 4 inches from the heat for 10 to 12 minutes, or until the pepper skin is charred (not just browned, but actually charred).

4. Stack the peppers pieces in a bowl and cover the bowl with a plate. This will slightly steam the peppers, making it easier to remove the skin.

5. When the peppers are cool enough to handle, peel off the charred skin.

1 In a medium nonstick saucepan, heat the oil over medium heat. Add the onion and garlic, and cook, stirring frequently, until the onion is golden brown and tender, about 10 minutes.

2 Stir in the lentils, tomato paste, salt, fennel seeds, and 2 cups of the water, and bring to a boil. Reduce to a simmer, cover, and cook 25 minutes.

3 Add the remaining ½ cup water and the pasta, and cook until the lentils are tender and the pasta is "al dente," about 10 minutes. *Makes 4 servings*

per serving: 190 calories, 2.9g total fat (0.4g saturated), 0mg cholesterol, 12g dietary fiber, 31g carbohydrate, 12g protein, 538mg sodium. **good source of:** fiber, folate, potassium, thiamin, vitamin B_6.

Marinated Roasted Peppers

Choose peppers of any color for this delicious side dish. Red, yellow, and orange peppers will be sweeter than green or black ones, but all are wonderful to have on hand. Roasted peppers can be served on their own, added to salads or sandwiches, or used to top a pizza.

> *4 large bell peppers*
> *3 tablespoons balsamic vinegar*
> *2 teaspoons olive oil*
> *¼ teaspoon salt*
> *1 clove garlic, thinly sliced*

1 Preheat the broiler. Roast the peppers and peel them (*see "Roasted Peppers," opposite page*).

2 Meanwhile, in a medium bowl, whisk together the vinegar, oil, and salt. Add the garlic. Add the roasted pepper pieces, tossing to combine. Cover and refrigerate for at least 1 hour or up to 3 days. Remove and discard the garlic before serving. *Makes 6 servings*

per serving: 48 calories, 1.7g total fat (0.2g saturated), 0mg cholesterol, 2g dietary fiber, 8g carbohydrate, 1g protein, 101mg sodium. **good source of:** vitamin B_6, vitamin C.

Roasted Jerusalem Artichokes, Potatoes & Herbs

Jerusalem artichokes, also known as sunchokes, have a nutty flavor and a creamy texture, almost like a potato. Their skin is very thin and does not need to be peeled, which is a good thing because these tubers can be very knobby.

> *⅓ cup water*
> *1 tablespoon olive oil*
> *2 teaspoons Dijon mustard*
> *1½ pounds Jerusalem artichokes, well scrubbed and cut into ½-inch-thick slices*
> *½ pound small white potatoes, cut into ½-inch-thick slices*
> *8 cloves garlic, unpeeled*
> *½ teaspoon rosemary, minced*
> *½ teaspoon thyme*
> *½ teaspoon salt*

1 Preheat the oven to 400°F. In a large bowl, whisk together the water, oil, and mustard until well combined. Add the Jerusalem artichokes, potatoes, garlic, rosemary, thyme, and salt. Toss well to coat.

2 Transfer the vegetables to a roasting pan large enough to hold them in a single layer. Roast for 35 to 40 minutes, shaking the pan occasionally, until the artichokes and potatoes are tender. *Makes 4 servings*

per serving: 192 calories, 3.8g total fat (0.5g saturated), 0mg cholesterol, 4g dietary fiber, 37g carbohydrate, 4g protein, 364mg sodium. **good source of:** niacin, potassium, thiamin, vitamin B_6.

Spinach, Mushroom & Red Pepper Sauté

This is a good basic recipe for sautéed spinach. You can substitute shredded Swiss chard, collard greens, or kale for the spinach. The sturdier greens may take a little longer to wilt.

> 2 teaspoons olive oil
>
> 1 small red onion, finely chopped
>
> 3 cloves garlic, minced
>
> 1 large red bell pepper, cut into ½-inch squares
>
> ½ pound mushrooms, thinly sliced
>
> 8 cups packed fresh spinach leaves
>
> ½ teaspoon salt
>
> ¼ teaspoon marjoram

1 In a nonstick Dutch oven or flameproof casserole, heat the oil over medium heat. Add the onion and garlic, and cook, stirring frequently, until the onion is soft, about 7 minutes.

2 Add the bell pepper and mushrooms, and cook, stirring frequently, until the vegetables are tender, about 7 minutes.

3 Add the spinach and sprinkle with the salt and marjoram. Cover and cook, stirring the spinach occasionally, until the spinach is wilted, about 4 minutes. *Makes 4 servings*

per serving: 67 calories, 2.6g total fat (0.4g saturated), 0mg cholesterol, 3g dietary fiber, 9g carbohydrate, 4g protein, 337mg sodium. **good source of:** beta carotene, fiber, folate, magnesium, potassium, vitamin B$_6$, vitamin C, vitamin E.

Peas with Lettuce & Fresh Mint

Braising peas with shredded lettuce is a dish the French modestly call French-style peas, or *petits pois à la française*. Of course the traditional French dish also includes a good deal of heavy cream and butter (*quelle surprise*), which we've eliminated in favor of olive oil.

> 2 teaspoons olive oil
>
> 2 cloves garlic, minced
>
> 3 cups shredded iceberg lettuce
>
> 2 pounds fresh peas, shelled, or 1 package (10 ounces) frozen peas, thawed
>
> ¼ cup chopped fresh mint
>
> ¾ teaspoon salt
>
> ½ cup water

1 In a large nonstick skillet, heat the oil over low heat. Add the garlic and cook until tender, about 2 minutes.

---

different spins

▶ **Spinach, Mushroom & Red Pepper Pizza** Follow the directions for *Spinach, Mushroom & Red Pepper Sauté*, but place the finished sauté on top of a crisp Italian bread shell. Scatter ⅓ cup of shredded part-skim mozzarella on top and bake at 450°F until the crust is crisp and the cheese has melted.

▶ **Caramelized Onion-Topped Potatoes** Follow the directions for *Smashed Potatoes (opposite page)*, but while the potatoes are cooking (step 2), in a large nonstick skillet, heat 2 teaspoons olive oil over medium heat.

Add 2 large onions, diced, and ½ teaspoon salt, and cook, stirring frequently, until the onions are golden brown and tender, about 20 minutes. Mash the potatoes as directed and serve topped with the onions.

▶ **Smashed Potatoes & Peas** Follow the directions for *Smashed Potatoes (opposite page)*, but increase the milk to ⅔ cup and add 1 cup of thawed frozen peas when mashing the potatoes in step 3. Stir in ¼ cup of minced scallions.

2 Stir in the lettuce, peas, mint, salt, and water, and cook, stirring frequently, until the lettuce has wilted and the peas are tender, about 5 minutes. *Makes 4 servings*

per serving: 84 calories, 2.6g total fat (0.4g saturated), 0mg cholesterol, 4g dietary fiber, 12g carbohydrate, 4g protein, 521mg sodium. good source of: fiber, folate, thiamin, vitamin C.

Summer Squash Sauté

"Sautéed" in its own juices along with garlic, shallots, and spices, summer squash picks up a lot of flavor. A small amount of butter added at the end enhances the buttery texture of the squash. If you've got a farmers' market near you, look for yellow squash that are bright and deeply colored; they are more flavorful and sweeter than their paler cousins.

3 cloves garlic, minced

3 shallots, minced

½ cup water

2 pounds yellow summer squash, shredded

½ teaspoon salt

½ teaspoon marjoram or oregano

¼ teaspoon pepper

⅛ teaspoon nutmeg

1¼ teaspoons butter

1 In a large nonstick skillet, heat the garlic, shallots, and water over low heat. Cook until the shallots are tender, about 3 minutes.

2 Add the summer squash, salt, marjoram, pepper, and nutmeg, and cook, stirring frequently, until the squash is tender, about 5 minutes.

3 Add the butter and cook just until melted, about 1 minute. *Makes 4 servings*

per serving: 67 calories, 1.7g total fat (0.9g saturated), 3mg cholesterol, 4g dietary fiber, 13g carbohydrate, 3g protein, 297mg sodium. good source of: fiber, folate, magnesium, potassium, thiamin, vitamin B₆, vitamin C.

Smashed Potatoes

Baking potatoes are fluffier and drier than Yukon Gold potatoes, but the combination makes a light, creamy, and extremely flavorful smash.

1 pound baking potatoes, well scrubbed and cut into 2-inch chunks

1 pound Yukon Gold potatoes

8 cloves garlic, peeled

4 cups water

1 teaspoon salt

½ cup milk

Add-ins (see below; optional)

1 In a large pot, combine the baking potatoes, Yukon Gold potatoes, garlic, water, and ¼ teaspoon of the salt. Bring to a boil over medium heat.

2 Reduce to a simmer and cook until the potatoes are tender, but not falling apart, about 20 minutes. Drain, reserving ¼ cup of the cooking liquid.

3 Return the potatoes to the pot and add the remaining ¾ teaspoon salt, the reserved potato cooking water, and the milk. With a potato masher, mash the potatoes until still quite lumpy.

4 Serve the potatoes as is, or stir in one of the following add-ins. *Makes 4 servings*

per serving: 229 calories, 1.2g total fat (0.7g saturated), 4mg cholesterol, 6g dietary fiber, 50g carbohydrate, 6g protein, 614mg sodium. good source of: fiber, magnesium, niacin, potassium, thiamin, vitamin B₆, vitamin C.

Spicy Corn & Cheese Stir in 1 cup shredded Manchego cheese, 1 cup corn kernels, and 1 minced jalapeño pepper.

Sun-Dried Tomatoes Stir in ¾ cup chopped sun-dried tomatoes.

Green Herbs Stir in 1 cup chopped cooked spinach, ¼ cup minced dill, and 2 tablespoons minced scallions.

Root Vegetables with Peanut Sauce

We added some other root vegetables here to complement the flavor of the burdock as well as fill out the dish, since burdock can be quite expensive.

1 burdock root (about 8 ounces), scrubbed and trimmed, but not peeled

1 medium parsnip (about 6 ounces)

1 carrot

1 white turnip (about 6 ounces)

1 clove garlic

3 tablespoons fresh lime juice

4 teaspoons creamy peanut butter

1 tablespoon reduced-sodium soy sauce

½ teaspoon honey

¼ teaspoon salt

1 Cut the burdock, parsnip, carrot, and turnip into matchstick strips. As you work, drop the burdock into a bowl of water with a little lemon juice or vinegar to prevent discoloration.

2 Drain the burdock. In a vegetable steamer, steam the burdock, parsnip, carrot, and turnip until crisp-tender, about 5 minutes.

3 In a small pot of boiling water, cook the garlic for 2 minutes to blanch. Drain, reserving 2 tablespoons of the cooking liquid. When cool enough to handle, mince the garlic.

4 In a medium bowl, combine the reserved cooking liquid, the garlic, lime juice, peanut butter, soy sauce, honey, and salt. Add the drained vegetables and toss until just combined. Serve warm or at room temperature. *Makes 4 servings*

per serving: 130 calories, 3g total fat (0.6g saturated), 0mg cholesterol, 6g dietary fiber, 25g carbohydrate, 4g protein, 339mg sodium. **good source of:** beta carotene, fiber, folate, magnesium, niacin, potassium, vitamin B$_6$, vitamin C.

Herb-Roasted Sweet Potato Skins

Save the scooped-out flesh from the sweet potatoes to make mashed sweet potatoes or sweet potato pie. Or use 1¾ cups of the mashed sweet potato flesh as a substitute for the 15-ounce can of pumpkin puree called for in the Pumpkin Cheesecake (*page 245*). **Serving suggestion:** This side dish would also make a great appetizer.

2 pounds small sweet potatoes

¼ cup grated Parmesan cheese

3 tablespoons chopped parsley

2 cloves garlic, minced

½ teaspoon oregano

½ teaspoon rosemary, minced

½ teaspoon salt

¼ teaspoon pepper

1 Preheat the oven to 400°F.

2 If the sweet potatoes are not small, halve them lengthwise to bake. Prick the sweet potatoes, place them on a baking sheet, and bake for 35 to 45 minutes, or until tender but not mushy. Remove from the oven and set on a rack to cool. (Alternatively, cook the sweet potatoes in the microwave.)

3 Meanwhile, in a medium bowl, combine the Parmesan, parsley, garlic, oregano, rosemary, salt, and pepper.

4 Preheat the broiler. When the potatoes are cool enough to handle, halve the whole ones (if using)

did you know?

Burdock is a brown-skinned root vegetable with white flesh that tastes like a cross between celery and artichokes. Popular in Japan (where it's called gobo), burdock can be found at Asian grocery stores and some health-food stores. Don't be put off if the outside of the root is dirty or muddy; just wash the root well (no need to peel). Like Jerusalem artichokes, burdock is very high in a type of carbohydrate called inulin, which can cause intestinal gas in certain individuals.

lengthwise. Scoop the sweet potato flesh out of the skins, leaving a wall ¼ inch thick. (Reserve the scooped out flesh for another use.) Cut each sweet potato shell lengthwise into ½-inch-wide wedges.

5 Add the skins to the herbed Parmesan mixture and gently toss to combine. Place the sweet potato skins on a baking sheet and broil 4 to 5 inches from the heat for 4 to 6 minutes, or until the cheese is melted. Serve hot. *Makes 4 servings*

per serving: 98 calories, 1.6g total fat (1g saturated), 4mg cholesterol, 3g dietary fiber, 18g carbohydrate, 4g protein, 248mg sodium. good source of: beta carotene.

Baked Apples & Sweet Potatoes with Crunchy Topping

No marshmallows on top of these sweet potatoes—just apples, apple juice, and a crisp, slightly sweetened oat topping.

> 3 teaspoons olive oil
>
> 5 cloves garlic, slivered
>
> ¾ cup apple juice
>
> 2 tablespoons fresh lemon juice
>
> 2 pounds sweet potatoes, peeled and thinly sliced
>
> 2 apples, cut into ½-inch-thick wedges
>
> ½ teaspoon salt
>
> ¼ teaspoon pepper
>
> ¼ cup old-fashioned rolled oats
>
> 4 teaspoons light brown sugar

1 Preheat the oven to 450°F. In a small nonstick skillet, heat 1 teaspoon of the oil over medium heat. Add the garlic and cook until soft, about 2 minutes. Add the apple juice and lemon juice and cook for 30 seconds.

2 Arrange the sweet potatoes and apples in a 7 x 11-inch glass baking dish. Sprinkle with the salt and pepper. Pour the apple juice mixture on top.

3 Cover with foil and bake for 25 minutes, or until the sweet potatoes are tender.

4 Meanwhile, in a small bowl, stir together the oats, brown sugar, and the remaining 2 teaspoons oil.

5 Sprinkle the oat mixture over the sweet potatoes, return to the oven, and bake until the topping is lightly browned and crisp, about 10 minutes. *Makes 6 servings*

per serving: 215 calories, 3g total fat (0.5g saturated), 0mg cholesterol, 4g dietary fiber, 46g carbohydrate, 3g protein, 212mg sodium. good source of: beta carotene, vitamin B$_6$, vitamin C.

Stir-Fried Sweet Potatoes

If you can find them, use white sweet potatoes (sometimes called Jersey sweets) in this dish. They have a somewhat firmer texture than orange-fleshed sweets.

> 1 tablespoon olive oil
>
> 2 pounds sweet potatoes, well scrubbed and cut into ½ x 3-inch sticks
>
> 3 cloves garlic, minced
>
> 1 tablespoon minced fresh ginger
>
> 2 tablespoons cider vinegar
>
> 2 teaspoons dark sesame oil
>
> ¾ teaspoon salt

1 In a large nonstick skillet, heat the olive oil over medium heat. Add the sweet potatoes and cook, stirring frequently, until not quite tender, about 7 minutes.

2 Add the garlic and ginger, and cook, stirring occasionally, for 2 minutes.

3 Add the vinegar, sesame oil, and salt, and toss until the sweet potatoes are well coated and cooked through. *Makes 6 servings*

per serving: 184 calories, 3.9g total fat (0.6g saturated), 0mg cholesterol, 5g dietary fiber, 35g carbohydrate, 3g protein, 306mg sodium. good source of: beta carotene, fiber, potassium, vitamin B$_6$, vitamin C.

Swiss Chard with Curry Spices

Washed Swiss chard has enough water clinging to its leaves to cook in its own steam.

1½ teaspoons olive oil

1 tablespoon water

3 cloves garlic, minced

1 teaspoon cumin

¾ teaspoon ground ginger

¾ teaspoon yellow mustard seeds

¼ teaspoon pepper

¼ teaspoon cardamom

2 bunches Swiss chard, washed and shredded (16 cups)

¼ teaspoon salt

1 In a nonstick Dutch oven, heat the oil and water over low heat. Add the garlic and cook until tender, about 2 minutes.

2 Add the cumin, ginger, mustard seeds, pepper, and cardamom, and stir to combine. Cook 1 minute or until fragrant.

3 Add the Swiss chard and salt. Cover and cook, stirring occasionally, until the chard is tender, about 5 minutes. Uncover and cook, stirring frequently, until most of the liquid has evaporated, about 3 minutes. *Makes 4 servings*

per serving: 53 calories, 2.3g total fat (0.3g saturated), 0mg cholesterol, 3g dietary fiber, 7g carbohydrate, 3g protein, 454mg sodium. **good source of:** beta carotene, magnesium, potassium, vitamin C, vitamin E, vitamin K.

Roasted Tomatoes with Garlic

When cooked slowly, even slightly unripe (or otherwise not terribly flavorful) plum tomatoes develop a concentrated tomato flavor. Because of their high flesh-to-seed ratio, plum tomatoes take extremely well to this preparation. Serve these alongside Simple Broiled Chicken (*page 108*), Parmesan-Crusted Crab Cakes (*page 73*), or Broiled Herb-Rubbed Pork Chops (*page 86*). The roasted tomatoes are so versatile, that they can also be served as part of an antipasto, added to a pasta sauce, or used on sandwiches. **Timing alert:** The tomatoes need to bake for 3 hours, but you can make them well ahead and refrigerate them.

3 tablespoons water

1 tablespoon olive oil

5 cloves garlic, minced

2 teaspoons coarse (kosher) salt

1 teaspoon sugar

¾ teaspoon basil

3 pounds plum tomatoes, halved lengthwise

1 Preheat the oven to 250°F. Line a jelly-roll pan with foil.

2 In a large bowl, whisk together the water, oil, garlic, salt, sugar, and basil. Add the tomatoes and toss to coat. Place the tomatoes, cut-sides up, on the foil-lined pan and bake for 3 hours, or until the tomatoes have collapsed and their skins have wrinkled.

roasting a whole head of garlic

Most people don't think of garlic as a vegetable, but it actually can be cooked and eaten as a sort of vegetable condiment. When garlic is cooked slowly in the oven, its pungency is tamed, though its delicious flavor is still in evidence. Roasted garlic is great spread on bread, added to salad dressings or dipping sauces, used as a sandwich spread, or eaten as a condiment with roast poultry or meat.

To roast garlic, preheat the oven to 400°F. Wrap a whole, unpeeled head (also called a bulb) of garlic in foil. Place it on a baking sheet, or in a small roasting pan, and roast until the garlic is soft, about 30 minutes. When cool enough to handle, unwrap the head of garlic, slice off one end (or cut the garlic head in half), and squeeze out the soft garlic inside.

3 Serve the tomatoes at room temperature or chilled. *Makes 4 servings*

per serving: 112 calories, 4.6g total fat (0.6g saturated), 0mg cholesterol, 4g dietary fiber, 18g carbohydrate, 3g protein, 972mg sodium. good source of: beta carotene, fiber, folate, niacin, potassium, riboflavin, thiamin, vitamin B$_6$, vitamin C, vitamin E.

Roasted White & Yellow Turnips

If you have access to a farmers' market, look for a variety of yellow turnip called yellow globe. It is especially sweet and tender. You certainly can use either all white or all yellow turnips instead of the combination.

¾ pound white turnips, peeled and cut into ½-inch-thick wedges

¾ pound yellow turnip (rutabaga), peeled and cut into ½-inch-thick wedges

2 carrots, cut into ½-inch-thick slices

½ cup chicken broth, homemade (page 252) or canned

1 tablespoon olive oil

5 cloves garlic, peeled and halved

¾ teaspoon salt

½ teaspoon rubbed sage

1 Granny Smith apple, cut into ½-inch-thick wedges

1 Preheat the oven to 400°F. In a vegetable steamer, steam the turnips and carrots until crisp-tender, about 5 minutes.

2 Transfer the turnips and carrots to a roasting pan. Add the broth, oil, garlic, salt, and sage, and toss to combine.

3 Cover and roast for 10 minutes. Uncover, add the apple, and roast, shaking the pan occasionally, for about 15 minutes, or until the vegetables are browned and tender. *Makes 4 servings*

per serving: 103 calories, 3.6g total fat (0.5g saturated), 0mg cholesterol, 5g dietary fiber, 17g carbohydrate, 2g protein, 587mg sodium. good source of: beta carotene, fiber, potassium, vitamin C.

Sautéed Winter Squash

Butternut and hubbard have the greatest amount of beta carotene of the commonly available varieties of winter squash.

⅓ cup golden raisins

½ cup hot water

2 teaspoons olive oil

1 medium red onion, cut into ½-inch chunks

3 cloves garlic, slivered

1½ pounds butternut or hubbard squash, peeled and cut into 1-inch chunks

¼ cup dry white wine

2 tablespoons red wine vinegar

1 tablespoon sugar

1 In a small bowl, combine the raisins and hot water, and set aside to soften.

2 In a large nonstick skillet, heat the oil over medium heat. Add the onion and garlic, and cook, stirring frequently, until the onion has colored, about 7 minutes.

3 Add the squash and cook, stirring often, until the squash begins to color, about 5 minutes.

4 Add the raisins and their soaking liquid, the wine, vinegar, and sugar. Bring to a simmer, cover, and cook until the vegetables are tender, about 10 minutes. *Makes 4 servings*

per serving: 138 calories, 2.5g total fat (0.4g saturated), 0mg cholesterol, 4g dietary fiber, 28g carbohydrate, 2g protein, 8mg sodium. good source of: beta carotene, magnesium, potassium, vitamin B$_6$, vitamin C.

Maple-Orange Baked Acorn Squash

Compact and sturdy, acorn squash serves as both food and plate. To turn this side dish into a main dish, spoon a serving of Southwestern Meatless Chili (*page 148*), Pork Vindaloo (*page 87*), or Hearty Turkey Stew (*page 132*) into the cavities of the baked squash halves.

½ teaspoon salt

½ teaspoon cardamom

½ teaspoon cinnamon

¼ teaspoon ground ginger

¼ teaspoon pepper

2 small acorn squash (¾ pound each), halved lengthwise and seeded

¼ cup maple syrup

⅔ cup orange juice

2 tablespoons orange marmalade

1 Preheat the oven to 450°F. In a small bowl, combine the salt, cardamom, cinnamon, ginger, and pepper.

2 Place the squash, cut-sides up, in a baking dish large enough to hold them in a single layer. Pour enough water into the pan to come halfway up the sides of the squash. Brush 1 tablespoon of the maple syrup over the cut-sides of the squash and sprinkle with the spice mixture. Cover with foil and bake for 25 minutes, or until the squash is tender. Leave the oven on.

3 Meanwhile, in a small saucepan, combine the remaining 3 tablespoons maple syrup, the orange juice, and marmalade, and bring to a boil over medium heat. Cook until the mixture is reduced to a syrup thick enough to coat the back of a spoon, about 5 minutes.

4 Remove the squash from the baking dish and discard the water. Return the squash to the dish, cut-sides up. Brush the squash with the maple-orange mixture and bake for 15 minutes, or until the squash is lightly browned around the edges.
Makes 4 servings

per serving: 162 calories, 0.3g total fat (0.1g saturated), 0mg cholesterol, 5g dietary fiber, 42g carbohydrate, 2g protein, 303mg sodium. **good source of:** fiber, potassium, thiamin, vitamin B_6, vitamin C.

salads

The word salad comes from the Latin verb *salare*, meaning to salt. A Roman salad consisted of fresh greens sprinkled with salt for flavor; hence the greens were *salata*, or salted. (Just as a side note, in Roman times salt was an expensive commodity and was used as a form of currency, giving us the English word salary.)

Salads have come a long way since then, and range from simple tossed salads—basically greens and a dressing—to grain and vegetable salads. By and large, salads are served chilled or at room temperature. And the so-called "side salad" (as opposed to a main-course salad) is intended to be an adjunct to a meal.

Side salads serve a number of functions in a meal. They can be served first, as a sort of appetite whetter. They can be served last (European style) as a bit of a palate cleanser before dessert. Or they can be served *with* the meal, as a side dish. The type of side salad you choose—and when you choose to serve it—should be governed by the flavors (and calories) in the rest of the meal.

did you know?

Not only do nut oils bring a delicate, fragrant touch to salad dressings, but they are also nutritious. Each type of nut oil has a slightly different nutritional profile, supplying more or less the same minerals, vitamins, and healthful fats found in the nuts themselves (with the exception of fiber, which is lost in the processing). Almond, hazelnut, macadamia, pecan, and pistachio oils provide the greatest amount of heart-healthy monounsaturated fats. And walnut oil is notable for its ample amounts of a type of fat called alpha-linolenic acid, which is similar to the beneficial omega-3 fats found in fish. Almond and hazelnut oils also supply the antioxidant vitamin E. Naturally, nut oils, like any oil, should be consumed in moderation because they also bring with them quite a lot of calories.

recipe creator
tossed salads

A tossed salad seems like it should be easy, but in fact there is an art to creating a balance between flavors, textures, and weights. Though this last consideration (weight) may seem odd, it's important to understand that a tossed salad needs to work as a cohesive whole, not a dish in which heavy ingredients sink to the bottom of the salad bowl. Choose from the following categories and follow these basic instructions: Prepare ½ cup of any salad dressing (*try one of the dressings on pages 253–255*). Place the dressing in the bottom of a large salad bowl. Add 4 cups SOFT GREENS, 2 cups STURDY GREENS, 2 cups PUNGENT GREENS (if you don't like pungent greens, just increase the amount of soft greens by 2 cups), and 2 cups ADD-INS, and toss. Sprinkle 1 or 2 GARNISHES over the top. *Makes 4 servings*

SOFT GREENS	STURDY GREENS	PUNGENT GREENS	ADD-INS	GARNISHES
▶ Leaf lettuce, torn	▶ Iceberg lettuce, torn	▶ Arugula, trimmed	▶ Carrots, 1 cup finely shredded	▶ Pecans or walnuts, ¼ cup chopped, toasted
▶ Boston lettuce, torn	▶ Romaine lettuce, torn	▶ Watercress, ends trimmed	▶ Red onion, ½ cup slivered	▶ Sunflower or pumpkin seeds, 3 Tbsp
▶ Bibb lettuce, torn	▶ Tatsoi	▶ Radicchio, torn	▶ Cilantro, ½ cup chopped	▶ Sesame seeds, 1 Tbsp toasted
▶ Mâche	▶ Red cabbage, shredded	▶ Chicory, torn	▶ Fresh dill, ¼ cup minced	▶ Feta, goat, or blue cheese, 3 Tbsp crumbled
▶ Baby spinach		▶ Belgian endive, sliced	▶ Chives or scallion greens, ¼ cup minced	▶ Parmesan cheese, 3 Tbsp grated
▶ Lamb's-quarters (wild spinach)		▶ Nasturtium leaves	▶ Fresh basil, ¼ cup slivered	▶ Cherry tomatoes, 1 cup halved
		▶ Escarole, torn		▶ Roasted peppers, 1 cup sliced or diced
		▶ Young dandelion greens, torn		

Asparagus with Confetti Dressing

Most salad dressings have very little in the way of nutrients (and usually quite a bit of fat). In this asparagus side salad we take the opportunity to boost the fiber and nutrient content of the tomato-lemon vinaigrette by adding bell peppers, carrot, cucumber, and onion. **Serving suggestion:** In addition to serving this as a side salad, this would make a very nice starter for a multicourse meal.

¼ cup tomato juice

3 tablespoons fresh lemon juice

1 tablespoon olive oil

2 teaspoons red wine vinegar

½ teaspoon salt

½ teaspoon black pepper

2 large red bell peppers, finely diced

½ cup shredded carrot

1 small cucumber, peeled, seeded, and diced

¼ cup finely chopped sweet onion, such as Vidalia

2 pounds asparagus

1 In a medium bowl, whisk together the tomato juice, lemon juice, oil, vinegar, salt, and black pepper. Add the bell peppers, carrot, cucumber, and onion, and stir to combine. Cover and let stand at room temperature for at least 15 minutes to blend the flavors.

2 In a vegetable steamer, steam the asparagus until crisp-tender, about 4 minutes.

3 Arrange the asparagus on a serving platter. Spoon the vegetable dressing over the asparagus. Serve at room temperature or chilled. *Makes 6 servings*

per serving: 66 calories, 2.7g total fat (0.4g saturated), 0mg cholesterol, 3g dietary fiber, 10g carbohydrate, 3g protein, 243mg sodium. good source of: beta carotene, fiber, folate, potassium, thiamin, vitamin B_6, vitamin C, vitamin E.

Roasted Pear Salad with Blue Cheese Dressing

Roasting pears intensifies their flavor while making them soft and tender. Choose firm pears, such as Bosc, for this recipe. The pears can be roasted in advance and refrigerated. Bring them to room temperature before serving.

2 pears, such as Bosc

½ cup dry white wine

4 teaspoons sugar

½ teaspoon tarragon

¼ teaspoon salt

⅔ cup buttermilk

2 tablespoons blue cheese, crumbled (1½ ounces)

1 tablespoon white wine vinegar

¼ teaspoon pepper

8 cups mixed salad greens

2 tablespoons chopped toasted pecans

1 Preheat the oven to 400°F. Halve the pears lengthwise, but do not peel them. Core the pears and slice them crosswise into ½-inch-thick slices.

2 In a 9-inch pie plate, stir together the wine, sugar, tarragon, and salt. Add the pears and stir to coat. Roast the pears until tender, turning them twice while they cook, about 20 minutes. (Timing will vary depending upon the firmness of the pears.)

3 Meanwhile, in a large bowl, whisk together the buttermilk, blue cheese, vinegar, and pepper. Add the mixed greens and toss to coat.

4 Arrange the greens on 4 serving plates. Top with the roasted pears and toasted pecans. *Makes 4 servings*

per serving: 199 calories, 6.4g total fat (2.5g saturated), 10mg cholesterol, 5g dietary fiber, 28g carbohydrate, 6g protein, 366mg sodium. good source of: beta carotene, fiber, folate, potassium, riboflavin, vitamin C.

Moroccan Carrot Salad

Warm spices, such as cumin, cinnamon, and coriander, are typical of many Moroccan dishes and marry well with the sweet carrots and currants in this salad. **Timing alert:** Although this salad is fine at room temperature, it's especially good served chilled, which will take at least 1 hour.

⅓ cup orange juice

⅓ cup fresh lemon juice

1 tablespoon plus 1 teaspoon honey

1 tablespoon olive oil

1 teaspoon cumin

1 teaspoon ground coriander

½ teaspoon salt

¼ teaspoon cinnamon

1 pound carrots, shredded

1 red bell pepper, cut into matchsticks

⅓ cup chopped cilantro

2 tablespoons dried currants

1 In a large bowl, whisk together the orange juice, lemon juice, honey, oil, cumin, coriander, salt, and cinnamon.

2 Stir in the carrots, bell pepper, cilantro, and currants, and toss to combine. Cover and refrigerate until well chilled, at least 1 hour. *Makes 4 servings*

per serving: 142 calories, 4g total fat (0.5g saturated), 0mg cholesterol, 5g dietary fiber, 27g carbohydrate, 2g protein, 334mg sodium. good source of: beta carotene, fiber, potassium, thiamin, vitamin B_6, vitamin C.

Caesar Salad

The Caesar Salad was invented in 1924 by Caesar Cardini, an Italian restaurateur in Tijuana, Mexico. The original, which included raw eggs, has undergone some modernization over the years. Shredding Parmesan from a block of cheese instead of using pregrated adds a nice touch to this classic American salad.

3 ounces whole-wheat Italian bread, cut into ½-inch cubes

¼ cup plain fat-free yogurt

1 tablespoon reduced-fat mayonnaise

3 tablespoons fresh lemon juice

1 tablespoon water

1½ teaspoons anchovy paste

½ teaspoon pepper

8 cups torn romaine lettuce

¼ cup grated Parmesan cheese

1 In a toaster oven or under the broiler, toast the bread cubes for about 1 minute, or until crisp.

2 In a large bowl, combine the yogurt, mayonnaise, lemon juice, water, anchovy paste, and pepper, whisking until smooth and blended.

3 Add the bread cubes, lettuce, and Parmesan, and toss to coat. *Makes 4 servings*

per serving: 123 calories, 4.2g total fat (1.3g saturated), 6mg cholesterol, 3g dietary fiber, 17g carbohydrate, 7g protein, 324mg sodium. good source of: beta carotene, calcium, fiber, folate, potassium, riboflavin, selenium, thiamin, vitamin C.

caesar salad as a main course

Anyone who has been to a restaurant in the past two decades has probably had a main-course adaptation of a Caesar Salad. All you have to do to convert this classic side dish to a main dish is top the salad with grilled or roasted meat, poultry, fish, or shellfish (figure on about 3 ounces of cooked per person). Here are several ideas for you to try:

- Jerk Pork Kebabs (*page 86*)
- Simple Broiled Flank Steak (*page 92*)
- Oven-Roasted Salmon Fillets (*page 46*)
- Grilled Mackerel (*page 57*)
- Zesty Lime-Broiled Shrimp (*page 68*)
- Simple Grilled Scallops (*page 71*)
- Simple Broiled Chicken (*page 108*)
- Spice-Rubbed Chicken (*page 110*)
- Cajun Grilled Duck (*page 137*)

Cucumber Salad with Mint-Scallion Dressing

This refreshing salad would make a delicious addition to a pita pocket sandwich of grilled chicken; it would also be great as a side dish for broiled fish. **Timing alert:** The yogurt for the dressing needs to drain for 1 hour, and once the salad is assembled, it should chill for about 1 hour.

> ⅔ cup plain fat-free yogurt
>
> 2½ pounds cucumbers (about 5), peeled halved, and seeded
>
> 1 teaspoon salt
>
> 1 tablespoon fresh lemon juice
>
> 1 tablespoon red wine vinegar
>
> 2 teaspoons olive oil
>
> 2 cloves garlic, minced
>
> 2 scallions, thinly sliced
>
> ¼ cup chopped fresh mint

1 Place a coffee filter or paper towel-lined sieve over a bowl and spoon in the yogurt. Let drain for 1 hour to thicken the yogurt slightly. Discard the whey.

2 Meanwhile, thinly slice the cucumbers crosswise. Place the cucumber slices in a colander and toss with ½ teaspoon of the salt. Place the colan-

der in the sink or on a plate and let stand for 30 minutes. Rinse under cold water and blot dry.

3 Transfer the thickened yogurt to a bowl and whisk in the lemon juice, vinegar, oil, garlic, and remaining ½ teaspoon salt.

4 Add the cucumbers to the yogurt mixture and toss gently to combine. Stir in the scallions and mint. Cover and refrigerate until well chilled, about 1 hour. *Makes 4 servings*

per serving: 73 calories, 2.7g total fat (0.4g saturated), 1mg cholesterol, 2g dietary fiber, 10g carbohydrate, 4g protein, 328mg sodium. good source of: calcium, folate, potassium, riboflavin, vitamin B$_{12}$, vitamin B$_6$, vitamin C.

Red Cabbage Slaw

Cabbage is the most classic slaw ingredient, but other crunchy vegetables (carrots) and fruits (apples) make good slaw companions. **Timing alert:** The salad should be chilled for at least 1 hour.

> ¾ cup plain fat-free yogurt
>
> ⅓ cup cider vinegar
>
> ¼ cup apple cider or juice
>
> 2 tablespoons reduced-fat mayonnaise
>
> ¾ teaspoon salt
>
> ¼ teaspoon celery seed
>
> 6 cups shredded red cabbage
>
> 2 carrots, shredded
>
> 2 Granny Smith apples, diced
>
> ¼ cup minced red onion
>
> ¼ cup minced fresh dill

1 In a large bowl, whisk together the yogurt, vinegar, cider, mayonnaise, salt, and celery seed.

2 Add the cabbage, carrots, apples, red onion, and dill, and toss well to combine. Cover and refrigerate the slaw until well chilled, about 1 hour. *Makes 4 servings*

per serving: 145 calories, 3.1g total fat (0.4g saturated), 3mg cholesterol, 5g dietary fiber, 28g carbohydrate, 5g protein, 554mg sodium. good source of: beta carotene, calcium, fiber, folate, indoles, magnesium, potassium, riboflavin, thiamin, vitamin B$_{12}$, vitamin B$_6$, vitamin C.

different spins

▶**Red Cabbage & Beet Slaw** Follow the directions for *Red Cabbage Slaw*, but omit the carrots and add 2 raw beets, peeled and shredded. Substitute ¼ cup parsley and 2 tablespoons minced chives for the dill.

▶**Pear & Cabbage Slaw** Follow the directions for *Red Cabbage Slaw*, but omit the celery seed. Substitute red wine vinegar for the cider vinegar and 2 Bartlett pears for the apples. Add ¼ cup chopped toasted walnuts or pecans.

Fresh Fennel Salad with Capers & Lemon

Look for firm, unwrinkled fennel bulbs, with fresh-looking green fronds. If you can't find the smaller capers (labeled "nonpareil"), you can use the bigger capers—often from Spain—but chop them up so they are not so overwhelming in the salad.

> 2 tablespoons chopped sun-dried tomatoes
>
> 3 tablespoons boiling water
>
> ¼ cup fresh lemon juice
>
> 4 teaspoons olive oil
>
> 1½ teaspoons Dijon mustard
>
> ¼ teaspoon salt
>
> 2 bulbs fennel (2½ pounds total)
>
> 2 teaspoons small (nonpareil) capers or large capers, coarsely chopped

1 In a medium heatproof bowl, combine the sun-dried tomatoes and boiling water. Let stand until the tomatoes have softened, 15 to 20 minutes (depending on the dryness of the tomatoes).

2 Add the lemon juice, oil, mustard, and salt to the sun-dried tomatoes.

3 Cut off the fennel stalks and fronds. Finely chop ¼ cup of the fronds and add to the bowl of dressing; discard the stalks. Cut the bulbs in half lengthwise and thinly slice crosswise.

4 Add the fennel and capers to the bowl and toss well to combine. Serve at room temperature. *Makes 4 servings*

per serving: 114 calories, 5.1g total fat (0.6g saturated), 0mg cholesterol, 7g dietary fiber, 17g carbohydrate, 3g protein, 377mg sodium. good source of: fiber, folate, niacin, potassium, vitamin C.

Marinated Tomato Salad

Sweet grape tomatoes are matched with silky persimmons, crunchy cucumbers, and red onion in a tart basil-mint puree for an altogether agreeable marinated salad. Be sure to use a fuyu persimmon, which is still firm when it's ripe—as opposed to a hachiya persimmon, which is inedible when it's still firm (it's not edible until it's very soft). **Timing alert:** The salad needs to marinate for at least 1 hour.

> ½ cup packed basil leaves
>
> 2 tablespoons coarsely chopped fresh mint
>
> 3 tablespoons red wine vinegar
>
> 3 tablespoons water
>
> 2 teaspoons olive oil
>
> ¼ teaspoon salt
>
> 1 pint grape or cherry tomatoes, halved
>
> 1 fuyu persimmon, cut into ½-inch cubes
>
> 1 small cucumber, peeled, halved, seeded, and diced
>
> ¼ cup minced red onion

1 In a blender or food processor, combine the basil, mint, vinegar, water, oil, and salt, and process to a smooth puree. Transfer the marinade to a medium bowl.

2 Add the tomatoes, persimmon, cucumber, and red onion, and toss to combine. Marinate at least 1 hour before serving. *Makes 4 servings*

per serving: 75 calories, 2.7g total fat (0.4g saturated), 0mg cholesterol, 3g dietary fiber, 13g carbohydrate, 1g protein, 300mg sodium. good source of: fiber, potassium, vitamin C.

Tangerine & Avocado Salad

A good substitute for tangerines in the salad would be 5 navel oranges, divided into sections and each section cut into thirds.

> 3 tablespoons fresh lime juice
>
> 4 teaspoons honey
>
> 1 tablespoon balsamic vinegar
>
> ½ teaspoon salt
>
> ⅛ teaspoon cayenne pepper
>
> 6 tangerines
>
> 1 Hass avocado, halved, pitted, peeled, and thinly sliced crosswise
>
> 3 tablespoons roasted sunflower seeds

1 In a large bowl, whisk together the lime juice, honey, vinegar, salt, and cayenne.

2 With a vegetable peeler, peel 3 long strips of zest from 1 tangerine. Cut the strips into ⅛-inch slivers. Peel the tangerines and separate into segments. Cut the segments crosswise into 2 or 3 pieces; discard any seeds.

3 Add the avocado, tangerines, and zest to the bowl and toss to combine. Chill until serving time.

---

how to pit an avocado

If you've never dealt with an avocado before, there are a couple of good tricks you can use to get the pit out. Start by cutting around the avocado lengthwise, slicing all the way up to the pit in the center. Then hold both halves of the avocado, twist in opposite directions, and pull apart. The pit will still be lodged in one half of the avocado. Place the avocado on a work surface, and tap the blade of a sharp, heavy knife into the pit. The blow should be forceful but light (you don't want the avocado to fly off the counter). Then, holding the avocado half in your hand, with the knife blade still stuck in the pit, twist the knife. This will twist the pit out of its berth in the avocado.

---

4 Sprinkle with the sunflower seeds just before serving. *Makes 4 servings*

per serving: 194 calories, 11g total fat (1.5g saturated), 0mg cholesterol, 5.8g dietary fiber, 26g carbohydrate, 3g protein, 299mg sodium. good source of: fiber, folate, potassium, thiamin, vitamin B_6, vitamin C, vitamin E.

Sweet Potato Salad with Mango-Curry Dressing

Instead of white potatoes and mayonnaise, this potato salad features sweet potatoes and a spicy-sweet curried dressing.

> 1½ pounds sweet potatoes, peeled and cut into ½-inch chunks
>
> ⅓ cup plain fat-free yogurt
>
> 1 tablespoon reduced-fat mayonnaise
>
> 3 tablespoons mango chutney, finely chopped
>
> 1½ teaspoons curry powder
>
> ¾ teaspoon cumin
>
> ½ teaspoon pepper
>
> ½ teaspoon salt
>
> 1 cup diced celery
>
> ⅓ cup minced red onion

1 In a vegetable steamer, steam the sweet potatoes until tender, about 10 minutes.

2 Meanwhile, in a salad bowl, blend the yogurt, mayonnaise, chutney, curry powder, cumin, pepper, and salt.

3 Add the sweet potatoes to the dressing along with the celery and onion, and toss gently until well coated. *Makes 4 servings*

per serving: 174 calories, 2.8g total fat (0.2g saturated), 2mg cholesterol, 4g dietary fiber, 35g carbohydrate, 4g protein, 486mg sodium. good source of: beta carotene, fiber, potassium, riboflavin, vitamin B_6, vitamin C.

Triple-Gold Potato Salad

The three golds in question are the buttery-fleshed Yukon Gold potatoes, roasted yellow corn, and yellow bell peppers. This salad is nice and spicy. If it's not fresh corn season, you can use frozen corn on the cob. Let it thaw before grilling.

> 2½ pounds Yukon Gold potatoes, cut into 1-inch chunks
>
> 4 cloves garlic, peeled
>
> 8 scallions, thinly sliced
>
> ⅓ cup fresh lime juice
>
> 3 tablespoons olive oil
>
> 2 chipotle peppers packed in adobo
>
> ¾ teaspoon salt
>
> 2 yellow bell peppers, cut lengthwise into flat panels
>
> 3 ears of corn, husked

1 In a vegetable steamer, steam the potatoes until tender, 7 to 10 minutes.

2 In a small pot of boiling water, cook the garlic for 2 minutes to blanch.

3 In a food processor, combine the garlic, scallions, lime juice, oil, chipotle peppers, and salt, and process until pureed. Transfer the dressing to a large bowl. Add the hot potatoes to the dressing, and toss to combine.

4 Meanwhile, preheat the broiler. Place the bell peppers, skin-side up, and the corn on the broiler pan and broil 6 inches from the heat, turning the corn as it browns, until the peppers are charred and the corn is lightly browned, about 10 minutes. When cool enough to handle, peel the peppers and cut into ½-inch squares. With a sturdy knife, cut the corn from the cob.

5 Add the peppers and corn to the bowl with the potatoes and toss well. Serve warm, at room temperature, or chilled. *Makes 8 servings*

per serving: 205 calories, 5.7g total fat (0.8g saturated), 0mg cholesterol, 4g dietary fiber, 38g carbohydrate, 4g protein, 231mg sodium. good source of: lutein, niacin, potassium, thiamin, vitamin B$_6$, vitamin C.

---

different *spins*

▶**Berry Salad with Feta** To make a more substantial luncheon salad, follow the directions for *Tri-Berry Salad*, but add ¼ cup minced red onion to the salad when tossing. Crumble ½ cup of feta cheese over the top along with the walnuts.

Tri-Berry Salad

This elevates the fruit salad to new heights. Serve it as an opener to a meal, or after the main course, European-style. It could even be a simple fruit dessert.

> ¼ cup orange juice
>
> 2 tablespoons red wine vinegar
>
> 2 tablespoons light brown sugar
>
> ¼ teaspoon pepper
>
> 3 cups halved strawberries
>
> 1 cup raspberries
>
> 1 cup blackberries
>
> ½ cup toasted walnuts, coarsely chopped

1 In a large bowl, whisk together the orange juice, vinegar, brown sugar, and pepper.

2 Add the strawberries, raspberries, and blackberries, and toss to coat.

3 Serve the berry mixture sprinkled with the toasted walnuts. *Makes 4 servings*

per serving: 169 calories, 7.3g total fat (0.6g saturated), 0mg cholesterol, 8g dietary fiber, 27g carbohydrate, 3g protein, 5mg sodium. good source of: anthocyanins, fiber, omega-3 fatty acids, vitamin C.

Tabbouleh

Tabbouleh is a Lebanese salad made with bulgur (a partially cooked cracked wheat), lemon juice, tomatoes, and a considerable amount of fresh parsley and mint.

> 1 cup fine or coarse bulgur
>
> 2½ cups boiling water
>
> ⅓ cup fresh lemon juice
>
> 1¼ cups chopped fresh parsley
>
> 3 scallions, thinly sliced
>
> ¼ cup chopped fresh mint
>
> 2 tablespoons olive oil
>
> ¾ teaspoon salt
>
> ¼ teaspoon allspice
>
> 2 cups grape or cherry tomatoes, halved

1 In a large heatproof bowl, combine the bulgur and boiling water. Let stand for 1 hour at room temperature. Drain and squeeze the bulgur dry.

2 Transfer the bulgur to a large salad bowl. Add the lemon juice and toss to combine. Let stand for 30 minutes.

3 Stir in the parsley, scallions, mint, oil, salt, and allspice. Add the tomatoes and toss to combine. Serve at room temperature or chilled. *Makes 4 servings*

per serving: 210 calories, 7.6g total fat (1.1g saturated), 0mg cholesterol, 8g dietary fiber, 34g carbohydrate, 6g protein, 461mg sodium. good source of: fiber, magnesium, niacin, potassium, vitamin C.

Wheatberry Salad with Peppers & Grapes

Wheatberries have a very satisfying texture. They are similar to barley in that they remain slightly chewy even when fully cooked.

> ¾ cup wheatberries
>
> 2½ cups water
>
> 2 red bell peppers, cut lengthwise into flat panels
>
> 1 green bell pepper, cut lengthwise into flat panels
>
> 3 tablespoons red wine vinegar
>
> 1 tablespoon walnut or olive oil
>
> ½ teaspoon salt
>
> 1 cup seedless red grapes, quartered
>
> 2 scallions, thinly sliced

1 In a medium saucepan, bring the wheatberries and water to a boil over high heat. Reduce to a simmer, cover, and cook until the wheatberries are tender but still slightly chewy, about 1 hour. Drain.

2 Meanwhile, preheat the broiler. Place the bell pepper pieces, skin-side up, on a broiler pan and broil 4 inches from the heat for 10 to 12 minutes, or until the skin is charred. When the peppers are cool enough to handle, peel them and cut into ½-inch squares.

---

different spins

▶**Chicken & Cheese Tabbouleh** For a main-course salad, follow the directions for *Tabbouleh*, and stir ½ pound cooked, diced chicken breast and 1 ounce crumbled feta cheese into the salad.

▶**Vegetarian Couscous Salad** For a main-course salad, follow the directions for *Couscous Salad (opposite page)*, but add 1½ cups each cooked chick-peas and halved cherry tomatoes. Increase the pumpkin seeds to 2 tablespoons.

▶**Shrimp & Feta Couscous Salad** For a main-course salad, follow the directions for *Couscous Salad (opposite page)*, but omit the pumpkin seeds and add ¾ pound of cooked medium shrimp and ⅓ cup of crumbled feta cheese.

▶**Crab & Sushi Rice Salad** For a main-course salad, follow the directions for *Sushi Rice Salad (opposite page)*, but add 1 cup of shredded cooked crabmeat or surimi (imitation crab) once the salad has chilled.

3 In a large bowl, whisk together the vinegar, walnut oil, and salt. Add the warm wheatberries, bell peppers, grapes, and scallions, and toss to combine. Serve warm, at room temperature, or chilled. *Makes 4 servings*

per serving: 217 calories, 4.5g total fat (0.7g saturated), 0mg cholesterol, 7g dietary fiber, 43g carbohydrate, 6g protein, 297mg sodium. good source of: beta carotene, fiber, niacin, potassium, selenium, thiamin, vitamin B$_6$, vitamin E.

Couscous Salad

Couscous makes an almost-instant pasta salad because it doesn't actually have to cook; it's merely steeped in boiling water to soften.

> 1⅓ cups couscous
>
> ¾ teaspoon salt
>
> 1 tablespoon plus 1 teaspoon olive oil
>
> 1 medium zucchini, cut into ¼-inch dice
>
> 1 teaspoon grated lemon zest
>
> ¼ cup fresh lemon juice
>
> 4 scallions, thinly sliced
>
> ¼ cup chopped fresh dill
>
> 1 tablespoon hulled pumpkin seeds (pepitas)

1 Prepare the couscous according to package directions, using ½ teaspoon of the salt. Add 1 tablespoon of the oil and fluff with a fork. Transfer to a large bowl.

2 Meanwhile, in a medium nonstick skillet, heat the remaining 1 teaspoon oil over medium heat. Add the zucchini and cook, stirring frequently, until tender but not mushy, about 3 minutes. Transfer to the bowl with the couscous.

3 Add the remaining ¼ teaspoon salt, the lemon zest, lemon juice, scallions, dill, and pumpkin seeds to the bowl. Toss to combine. *Makes 4 servings*

per serving: 223 calories, 4g total fat (0.6g saturated), 0mg cholesterol, 3g dietary fiber, 40g carbohydrate, 7g protein, 298mg sodium.

Sushi Rice Salad

For many people, the best part of sushi is the vinegared rice that goes into it. The type of rice used to make sushi is a short-grain rice with a slightly higher starch content than that of long-grain rices, which helps it stick together when it's formed into a log or a roll. Here's a salad based on the flavors of sushi (rice vinegar, wasabi, pickled ginger), along with a good helping of spinach. Look for sushi rice at Asian markets and some supermarkets. Of course you could make this salad with regular long-grain rice, as well.

> 1 cup sushi rice
>
> 1⅓ cups water
>
> ⅓ cup rice vinegar
>
> 2 tablespoons sugar
>
> 1 teaspoon wasabi powder
>
> ½ teaspoon salt
>
> 1 tablespoon chopped pickled ginger
>
> 1 carrot, cut into ¼-inch dice
>
> 8 cups fresh spinach leaves, shredded
>
> 2 teaspoons sesame seeds

1 In a medium saucepan, combine the rice and water. Bring to a boil, reduce to a simmer, cover, and cook for 15 minutes. Remove from the heat and let stand, covered, for 10 minutes.

2 Meanwhile, in a large bowl, whisk together the vinegar, sugar, wasabi powder, and salt. Add the warm rice, pickled ginger, and carrot, and fluff with a fork.

3 Add the spinach and sesame seeds, and toss to combine. Serve at room temperature or chilled. *Makes 4 servings*

per serving: 244 calories, 1.5g total fat (0.2g saturated), 0mg cholesterol, 3g dietary fiber, 52g carbohydrate, 5g protein, 408mg sodium. good source of: beta carotene, folate, lutein, niacin, riboflavin, selenium, thiamin.

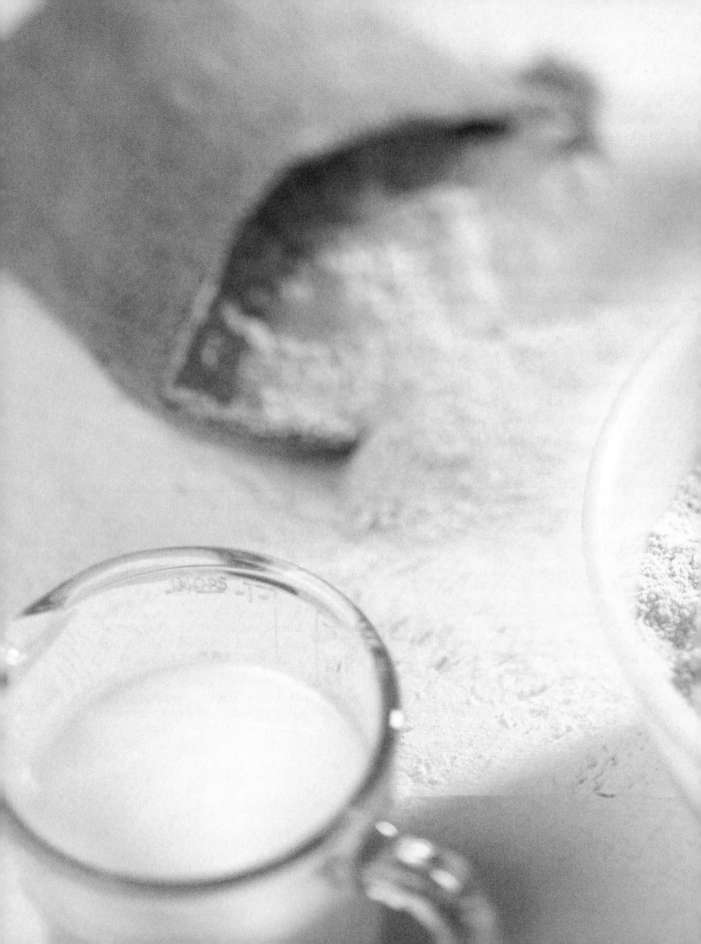

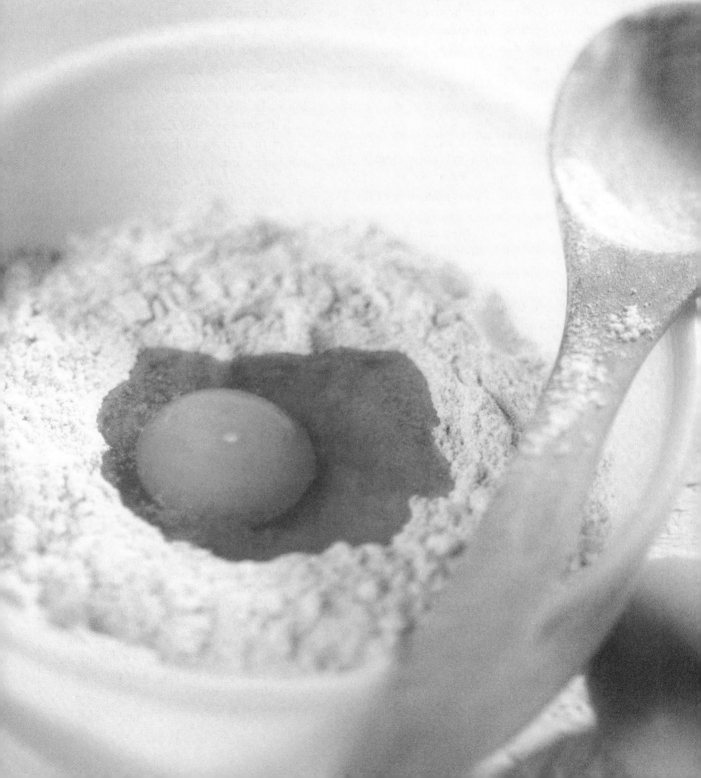

breads & muffins

The beauty of bread is its simplicity. Flour and liquid are the main ingredients, along with a leavener. These basics yield a nourishing and tasty food—one that is high in protein and B vitamins, and comes in a wide variety of shapes, textures, and flavors. Add optional ingredients, such as salt, sweeteners, and fats, and the varieties of bread become truly innumerable.

Although there are also unleavened breads (tortillas and matzo, for example), this chapter concerns itself with leavened breads, the two main types being yeast breads and quick breads.

yeast breads

Though the ingredients in bread are simple, their interaction is complex. Each component plays a specific role in the flavor and texture of the finished product.

Flour is, of course, the main ingredient. For raised breads, wheat flour is ideal: It is uniquely suited for bread-making, because when mixed with liquid, some of its proteins combine to form gluten. Gluten works with yeast and starch to form a network of cells elastic enough to expand during the leavening process, yet strong enough to contain the gases produced by the yeast, so that the resulting bread is light.

Other types of grains can produce gluten, but not to the extent that wheat can. Rye, the next-best gluten producer, is a poor second to wheat. Breads made solely from low-gluten flours will be dense and heavy. As a result, most raised breads contain at least some wheat flour.

Liquid is used in raised breads to help dissolve and distribute the yeast throughout the flour, and is necessary for the formation of gluten and the gelatinization of starch. Many kinds of liquid can be used; all have a different effect on the dough's development. Water produces a bread with a crisp, thick crust. Milk, another popular choice, produces a bread with a tender, brown crust and helps keep bread fresh. Other liquids—such as the water that potatoes have been cooked in, buttermilk, sour cream,

yogurt, fruit juice, vegetable juice, or beer—have different effects on the texture and flavor of the bread.

Yeast is a single-cell fungus that will multiply rapidly, given the right conditions. Yeast leavens bread because it ferments the simple carbohydrates naturally present in the flour, producing carbon dioxide and alcohol as waste products. Bread rises when the gluten traps the carbon dioxide in the dough. (The alcohol is largely evaporated during baking.) Yeast is also responsible for bread's characteristic flavor and aroma.

Salt not only adds flavor to bread, but also affects the actions of the yeast and gluten. It is possible to make bread without any salt at all, but a small amount of salt will help strengthen the gluten, make the dough easier to handle, and prevent the yeast from multiplying too rapidly.

Sweeteners—sugar, honey, molasses, corn syrup, and maple sugar—are optional ingredients in bread. Their main function is to provide a readily available form of energy for the yeast at the start of the process, thus helping the bread to rise faster (though dough containing a lot of sugar will take longer to rise because the sugar acts as a preservative, slowing the action of the yeast). Sweeteners also contribute flavor, help to keep the bread tender by retaining moisture, and aid in browning.

how to tell when yeast bread is done

The first clue you have to your yeast bread being done is its top: It should be golden brown. But the top may get brown before the inside is cooked—if your oven is too hot, for example. So, as a second test for doneness, you actually turn the loaf over (or out of the pan) and tap it on the bottom. A properly risen yeast bread will sound hollow. This is a judgment that may be hard to make until you have heard the "thud" of an underdone loaf.

bread enhancements

One of the best reasons to make your own breads or muffins is that you can improve the nutritional profile by not only subtracting the amount of fat and sugar used in many commercial products, but also by adding in a variety of ingredients that bring their own health benefits. Here are some examples of what you can add:

▶**Fruit** Dried fruit adds flavor, moisture, texture, and concentrated nutrients. Certain fruits, such as mashed bananas, applesauce, or pureed dried plums (prunes), can replace some of the fat in a muffin or quick-bread recipe. Other soft fruit, like berries, provide taste, texture, and fiber.

▶**Vegetables** Shredded vegetables, such as carrots, zucchini, and beets, keep breads moist and add fiber and nutrients.

▶**Seeds and nuts** Flax, poppy, sesame, sunflower, and pumpkin seeds, and all types of nuts, provide crunch, flavor, and minerals. For the most flavor, toast the seeds or nuts before adding them.

▶**Whole grains** Brown rice, wheatberries, barley, bulgur, and triticale can be cooked and added to doughs for their nutritional benefits and to provide a chewy texture. Add up to 1 cup of cooked grain for every 4 cups of flour.

▶**Other flours** In recipes calling for all-purpose flour, one-fourth of it can be replaced with whole-grain and other flours. Some good choices are whole-wheat, oat, and rye flours.

▶**Oats** Rolled oats that have been toasted give bread a nutty flavor. You can also grind oats in a food processor and use them in place of oat flour.

▶**Bran** For added fiber (if you aren't using whole-grain flour), add up to ⅓ cup of wheat or oat bran for every 4 cups of all-purpose flour.

▶**Wheat germ** For B vitamins and a nutty flavor, use up to ¼ cup of wheat germ for every 4 cups of flour.

▶**Soy protein powder** This powder, available at health-food stores, gives bread a protein and isoflavone boost. Add up to 3 tablespoons of unflavored powder for every 4 cups of flour.

▶**Nonfat dry milk powder** This fat-free powder adds extra calcium to homemade loaves without any added fat. Add up to ¼ cup for every 4 cups of flour.

Fat is another optional ingredient that is frequently used in commercial breads. Fat adds flavor, makes the loaf more tender, and helps the bread brown better. It also helps to increase the dough's elasticity so it can expand even more without letting carbon dioxide escape, thereby producing a loaf with greater volume.

quick breads

Quick breads are leavened with baking powder, baking soda, or both. They are called quick breads because no rising time is required. At baking temperatures, the leavener reacts with water and acid in the batter or dough to form carbon dioxide, and the quick bread rises.

Like yeast breads, quick breads are made from flour, liquid, and sometimes salt, but they usually contain eggs, sugar, and fat as well. There are three types of quick bread mixtures that differ in the proportions of ingredients:

Pour batters Pour batters—as their name suggests—are thin enough to be poured and are usually made with an even ratio of flour to liquid. Examples include pancakes, waffles, and popovers.

Drop batters These batters have a higher proportion of flour to liquid than pour batters. They are thick and need to be spooned into the baking pan or "dropped" onto a baking sheet. Muffins, tea breads, and some biscuits are made from drop batters.

Soft doughs Thicker than drop batters, these doughs have the highest proportion of flour to liquid of the quick breads. They are firm enough to handle, but they should be handled gently to keep them from getting tough. The doughs are generally patted out and then cut into shapes, as for scones and so-called rolled biscuits.

Golden-Crust Pizza

Using carrot juice as the liquid in a basic yeast-risen pizza dough adds a wonderful golden color and a good amount of beta carotene. You can make the basic tomato-and-cheese-topped pizza below, or try one of the additional toppings (*recipes follow*). The nutrition analysis is for the plain jane version. **Timing alert:** You can prepare the dough through step 4, punch it down, wrap it, and freeze it. The dough can be frozen up to a month before using. When you're ready to make the pizza, bring the dough to room temperature and then roll it out as directed in step 5. Proceed with the topping and baking.

1 package (¼ ounce) active dry yeast

1 teaspoon sugar

¼ cup lukewarm water (105° to 115°F)

3½ cups flour plus extra for kneading

1¼ cups carrot juice

1 tablespoon olive oil

¾ teaspoon salt

2 tablespoons yellow cornmeal

2 cups storebought marinara sauce

Toppings (optional; recipes follow)

1 cup shredded part-skim mozzarella (4 ounces)

1 cup shredded fat-free mozzarella (4 ounces)

1 In a large bowl, sprinkle the yeast and sugar over the lukewarm water. Let sit until foamy, about 5 minutes.

2 Stir in ½ cup of the flour, cover, and let stand in a draftfree spot until doubled in bulk, about 30 minutes.

3 Stir in the carrot juice and oil until well combined. Add the remaining 3 cups flour and the salt, and stir until the dough comes together. Transfer the dough to a floured work surface and knead until the dough is smooth and elastic, about 10 minutes. (As you knead, use more flour for your hands and work surface to keep the dough from sticking.)

4 Spray a large bowl with nonstick cooking spray. Add the dough, turning to coat. Cover with a damp cloth and let stand in a warm draftfree spot until almost doubled in bulk, about 45 minutes.

different spins

▶ **Mexican Pizza** Follow the directions for *Golden-Crust Pizza*, but substitute 3 cups of thick bottled salsa for the marinara sauce. Top with 2 cups corn kernels and 1 bottled jalapeño pepper, minced, in step 6. Substitute reduced-fat Monterey jack cheese for the mozzarella.

▶ **Apple & Fontina Cheese Pizza** Follow the directions for *Golden-Crust Pizza,* and in step 6, top the pizza with 2 thinly sliced Granny Smith apples. Substitute shredded fontina for the part-skim mozzarella (but keep the fat-free mozzarella).

5 Preheat the oven to 500°F. Punch the dough down and turn it out onto a lightly floured surface. Roll the dough out to an 11 x 17-inch rectangle. Sprinkle a large baking sheet with the cornmeal. Place the dough on top.

6 Spoon the marinara sauce evenly over the dough. If using a topping, add it here. Bake on the lowest shelf of the oven for 10 minutes.

7 Scatter the cheeses over the top and bake for 10 minutes longer, or until the cheeses have melted and the crust is crisp and brown. *Makes 8 slices*

per slice: 333 calories, 5.9g total fat (2g saturated), 10mg cholesterol, 3g dietary fiber, 54g carbohydrate, 15g protein, 664mg sodium. good source of: beta carotene, calcium, folate, niacin, riboflavin, selenium, thiamin.

Bell Pepper & Onion Topping In a medium skillet, combine 1 thinly sliced bell pepper (red, yellow, or green), 1 thinly sliced small red onion, ¼ cup water, 1 tablespoon balsamic vinegar, and ½ teaspoon oregano. Cook over medium heat until softened.

Spicy Mushroom Topping In a medium nonstick skillet, sauté 2 cups sliced mushrooms (shiitake, cremini, or button) in 2 teaspoons olive oil along with 3 cloves minced garlic and a pinch of red pepper flakes.

Sausage & Broccoli Rabe Topping In a medium nonstick skillet, cook 2 cups chopped broccoli rabe, 2 cloves of slivered garlic, and 2 links of hot

Italian-style turkey sausage in ½ cup water over medium heat until the broccoli rabe is softened. Drain off any excess liquid. Cut the sausage into thin slices. Sprinkle the sauce-topped pizza dough (step 6) with the cooked broccoli rabe, the sausage slices, and ¼ cup golden raisins.

Bean & Corn Topping Sprinkle the sauce-topped pizza dough (step 6) with 1 cup corn kernels, 1 cup cooked (or canned) black beans, ⅓ cup chopped cilantro, and 2 sliced scallions.

Seed-Topped Flatbreads

This dough is allowed to rest for about 30 minutes before it gets rolled out. This is to relax the gluten in the dough, so that it doesn't spring back when you're trying to roll it out.

2 cups flour plus extra for kneading

2 teaspoons baking powder

¾ teaspoon salt

⅔ cup water

1 tablespoon olive oil

1 large egg white lightly beaten with 1 tablespoon water

2 tablespoons hulled pumpkin seeds (pepitas)

1 tablespoon hulled sunflower seeds

1 teaspoon sesame seeds

½ teaspoon poppy seeds

3 tablespoons grated Parmesan cheese

1 In a medium bowl, combine the flour, baking powder, and salt. In a small bowl, combine the water and oil. Make a well in the center of the flour mixture and gradually stir in the liquid. Stir until almost combined, then turn the dough out onto a lightly floured work surface and knead a few times until the dough is smooth. Add a little more flour to the work surface if the dough is sticking.

2 Spray a bowl with nonstick cooking spray. Add the dough, turning it in the bowl to coat. Cover and let rest for 30 minutes.

3 Preheat the oven to 400°F. Cut the dough into 6 pieces. Roll each piece out to a 5-inch round. Place on a large baking sheet lined with parchment paper or sprayed with nonstick cooking spray.

4 Brush the tops of the dough rounds with the egg white mixture. Scatter the pumpkin seeds, sunflower seeds, sesame seeds, and poppy seeds over the tops. Sprinkle the Parmesan over the seeds.

5 Bake for 5 minutes, or until golden brown and lightly crisped. *Makes 6 breads*

per bread: 214 calories, 5.8g total fat (1.2g saturated), 2mg cholesterol, 1g dietary fiber, 33g carbohydrate, 7g protein, 425mg sodium. good source of: folate, niacin, selenium, thiamin.

seeds of health

Seeds, like nuts, have seen their nutritional reputation rise in recent years. Ounce for ounce, they're high in calories, but also rich in healthy fat, as well as a variety of nutrients. Many common foods that we eat—including legumes, nuts, and grains—are actually seeds. Many seeds (such as sesame, sunflower, safflower, rape, and cotton) are grown for their oil. Some (such as sesame, poppy, and pumpkin) are used as snacks and flavorings. Others (such as pear, orange, and apple) are too hard and tasteless to eat, though some people do eat them.

Any seed consists of an outer layer that covers stored food, along with the embryo of a new plant. Besides healthy polyunsaturated and monounsaturated fats, seeds are rich in vitamins, minerals, and fiber. They also contain phytochemicals, some of which may have cardioprotective or anticancer effects. Since they come from plants, they contain no cholesterol. Some seeds, notably sunflower, are among the best sources of vitamin E. Flaxseeds are rich in alpha-linolenic acid, a fat similar to the omega-3s in fish. Rape seeds, from which canola oil is made, also contain alpha-linolenic acid, as do hemp seeds.

Sunshine Bread

Roasted sunflower seeds and ground flaxseeds lend crunch and nuttiness to this quick bread. If you have any flaxseed oil on hand, use a combination of 1 tablespoon of flaxseed oil and 3 tablespoons of olive oil in the batter, instead of all olive oil.

> ½ cup flaxseeds
>
> 1 cup all-purpose flour
>
> ¾ cup whole-wheat flour
>
> ½ cup yellow cornmeal
>
> 1 tablespoon sugar
>
> 2 teaspoons baking powder
>
> ¾ teaspoon salt
>
> 1 large egg
>
> 1 large egg white
>
> 1 cup low-fat (1%) or fat-free milk
>
> ¼ cup extra-light olive oil
>
> ⅓ cup roasted, salted sunflower seeds

1 Preheat the oven to 350°F. Spray an 8½ x 4½-inch loaf pan with nonstick cooking spray. Dust with flour.

2 In a mini-food processor, spice mill, or coffee grinder, grind the flaxseeds until finely ground.

3 In a large bowl, combine the ground flaxseeds, all-purpose flour, whole-wheat flour, cornmeal, sugar, baking powder, and salt. In a small bowl, combine the whole egg, egg white, milk, and olive oil. Make a well in the flour mixture and add the milk mixture. Stir until just combined. Stir in the sunflower seeds.

4 Scrape the batter into the loaf pan. Bake 45 minutes, or until a toothpick inserted in the cen-ter comes out clean. Cool in the pan on a rack for 5 minutes, then turn out of the pan onto the rack to cool completely. *Makes 10 slices*

per slice: 205 calories, 11g total fat (1.3g saturated), 22mg cholesterol, 2g dietary fiber, 21g carbohydrate, 6g protein, 330mg sodium. good source of: riboflavin, selenium, thiamin, vitamin E.

---

did you know?

Of all nuts, walnuts are special because they contain the heart-healthy polyunsaturated fat called alpha-linolenic acid. A study at University of California, Davis confirmed that walnuts help reduce blood cholesterol, especially the small dense LDL cholesterol that is most likely to damage coronary arteries. The walnuts (1½ ounces a day) were beneficial whether the initial diet was low-fat or not. Though walnuts, like all nuts, are high in calories, subjects who ate them did not gain weight.

Walnut-Oat Batter Bread

Batter bread is bread that is made of a yeast-leavened dough that is wetter than normal bread doughs and is "kneaded" by being vigorously stirred with a wooden spoon. If at all possible, make this bread with walnut oil for the extra measure of flavor (and alpha-linolenic acid, a type of omega-3 fatty acid) it will bring. **Timing alert:** The bread will take about 3 hours.

> 4 cups old-fashioned rolled oats
>
> 1 package (¼ ounce) active dry yeast
>
> 2¼ cups lukewarm water (105° to 115°F)
>
> 1 tablespoon brown sugar
>
> 1¾ cups all-purpose flour
>
> ¾ cup whole-wheat flour
>
> ¼ cup nonfat dry milk powder
>
> ⅓ cup molasses
>
> 1 tablespoon olive or walnut oil
>
> 2 teaspoons salt
>
> ½ cup walnuts, coarsely chopped

1 Preheat the oven to 350°F. Place the oats on a baking sheet, and bake, stirring once or twice, for 7 minutes, or until lightly browned and fragrant. (Turn the oven off.) Transfer 2 cups of the oats to a food processor and pulse on and off until they have the consistency of flour.

2 In a large bowl, combine the yeast, ¼ cup of the lukewarm water, and the brown sugar. Let stand until foamy, about 5 minutes.

3 Add the remaining 2 cups lukewarm water, the ground oats, whole oats, all-purpose flour, whole-wheat flour, milk powder, molasses, oil, and salt to the yeast mixture and stir to combine. Stir in the

walnuts. With a wooden spoon, stir until well combined. Cover with a dampened towel and let stand in a warm draftfree spot until doubled in bulk, about 1 hour.

4 Spray two 8½ x 4½-inch loaf pans with nonstick cooking spray. Punch the dough down, divide in half, and transfer to the loaf pans. Cover with a dampened towel and let stand in a warm draft-free spot until doubled in bulk, about 30 minutes.

5 Preheat the oven to 350°F. Bake the bread for 45 minutes, or until the top is richly browned and the bottom sounds hollow when tapped. Turn the loaves out of the pans onto a wire rack to cool completely. *Makes 20 slices*

per slice: 161 calories, 3.5g total fat (0.5g saturated), 0mg cholesterol, 3g dietary fiber, 28g carbohydrate, 5g protein, 241mg sodium. **good source of:** omega-3 fatty acids, selenium, thiamin.

6-Grain Bread

The English language uses a number of different terms for whole grains, including kernel, groat, and corn. In the case of wheat, the whole grain is called a berry. Wheatberries are unhulled grains, which gives them a chewy texture and also means that they have to be cooked to soften them enough to use in this bread. **Timing alert:** From start to finish, this bread will probably take about 5½ hours.

> ½ cup wheatberries
>
> 2 tablespoons flaxseeds
>
> ¼ cup lukewarm water (105° to 115°F)
>
> 4 tablespoons honey
>
> 1 package (¼ ounce) active dry yeast
>
> 2 tablespoons olive oil
>
> 1½ cups whole-wheat flour
>
> 1 cup all-purpose flour plus extra for kneading
>
> ½ cup oat flour
>
> ½ cup rye flour
>
> ½ cup wheat bran
>
> ⅓ cup hulled sunflower seeds
>
> 3 tablespoons yellow cornmeal
>
> 2 teaspoons salt

1 In a small saucepan, combine the wheatberries and water to cover by several inches. Bring to a boil, reduce to a simmer, and cook until the wheatberries are tender, but still slightly crunchy, about 1 hour. Drain, reserving 1½ cups of the cooking liquid; keep it lukewarm for use in step 4. (You can cook the wheatberries the day before, drain them and store them separately from their cooking liquid. Warm the liquid to lukewarm before using.)

2 Meanwhile, in a mini-food processor, spice mill, or coffee grinder, grind the flaxseeds until powdery. Transfer the ground flax to a large bowl.

3 In a small bowl, stir together the lukewarm water and 1 tablespoon of the honey. Sprinkle the yeast over the top and let stand until foamy, about 5 minutes.

4 Add the yeast mixture to the ground flax. Add the reserved 1½ cups lukewarm wheatberry cooking liquid, the remaining 3 tablespoons honey, the oil, whole-wheat flour, all-purpose flour, oat flour, rye flour, wheat bran, sunflower seeds, cornmeal, and salt, and stir to combine. Stir in the wheatberries. The dough will be somewhat sticky.

5 Transfer the dough to a floured work surface and knead until the dough is smooth and elastic, about 10 minutes. (As you knead, use more flour for your hands and work surface to keep the dough from sticking.) Spray a large bowl with nonstick cooking spray. Add the dough, turning to coat. Cover with a dampened towel and let stand in a warm, draftfree spot until doubled in bulk, about 1½ hours.

6 Punch the dough down, cover, and let rise until doubled in bulk, about 1 hour.

7 Preheat the oven to 350°F. Spray a 9 x 5-inch loaf pan with nonstick cooking spray. Transfer the dough to the pan. Cover and let rise until the dough fills the pan, about 30 minutes.

8 Bake the loaf for 55 minutes, or until the top is well browned and the bottom sounds hollow when tapped. Turn the loaf out of the pan onto a wire rack to cool completely before slicing. *Makes 16 slices*

per slice: 167 calories, 4.1g total fat (0.5g saturated), 0mg cholesterol, 5g dietary fiber, 29g carbohydrate, 5g protein, 293mg sodium. **good source of:** fiber, omega-3 fatty acids, selenium, thiamin.

Peppery Potato Bread with Cheddar & Scallions

If you'd like, you can make instant mashed potatoes and skip step 1 of the recipe (you need 1 cup of mashed). Then in step 2, use plain lukewarm water (105° to 115°F) in place of the potato cooking water. You will also need to blanch the garlic in boiling water for 2 minutes before mincing.

> ¾ pound baking potatoes, peeled and thinly sliced
>
> 3 cups water
>
> 2 cloves garlic, peeled
>
> 1 package (¼ ounce) active dry yeast
>
> 1 teaspoon sugar
>
> 1 tablespoon olive oil
>
> 1 tablespoon Dijon mustard
>
> 2½ cups all-purpose flour
>
> 1 cup rye flour
>
> 1¼ teaspoons salt
>
> ½ teaspoon cayenne pepper
>
> ¾ cup shredded extra-sharp Cheddar cheese (3 ounces)
>
> 4 scallions, thinly sliced

1 In a medium saucepan, bring the potatoes, water, and garlic to a boil over medium heat. Cook until the potatoes are tender, about 15 minutes. Drain, reserving 1¼ cups of the potato cooking liquid. With a potato masher, mash the potatoes and garlic until smooth. Measure out 1 cup of mashed potatoes and transfer to a large mixing bowl (discard—or eat—any remainder).

2 Transfer ¼ cup of the potato cooking liquid to a small bowl and let cool to lukewarm (105° to 115°F). Sprinkle the yeast and sugar over the lukewarm liquid and let stand until foamy, about 5 minutes.

3 Meanwhile, add the remaining 1 cup potato cooking liquid, the oil, and mustard to the mashed potatoes and stir to combine. Add the all-purpose flour, rye flour, salt, and cayenne, mixing until well combined.

4 Add the yeast mixture and stir until well combined. In an electric mixer fitted with a dough hook, beat the dough until soft and silky. (If you don't have a dough hook, use a wooden spoon.) Beat in the Cheddar and scallions. The dough will be sticky.

5 Spray a large bowl with nonstick cooking spray. Add the dough to the bowl, turning to coat. Cover the bowl with a dampened towel and let rise in a warm draftfree spot until doubled in bulk, about 45 minutes.

6 Preheat the oven to 400°F. Spray two 8½ x 4½-inch loaf pans with nonstick cooking spray. Punch the dough down, divide in half, and place in the pans. There is no need to shape the dough, it will simply fill the pans. Cover and let rise in a warm draftfree spot for 15 minutes. Bake for 30 to 35 minutes, or until browned.

7 Turn the bread out of the pans onto a wire rack and cool completely before slicing. *Makes 16 slices*

per slice: 141 calories, 3.1g total fat (1.3g saturated), 6mg cholesterol, 2g dietary fiber, 24g carbohydrate, 5g protein, 240mg sodium. good source of: folate, niacin, riboflavin, selenium, thiamin.

Angel Biscuits

Angel biscuits are also called Bride's Biscuits, because the extra leavening power of yeast makes them virtually foolproof—perfect for the new bride or beginner cook. A bit of whole-wheat flour is a health improvement over the original refined-flour version.

> 1 teaspoon active dry yeast
>
> 2 teaspoons sugar
>
> ¼ cup lukewarm water (105° to 115°F)
>
> 1½ cups all-purpose flour
>
> ½ cup whole-wheat flour
>
> 2 teaspoons baking powder
>
> ½ teaspoon baking soda
>
> ¼ teaspoon salt
>
> 2 tablespoons unsalted butter
>
> ¾ cup buttermilk, at room temperature

1 In a small bowl, sprinkle the yeast and 1 teaspoon of the sugar over the water. Let stand until the mixture is foamy, about 5 minutes.

2 Meanwhile, in a large bowl, combine the remaining 1 teaspoon sugar, the all-purpose flour, whole-wheat flour, baking powder, baking soda, and salt, and stir well to combine. With a pastry blender or 2 knives, cut in the butter until the mixture resembles coarse meal.

3 Stir the buttermilk into the yeast mixture. Make a well in the center of the flour mixture, pour in the buttermilk-yeast mixture, and stir until just combined. Cover with a dampened towel and let stand in a warm draftfree spot until doubled in bulk, about 45 minutes.

4 Punch the dough down, cover, and let rest for 10 minutes. On a lightly floured surface, with floured hands, pat the dough out to a ¾-inch thickness. With a 2-inch round biscuit cutter, cut out biscuits. Gather the scraps, repat about ¾ inch thick, and cut out more biscuits. (Repeat until all the dough is cut out.) Place the biscuits, 2 inches apart, on a nonstick baking sheet. Cover loosely and let stand for 15 minutes or until puffed.

5 Meanwhile, preheat the oven to 400°F. Bake the biscuits for 15 to 17 minutes, or until lightly golden. *Makes 12 biscuits*

per biscuit: 101 calories, 2.3g total fat (1.3g saturated), 6mg cholesterol, 1g dietary fiber, 17g carbohydrate, 3g protein, 156mg sodium. good source of: folate, niacin, riboflavin, selenium, thiamin.

---

did you know?

Working closely with calcium and vitamin D, magnesium helps form and maintain bones and teeth. By helping to keep bones strong, an adequate magnesium intake may help prevent osteoporosis. Though few Americans are truly deficient in magnesium, many consume less than the recommended levels (310 to 420 mg a day). Sunflower seeds are one of the top sources of dietary magnesium: An ounce of seeds contains 100 mg.

Sunflower & Sesame Drop Biscuits

Traditional biscuits are made with all butter, a combination of butter and lard, or butter and solid vegetable shortening. Here we've used a small amont of butter for flavoring and monounsaturated olive oil for the remainder of the fat.

> 1½ cups flour
> 1¼ teaspoons baking powder
> ½ teaspoon baking soda
> ½ teaspoon salt
> 1 teaspoon sugar
> 3 tablespoons dry-roasted sunflower seeds
> 1 tablespoon sesame seeds
> 1 tablespoon cold unsalted butter
> 3 tablespoons olive oil
> ¾ cup plus 2 tablespoons buttermilk

1 Preheat the oven to 425°F. Spray a large baking sheet with nonstick cooking spray.

2 In a large bowl, stir together the flour, baking powder, baking soda, salt, and sugar. Stir in the sunflower seeds and sesame seeds.

3 With a pastry blender or two knives, cut in the butter and oil until the mixture resembles coarse meal. Stir in the buttermilk until the mixture forms a soft dough. Do not overmix.

4 Drop the dough by well-rounded tablespoons 2 inches apart onto the baking sheet. Bake for 12 minutes, or until the biscuits are golden brown and crusty. *Makes 12 biscuits*

per biscuit: 120 calories, 6.1g total fat (1.3g saturated), 3mg cholesterol, 1g dietary fiber, 14g carbohydrate, 3g protein, 193mg sodium. good source of: selenium, thiamin, vitamin E.

Peppery Corn Crackers

These crisp and spicy corn crackers are not made with wheat flour, but if you're sensitive to gluten, you should be aware that oat flour does have some.

1 cup yellow cornmeal
⅓ cup oat flour
1 teaspoon salt
½ teaspoon baking soda
¼ teaspoon cayenne pepper
¼ cup plain fat-free yogurt
3 tablespoons milk
2 tablespoons extra-light olive oil

1 Preheat the oven to 350°F. Spray a baking sheet with nonstick cooking spray.

2 In a medium bowl, combine the cornmeal, oat flour, salt, baking soda, and cayenne. In a small bowl, combine the yogurt, milk, and oil. Add the yogurt mixture to the cornmeal mixture and stir until a soft dough forms.

3 Place the dough on the prepared baking sheet and pat into a square shape. Place a sheet of wax paper over the dough. Roll into a 10-inch square, a scant ¼ inch thick. Make sure the center is as thin as the edges. Remove the wax paper. If necessary, trim the dough to form a square. Cut the dough into 2½ x 2-inch rectangles (but leave the crackers just where they are, on the baking sheet).

4 Bake for 20 minutes, or until golden brown and crisp. Cool the crackers for 5 minutes on the baking sheet before transferring to a wire rack to cool completely. Store in an airtight container. *Makes 20 crackers*

per cracker: 47 calories, 1.7g total fat (0.3g saturated), 0mg cholesterol, 1g dietary fiber, 7g carbohydrate, 1g protein, 119mg sodium.

Oniony Cornbread

Cornbread is a delicious side dish, but also makes a good base for stuffings, such as Apple & Onion Cornbread Stuffing (*page 126*); but see the cooking instructions below.

1¼ cups flour
¾ cup yellow cornmeal
1 tablespoon sugar
1½ teaspoons baking powder
½ teaspoon baking soda
½ teaspoon salt
¼ teaspoon cayenne pepper
1⅓ cups buttermilk
2 tablespoons extra-light olive oil
1 large egg
1 large onion, grated

1 Preheat the oven to 400°F. Spray an 8-inch square baking pan with nonstick cooking spray.

2 In a large bowl, stir together the flour, cornmeal, sugar, baking powder, baking soda, salt, and cayenne.

3 In a separate bowl, whisk together the buttermilk, oil, and egg. Make a well in the center of the flour mixture and pour in the buttermilk mixture. Add the grated onion and stir until combined.

4 Spoon the batter into the baking pan. Bake for 20 minutes, or until a toothpick inserted in the center comes out clean. *Makes 9 squares*

per square: 167 calories, 4.3g total fat (0.8g saturated), 25mg cholesterol, 2g dietary fiber, 27g carbohydrate, 5g protein, 284mg sodium. **good source of:** selenium, thiamin.

cornbread for stuffings

Since bread-type stuffings do better when they are slightly dried out, bake the cornbread in a shallower pan. Spray a 9 x 13-inch baking pan with nonstick cooking spray and spread the batter out. Bake at 400°F for 25 minutes, or until the cornbread is set. .

Date & Walnut Bread

If you remember date-nut bread from your youth, this recipe will take you right back. To complete the nostalgia, serve the bread spread lightly with reduced-fat or fat-free cream cheese.

2 cups pitted dates (10 ounces), chopped

1 cup boiling water

1½ cups old-fashioned rolled oats

1 cup walnuts

1½ cups flour

1 teaspoon salt

1 teaspoon baking powder

½ teaspoon baking soda

½ cup packed light brown sugar

½ cup molasses

2 tablespoons extra-light olive oil

1 large egg

1 large egg white

1 Preheat the oven to 350°F. Spray two 8½ x 4½-inch loaf pans with nonstick cooking spray.

2 In a medium heatproof bowl, combine the dates and boiling water. Let stand while you prepare the remaining ingredients.

3 Place the oats in a baking pan and bake for 10 minutes, or until crisp and golden brown. Bake the walnuts in a separate pan for 7 minutes, or until lightly crisped. When cool enough to handle, coarsely chop the walnuts. Transfer the oats to a food processor and process until finely ground.

4 In a large bowl, stir together the flour, salt, baking powder, baking soda, and ground oats.

5 Add the brown sugar, molasses, oil, whole egg, and egg white to the bowl with the dates (and soaking water), and stir to combine.

6 Make a well in the center of the flour mixture. Add the date mixture and walnuts, and stir just until moistened. Spoon the batter into the pans. Bake for 55 minutes, or until a toothpick inserted in the center of a loaf comes out clean. Cool them for 5 minutes in the pans on a rack, then turn out onto the rack to cool completely. *Makes 24 slices*

per slice: 164 calories, 4.5g total fat (0.6g saturated), 9mg cholesterol, 2g dietary fiber, 30g carbohydrate, 3g protein, 152mg sodium. good source of: omega-3 fatty acids.

Cranberry-Ginger Tea Bread

These can also be made in three 5½ x 3-inch mini loaf pans (bake for about 45 minutes)—perfect for gift giving.

1 cup old-fashioned rolled oats

1¾ cups flour

1 cup sugar

1½ teaspoons baking powder

½ teaspoon baking soda

½ teaspoon salt

1 large egg

2 large egg whites

⅔ cup buttermilk

¼ cup extra-light olive oil

2 cups (8 ounces) fresh or frozen cranberries, coarsely chopped

⅓ cup crystallized ginger, coarsely chopped

1 Preheat the oven to 350°F. Spray a 9 x 5-inch loaf pan with nonstick cooking spray; set aside.

2 On a baking sheet, toast the oats until brown and fragrant, about 10 minutes. Transfer to a food processor and pulse until finely ground. Transfer to a large bowl. Add the flour, sugar, baking powder, baking soda, and salt.

3 In a medium bowl, whisk together the whole egg, egg whites, buttermilk, and oil until well combined. Stir the egg mixture into the flour mixture until just combined. Fold in the the cranberries and ginger.

4 Spoon the batter into the loaf pan, smooth the top, and bake for 1 hour or until a toothpick inserted in the center comes out clean. Transfer to a wire rack and cool the loaf in the pan for 10 minutes. Then turn out of the pan and cool completely on the rack before slicing. *Makes 16 slices*

per slice: 168 calories, 4.3g total fat (0.7g saturated), 14mg cholesterol, 1g dietary fiber, 30g carbohydrate, 3g protein, 156mg sodium. good source of: selenium.

Banana-Apricot Bread

For an easy variation on this bread, use dark or golden raisins instead of the diced dried apricots.

⅔ cup diced dried apricots

½ cup boiling water

2 cups all-purpose flour

½ cup whole-wheat flour

1¾ teaspoons baking powder

½ teaspoon ground cardamom

½ teaspoon salt

1 cup mashed bananas (about 3)

½ cup honey

½ cup low-fat (1%) or fat-free milk

2 tablespoons walnut oil

⅔ cup chopped almonds, toasted

1 Preheat the oven to 350°F. Spray a 9 x 5-inch loaf pan with nonstick cooking spray. Dust with flour, shaking off the excess.

2 In a small heatproof bowl, combine the apricots and boiling water, and let stand for 10 minutes.

3 Meanwhile, in a medium bowl, stir together the all-purpose flour, whole-wheat flour, baking powder, cardamom, and salt.

4 In a large bowl, stir together the bananas, honey, milk, and oil. Drain the apricots, discarding the soaking liquid. Stir the apricots into the banana mixture along with the toasted almonds. Stir in the flour mixture until just combined.

5 Spoon the batter into the loaf pan and bake for 1 hour, or until a toothpick inserted in the center comes out clean. Transfer to a wire rack and cool in the pan for 10 minutes. Turn out onto a rack to cool completely. *Makes 20 slices*

per slice: 144 calories, 4g total fat (0.4g saturated), 0mg cholesterol, 2g dietary fiber, 25g carbohydrate, 3g protein, 83mg sodium. good source of: omega-3 fatty acids, riboflavin, selenium, thiamin.

Butternut-Cherry Tea Bread

Butternut squash are generally larger than 1¼ pounds, so you can either cut off a chunk of a squash, or roast the whole squash and use only 1¼ cups of the roasted squash in the bread. Serve any leftover squash as a vegetable side dish, or use it in place of pumpkin puree in a recipe. The pumpkin pie spice blend called for below is intended to be a convenience, but if you don't have any, you can simply substitute ¾ teaspoon cinnamon, ½ teaspoon ground ginger, and ⅛ teaspoon each allspice and cloves.

1 piece butternut squash (1¼ pounds), halved lengthwise and seeded

½ cup water

1¾ cups flour

2 tablespoons yellow cornmeal

1½ teaspoons pumpkin pie spice

1 teaspoon baking powder

½ teaspoon baking soda

½ teaspoon salt

½ cup packed light brown sugar

3 tablespoons extra-light olive oil

1 large egg

2 large egg whites

½ cup buttermilk

½ cup dried cherries, cranberries, or raisins

1 Preheat the oven to 400°F. Place the squash, cut-sides down, in a small baking pan. Add the water, cover, and bake for 30 minutes, or until the squash is tender. Reduce the oven temperature to 350°F. When cool enough to handle, scoop the squash flesh into a bowl and mash with a fork. Measure out 1¼ cups (save any remainder for another use).

2 In a medium bowl, stir together the flour, cornmeal, pumpkin pie spice, baking powder, baking soda, and salt.

3 In a large bowl, with an electric mixer, beat together the brown sugar and oil until well combined. Add the whole egg and egg whites, one at a time, beating well after each addition. Beat in the

recipe creator
fruit muffins

In the past couple of decades, the line between muffin and cupcake has been seriously blurred. A real muffin should be only vaguely sweet and relatively low in fat. A basic recipe also provides ample opportunity to improve the health profile of a muffin by adding fruits, nuts, and whole grains. Choose from the 5 categories below and follow these basic instructions: In a large bowl, combine 1½ cups all-purpose flour with 1 FLOUR ADD-IN, 1 SWEETENER, 1½ teaspoons baking powder, ½ teaspoon baking soda, and ½ teaspoon salt. In a small bowl, combine 1 LIQUID, 1 OIL, and 2 large egg whites. Make a well in the center of the dry ingredients and stir in the liquid mixture. Fold in 1 FRUIT and 1 SEED/NUT (if desired). If using frozen fruit, do not thaw before adding to the batter. Spoon into 12 paper-lined 2½-inch muffin cups. Bake at 375°F for 17 to 20 minutes, or until a toothpick inserted in the center of a muffin comes out clean. Remove from the pan and let cool on a wire rack. *Makes 12 muffins*

FLOUR ADD-INS	SWEETENERS	LIQUIDS	OILS	FRUITS	SEEDS/NUTS*
▶ ½ cup all-purpose flour (for a total of 2 cups)	▶ Granulated sugar, ⅓ cup	▶ Low-fat (1%) or fat-free milk, 1 cup	▶ Extra-mild olive oil, 2 Tbsp	▶ Dried cherries or cranberries, 1 cup	▶ Sunflower seeds, ½ cup chopped
▶ ½ cup whole-wheat flour	▶ Light brown sugar, ⅓ cup packed	▶ Buttermilk, 1 cup	▶ Walnut oil, 2 Tbsp	▶ Raisins or dried currants, 1 cup	▶ Pecans, ½ cup chopped
▶ ½ cup cornmeal	▶ Granulated maple sugar, ⅓ cup	▶ Plain low-fat yogurt, 1 cup	▶ Hazelnut oil, 2 Tbsp	▶ Chopped mixed dried fruit, 1 cup	▶ Pistachios, ½ cup chopped
▶ ½ cup oat or wheat bran + 3 Tbsp ground flaxseeds			▶ Flaxseed oil, 2 Tbsp	▶ Fresh or frozen blueberries, 1 cup	▶ Walnuts, ½ cup chopped
▶ ½ cup whole-wheat flour + 3 Tbsp wheat germ			▶ Dark sesame oil, 2 Tbsp	▶ Fresh or frozen raspberries, 1 cup	▶ Almonds, ½ cup chopped
			▶ Canola oil, 2 Tbsp	▶ Pears, 1 cup finely chopped	▶ Pumpkin seeds, ½ cup chopped
				▶ Apples, 1 cup finely chopped	* optional

1¼ cups mashed squash and the buttermilk. Fold in the flour mixture. Fold in the cherries.

4 Spray an 8½ x 4½-inch loaf pan with nonstick cooking spray. Spoon the batter into the loaf pan and bake for 1 hour, or until a toothpick inserted in the center comes out clean. Cool for 10 min-utes in the pan, then turn the bread out of the pan onto a wire rack to cool completely. *Makes 12 slices*

per slice: 177 calories, 4.1g total fat (0.7g saturated), 18mg cholesterol, 2g dietary fiber, 32g carbohydrate, 4g protein, 220mg sodium. good source of: selenium.

Wild Rice Philpy

The moist rice bread called philpy comes from the Carolinas and dates back to Colonial times when one of the area's principal cash crops was rice. Here, instead of the traditional white rice, we've made a philpy with wild rice (which is technically a grass and not a rice) for an interesting crunch. You could also use ¾ cup of leftover cooked regular rice or a wild rice blend. Serve the bread just as you would cornbread.

¼ cup wild rice
¾ cup flour
¾ teaspoon salt
¾ teaspoon baking powder
½ teaspoon baking soda
1 cup buttermilk
1 large egg

1 In a medium saucepan of boiling water, cook the wild rice until very tender, about 50 minutes. Drain, transfer to a medium bowl, and let cool for 5 minutes.

2 Meanwhile, in a small bowl, stir together the flour, salt, baking powder, and baking soda.

3 Preheat the oven to 400°F. Spray an 8-inch cake pan with nonstick cooking spray. Mash the rice with a potato masher until about one-fourth of the grains are broken up. Stir in the buttermilk.

4 Add the egg and stir until well combined. Stir in the flour mixture. Spoon the batter into the pan and bake for 20 to 25 minutes, or until the top is lightly golden and a toothpick inserted in the center comes out clean. *Makes 8 servings*

per serving: 80 calories, 1.1g total fat (0.4g saturated), 28mg cholesterol, 1g dietary fiber, 14g carbohydrate, 4g protein, 359mg sodium. good source of: riboflavin, selenium, thiamin.

different spins

▶ **Breakfast Philpy** Follow the directions for *Wild Rice Philpy* and add ¾ cup of dried cranberries, cherries, or raisins in step 3.

pancakes

There's a wealth of storebought pancake mixes available, so the only reason to make your own is if you can truly make a nutritional difference. Here's a collection of unusual mixes. Each of the pancake mixes will make a total of 4 to 5 cups, with each cup making about 8 pancakes. Here are the basic instructions for making one batch of 8 pancakes:

For Buckwheat Mix and Masa Harina Mix Scoop out 1 cup of pancake mix and place it in a large bowl. Make a well in the center of the mix and stir in 1 egg yolk, ¾ cup cold water, and 2 teaspoons mild olive oil. Beat 2 egg whites until stiff peaks form, and fold the beaten egg whites into the batter. For each pancake, use a generous ⅓ cup of batter. (For a quicker version, you can omit the whipping of the egg whites and just stir 1 whole egg and 1 egg white into the pancake mix. The resulting pancakes will be flatter; and the yield will be about 7 pancakes.)

For the Toasted Wheat Mix The instructions are the same as above, but start with 1¼ cups of mix and use a generous ¼ cup of batter for each pancake.

Buckwheat & Currant Pancake Mix

The dry mix recipe makes a total of 4 cups, enough for four batches of 8 pancakes.

2 cups whole-wheat flour
1 cup buckwheat flour
½ cup nonfat dry milk powder
¼ cup yellow cornmeal
2 tablespoons light brown sugar
5 teaspoons baking powder
1 teaspoon salt
¼ cup dried currants

In a large bowl, stir together the whole-wheat flour, buckwheat flour, nonfat dry milk, cornmeal, brown sugar, baking powder, and salt. Stir until well combined. Add the currants and mix again. Store the mix in the refrigerator or freezer. *Makes 32 pancakes*

per pancake: 74 calories, 2g total fat (0.4g saturated), 27mg cholesterol, 2g dietary fiber, 11g carbohydrate, 3g protein, 131mg sodium. good source of: selenium.

grinding flaxseeds

Although unground flaxseeds would add texture to dough, to get the benefit of their nutrients, the seeds need to be ground (otherwise they pass through the body undigested). Use a spice grinder or a coffee grinder to do this. It's better to grind your own flaxseeds than to buy pre-ground flax meal, because the oils in the flax meal may have gone rancid.

Masa Harina Pancake Mix

Masa harina, a ground-hominy flour used for making tortillas, is available at many supermarkets. Buttermilk powder, too, is available at many supermarkets, but if you can't find it, use nonfat dry milk powder, omit the baking soda, and increase the baking powder to 5 teaspoons. Be warned that the cocoa, which gives the pancakes a rich flavor, also gives them a sort of gray color: But just close your eyes, because they are delicious. The dry mix recipe makes a total of 4 cups, enough for four batches of 8 pancakes.

> 3 cups masa harina
> ½ cup buttermilk powder
> ¼ cup unsweetened cocoa powder
> 6 tablespoons packed light brown sugar
> 4 teaspoons baking powder
> 1½ teaspoons baking soda
> 1 teaspoon cinnamon
> ½ teaspoon salt

In a large bowl, stir together the masa harina, buttermilk powder, cocoa powder, brown sugar, baking powder, baking soda, cinnamon, and salt. Store the mix in the refrigerator or freezer. *Makes 32 pancakes*

per pancake: 76 calories, 2.4g total fat (0.5g saturated), 27mg cholesterol, 1g dietary fiber, 12g carbohydrate, 3g protein, 143mg sodium.

Toasted Wheat & Flaxseed Pancake Mix

The dry mix recipe makes a total of 5 cups, enough for four batches of 8 pancakes.

> ½ cup flaxseeds
> 1½ cups whole-wheat flour
> 1½ cups brown rice flour
> ½ cup toasted wheat germ
> ½ cup nonfat dry milk powder
> 2 tablespoons maple sugar or light brown sugar
> 5 teaspoons baking powder
> 1 teaspoon baking soda
> 1 teaspoon salt

1 In a mini-food processor, coffee mill, or spice grinder, finely grind the flaxseeds.

2 In a large bowl, whisk together the whole-wheat flour, brown rice flour, wheat germ, dry milk powder, maple sugar, baking powder, baking soda, salt, and ground flaxseeds. Store the mix in the refrigerator or freezer. *Makes 32 pancakes*

per pancake: 81 calories, 2g total fat (0.4g saturated), 27mg cholesterol, 2g dietary fiber, 13g carbohydrate, 4g protein, 160mg sodium. good source of: omega-3 fatty acids, selenium.

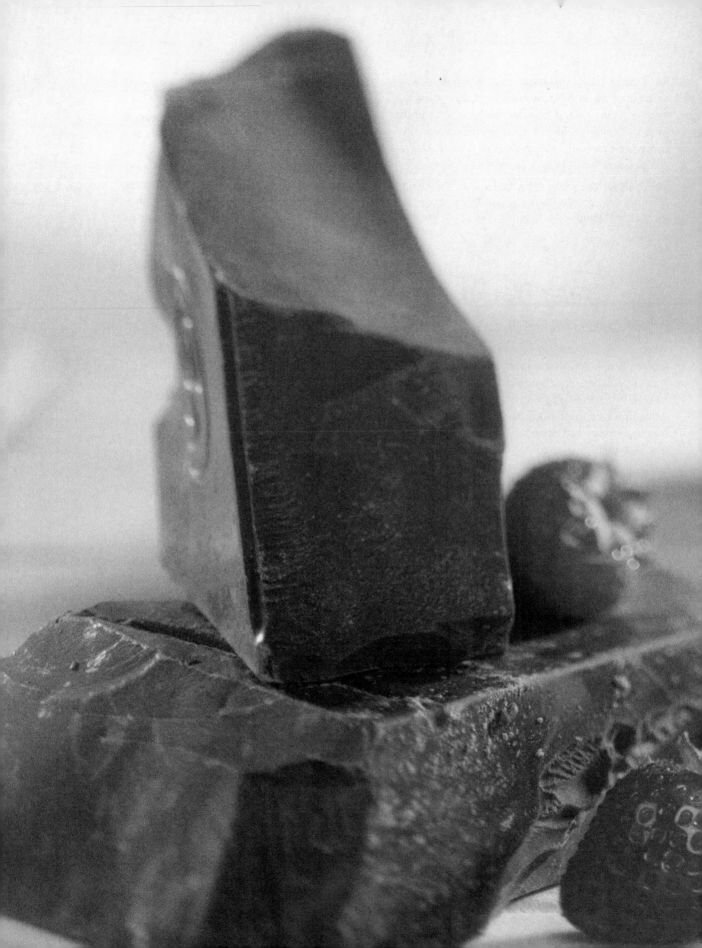

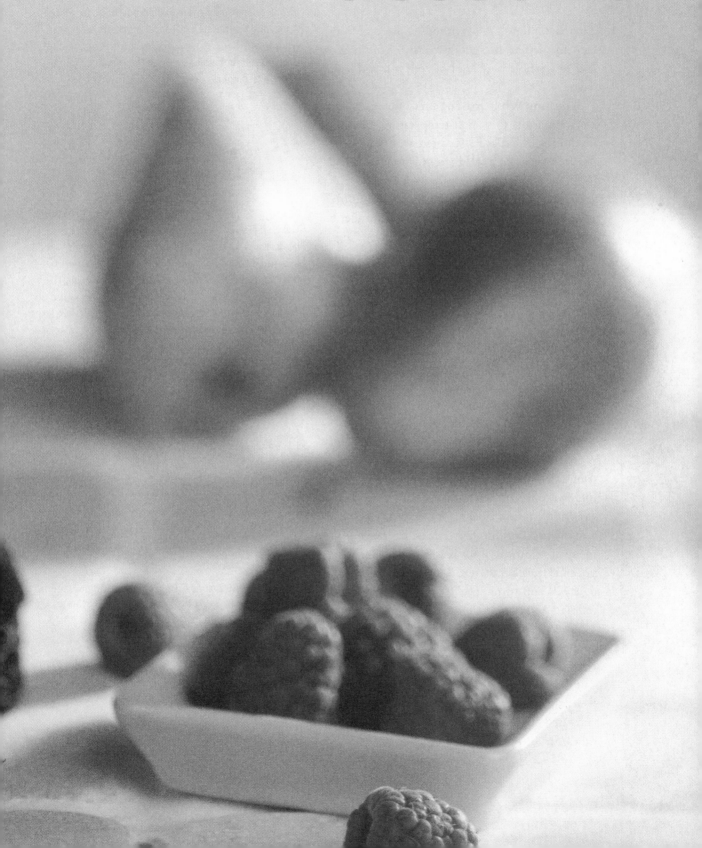

desserts

fruit

There's nothing wrong with just a piece of fresh fruit for dessert, but gently cooked fruit brings you to a whole new level of concentrated fruit flavor.

Roasting While roasting isn't often associated with fruit, this high-temperature method intensifies fruit flavor. Roasted fruit can be a dessert or part of a salad (*see Roasted Pear Salad with Blue Cheese Dressing, page 200*).

Baking Baked fruit can be simply baked (*see Baked Green Apples, page 229*), or baked under a topping, as for crisps (*see Cherry-Raspberry Crisp, page 230*) and cobblers (see *Buttermilk Biscuit-Topped Apple Cobbler, page 230*). Of course, fruit is also traditionally baked in pies (*see Spiced Blueberry Pie, page 240, and One-Crust Apple Pie, page 239*).

Broiling/grilling Most large fruits (pineapple, nectarines, peaches) can be broiled or grilled. Halve or thickly slice the fruit and brush with fruit juice or maple syrup, or sprinkle with a little sugar, and cook until lightly browned.

Poaching Hard fruits (such as apples and pears) can be cooked gently in liquid—wine, fruit juice, or cider. The poaching liquid can then be cooked down to make a sauce (*see Wine-Poached Pears with Goat Cheese, opposite page*).

Stewing Both fresh and dried fruit take well to stewing. Stewed fruit is somewhat similar to poached fruit, but there is less liquid and the fruit collapses and turns into a chunky sauce, often referred to as a compote (*see Orange-Apricot Compote and Rhubarb Compote, both on page 228*). Applesauce is also a type of compote (*see Cranberry-Ginger Applesauce, opposite page*).

Fruit sauces Made from any number of fruits, simple sauces can be pureed or left chunky and used to top frozen yogurt or angel food cake. *(See "Recipe Creator," page 231.)*

> ### did you know?
> Black pepper may seem like an odd thing to put on fruit, but the pungency of the spice helps set up your taste buds to appreciate the flavors of the fruit. Other hot spices—such as allspice, cinnamon, and ginger—perform a similar function.

Strawberries with Balsamic Vinegar & Pepper

Strawberries combined with balsamic vinegar is a classic Italian dessert and presumes a mellow, aged balsamic. However, if you are using an unaged balsamic, begin by adding 1 teaspoon of vinegar, then tasting and adding more if desired. The amount of vinegar you use will also depend on the sweetness of the berries. **Serving suggestion:** You can serve the berries as is, or use it as a topping for frozen yogurt.

3 cups sliced strawberries
⅓ cup packed light brown sugar
½ teaspoon vanilla extract
2 teaspoons balsamic vinegar
⅛ teaspoon pepper

1 In a medium bowl, combine the strawberries, brown sugar, and vanilla. Toss to combine. Cover and let stand for 20 minutes, stirring occasionally.

2 Just before serving, stir in the vinegar and pepper. *Makes 4 servings*

per serving: 109 calories, 0.5g total fat (0g saturated), 0mg cholesterol, 3g dietary fiber, 27g carbohydrate, 1g protein, 9mg sodium. good source of: fiber, vitamin C.

Wine-Poached Pears with Goat Cheese

A melon baller is the perfect tool for scooping out the core from the pear half, conveniently creating a perfect, bowl-shaped hollow to hold the creamy goat cheese filling. If you don't have a melon baller, use a small spoon and try not to remove too much pear flesh. **Timing alert:** The pears need to chill for 2 hours.

1½ cups dry red wine

⅓ cup sugar

1 cinnamon stick, split lengthwise

1 vanilla bean, split lengthwise, or
½ teaspoon vanilla extract

¼ teaspoon cracked black peppercorns

4 firm-ripe pears, such as Bosc or Bartlett, peeled, halved, and cored

¼ cup soft goat cheese (1 ounce)

¼ cup fat-free cream cheese

1 In a large nonaluminum skillet, combine the wine, sugar, cinnamon stick, vanilla bean (if using extract, do not add it yet), and peppercorns. Bring to a boil over medium heat. Add the pears, reduce to a simmer, and place a piece of wax paper directly over the pears (to keep them from discoloring). Simmer until the pears are just tender when pierced with a knife, 7 to 10 minutes. (Timing may vary depending upon the ripeness of the pears.) With a slotted spoon, transfer the pears to a shallow bowl or pan.

2 Bring the wine mixture to a boil over high heat. Boil until the liquid is reduced to a syrup thick enough to coat the back of a spoon, about 7 minutes. Strain and discard the solids. Cool to room temperature (add extract if using), then pour over the pears. Cover and refrigerate until the pears are well chilled, about 2 hours.

3 In a small bowl, mash the goat cheese with the cream cheese until well blended. Place the pears and syrup on 4 serving plates. Spoon the softened cheese mixture into the hollow of each pear half and serve. *Makes 4 servings*

per serving: 267 calories, 2.7g total fat (1.4g saturated), 5mg cholesterol, 4g dietary fiber, 45g carbohydrate, 5g protein, 115mg sodium. good source of: fiber.

Cranberry-Ginger Applesauce

Choose any combination of apples you like. If you use red apples, the peel will heighten the blush that the cranberries give to the sauce.

2½ pounds apples (about 7 medium)

½ cup cranberries, fresh or frozen

3 pieces fresh ginger, each ⅓ inch thick x 1½ inches in diameter

Grated zest of 1 lemon

1 Core the apples and cut into wedges, but do not peel.

2 In a medium saucepan, combine the apples, cranberries, ginger, and lemon zest. Cover and cook over medium-low heat, stirring occasionally, until the apples have given up juice and are at a steam-boil, 7 to 10 minutes.

3 Reduce the heat to low and simmer, stirring occasionally, until the apples have totally collapsed and no longer hold their shape, about 10 minutes.

4 Pass the apples through a food mill or coarse sieve to remove the skin. Discard the skin and ginger. Serve at room temperature or chilled. *Makes about 3 cups*

per ½ cup: 117 calories, 0.7g total fat (0.1g saturated), 0mg cholesterol, 6g dietary fiber, 30g carbohydrate, 0g protein, 0mg sodium. good source of: fiber, quercetin, vitamin C.

did you know?

Pears and apples may reduce the risk of lung disease, such as chronic bronchitis and emphysema, according to a Dutch study. These fruits are rich in compounds called catechins and other flavonoids, which act as antioxidants and may help protect the lungs. Fruit was found to be protective even after smoking (and other factors) were taken into consideration.

Orange-Apricot Compote

Dried fruit compotes make quick, simple fruit desserts. You can eat them warm or chilled, by themselves or with yogurt or frozen yogurt. They also make a great substitute for jam on toast or pancakes. If you prefer tart fruit, do not add the sugar until step 2, after you've cooked the apricots. Then add half the sugar, stir to dissolve, and taste again before adding any more sugar.

> ½ cup apricot nectar
>
> ½ cup orange juice
>
> ¼ cup sugar
>
> 2 tablespoons fresh lemon juice
>
> ¼ teaspoon cardamom
>
> 2 cups (12 ounces) dried apricots

1 In a medium nonaluminum saucepan, bring the apricot nectar, orange juice, sugar, lemon juice, and cardamom to a boil.

2 Add the apricots and simmer until tender, about 20 minutes. Serve warm, at room temperature, or chilled. *Makes 6 servings*

per serving: 190 calories, 0.3g total fat (0g saturated), 0mg cholesterol, 5g dietary fiber, 49g carbohydrate, 2g protein, 7mg sodium. good source of: beta carotene, fiber, potassium.

Rhubarb Compote

Because rhubarb has so much water in it, it will completely fall apart when cooked if you're not careful. So, if you want a chunky sauce, keep an eye on it and stop the cooking process once the rhubarb is softened but still chunky. It's especially important to watch it if you're using out-of-season hothouse rhubarb, because it's not as hardy as field-grown. **Serving suggestion:** Serve this fruit compote on its own, dolloped with lightly sweetened low-fat yogurt, or as a topping for frozen yogurt.

> ⅓ cup frozen pineapple juice concentrate
>
> ½ cup packed light brown sugar
>
> 3 tablespoons finely chopped fresh ginger
>
> 1 vanilla bean, split lengthwise, or
>   ½ teaspoon vanilla extract
>
> ¼ teaspoon salt
>
> 6 cups sliced rhubarb (2 pounds), cut into
>   1-inch lengths

1 In a medium, heavy-bottomed nonaluminum saucepan, combine the pineapple juice concentrate, brown sugar, ginger, vanilla bean (if using extract, do not add it yet), and salt. Cook over low heat until the sugar has melted.

2 Stir in the rhubarb and bring to a simmer. Cover and cook, stirring frequently, until the rhubarb is tender and the compote is chunky, about 15 minutes. Transfer to a medium bowl and

different spins

▶**Mango-Peach Compote** Follow the directions for *Orange-Apricot Compote*, but use mango nectar instead of apricot nectar, pineapple juice instead of orange juice, and halved dried peaches instead of apricots. Reduce the sugar to 2 tablespoons. Omit the cardamom and stir in 2 teaspoons grated lemon zest.

▶**Cherry-Plum Compote** Follow the directions for *Orange-Apricot Compote*, but use red wine instead of apricot nectar, and cinnamon instead of the cardamom. Substitute 1⅓ cups small pitted dried plums (prunes) and ⅔ cup dried cherries for the apricots.

▶**Pear & Golden Raisin Compote** Follow the directions for *Orange-Apricot Compote*, but use pear nectar instead of apricot nectar, and white wine instead of orange juice. Omit the cardamom and use ½ teaspoon ground ginger and ⅛ teaspoon black pepper. Use a combination of 1⅓ cups dried pears and ⅔ cup golden raisins instead of the apricots.

cool to room temperature. If you're using vanilla extract, stir it in now.

3 Once cooled, remove the vanilla bean. Serve warm, at room temperature, or chilled. *Makes 4 servings*

per serving: 187 calories, 0.4g total fat (0.1g saturated), 0mg cholesterol, 4g dietary fiber, 46g carbohydrate, 2g protein, 164mg sodium. good source of: potassium, vitamin C.

Baked Green Apples

Serve these either warm, at room temperature, or chilled. If you like, serve with a dollop of plain fat-free yogurt.

⅓ cup dried cherries, coarsely chopped

⅓ cup walnuts, coarsely chopped

2 tablespoons brown sugar

1 tablespoon fresh lemon juice

4 Granny Smith apples

½ cup apple cider or apple juice

¼ teaspoon cinnamon

1 Preheat the oven to 350°F. In a small bowl, stir together the cherries, walnuts, brown sugar, and lemon juice.

2 With an apple corer or a vegetable peeler, core the apples from the stem end, stopping about ½ inch from the bottom of the apple. Core out the hollow until it's about the width of a quarter. Fill the hollow with the cherry mixture.

3 In a baking pan just large enough to hold the apples snugly, stir together the apple cider and cinnamon. Place the apples, open-side up, in the apple juice mixture. Cover the apples with foil.

4 Bake for 25 minutes, or until the apples are tender but not falling apart. To serve, spoon the pan juices over the apples. *Makes 4 servings*

per serving: 188 calories, 5.4g total fat (0.5g saturated), 0mg cholesterol, 4g dietary fiber, 35g carbohydrate, 2g protein, 8mg sodium. good source of: fiber.

Lemon-Honey Quince

Fresh quince have a wonderful, perfumy aroma, sort of like super-fragrant pears (which quince vaguely resemble). Quince cooked with a little honey, lemon juice, and vanilla makes a deliciously simple fruit dessert. **Serving suggestion:** Serve topped with plain yogurt or a scoop of low-fat frozen yogurt. To turn this into a fruit condiment for meat or poultry, add ½ teaspoon of rosemary or sage to the quince as they cook.

1½ cups apple cider or apple juice

3 tablespoons honey

2 tablespoons fresh lemon juice

1 cinnamon stick

1 vanilla bean, split, or ½ teaspoon vanilla extract

¼ teaspoon pepper

2 pounds quince, peeled and cut into 8 wedges each

1 In a large skillet, bring the apple cider, honey, lemon juice, cinnamon stick, vanilla bean (if using extract, do not add it yet), and pepper to a boil over medium heat.

2 Add the quince, reduce to a simmer, and cook until the quince are tender (some will break up, don't be concerned), about 30 minutes. Remove from the heat. If you're using vanilla extract, stir it in now.

3 Serve warm, at room temperature, or chilled. Before serving, remove the cinnamon stick and vanilla bean. *Makes 4 servings*

per serving: 227 calories, 0.2g total fat (0g saturated), 0mg cholesterol, 5g dietary fiber, 60g carbohydrate, 1g protein, 19mg sodium. good source of: fiber, potassium, vitamin C.

Cherry-Raspberry Crisp

Dark red fruit like raspberries and cherries have good amounts of the antioxidant phytochemicals called anthocyanins. You can use either sweet or sour cherries in this crisp.

- ¼ cup granulated sugar
- 2 tablespoons plus ¼ cup flour
- 1 teaspoon cinnamon
- ½ teaspoon pepper
- ½ teaspoon salt
- ⅛ teaspoon allspice
- 2 bags (12 ounces each) frozen pitted cherries
- 1 cup fresh or frozen unsweetened raspberries, thawed
- ½ cup old-fashioned rolled oats
- ¼ cup packed light brown sugar
- 2 tablespoons extra-light olive oil

1 Preheat the oven to 400°F. In a large bowl, stir together the granulated sugar, 2 tablespoons of the flour, the cinnamon, pepper, ¼ teaspoon of the salt, and the allspice. Add the cherries and raspberries, tossing to coat. Transfer to a 9-inch pie plate. Set aside.

2 In a medium bowl, stir together the remaining ¼ cup flour, remaining ¼ teaspoon salt, the oats, and brown sugar. With a pastry blender or two knives, cut in the oil until the mixture resembles coarse crumbs. Sprinkle the mixture over the fruit.

3 Bake for 25 minutes, or until the fruit is bubbling and piping hot and the topping is golden brown and crisp. *Makes 6 servings*

per serving: 259 calories, 5g total fat (0.7g saturated), 0mg cholesterol, 2g dietary fiber, 53g carbohydrate, 4g protein, 198mg sodium. good source of: anthocyanins, quercetin.

Buttermilk Biscuit-Topped Apple Cobbler

Biscuit toppings are generally made with all butter or a combination of butter and solid vegetable shortening. This one is made with a combination of butter and olive oil, so you're getting lots of rich flavor, but with less saturated fat. **Timing alert:** The dough needs to chill for 30 minutes before baking.

- ½ cup whole-wheat flour
- ½ cup plus 1 tablespoon all-purpose flour
- ⅔ cup plus 1 tablespoon sugar
- 2 teaspoons grated lemon zest
- 1 teaspoon baking powder
- ½ teaspoon baking soda
- ½ teaspoon salt
- 2 tablespoons cold unsalted butter, cut up
- 1 tablespoon extra-light olive oil
- ¼ cup buttermilk
- 3 pounds Granny Smith apples (about 6), peeled and thinly sliced
- 1 tablespoon fresh lemon juice
- 1 teaspoon cinnamon

1 In a large bowl, stir together the whole-wheat flour, ½ cup of the all-purpose flour, 1 tablespoon of the sugar, the lemon zest, baking powder, baking soda, and ¼ teaspoon of the salt. With a pastry blender or 2 knives, cut in the butter and olive oil until the mixture resembles coarse meal.

2 Stir in the buttermilk until the dough almost comes together. (Add up to 1 tablespoon more buttermilk, 1 teaspoon at a time, if the dough is too dry.) Pat the dough into a disk, wrap in plastic wrap, and chill for 30 minutes.

3 Meanwhile, in a large bowl, combine the apples, the remaining ⅔ cup sugar, and remaining 1 tablespoon all-purpose flour, and toss well to coat. Add the lemon juice, cinnamon, and the remaining ¼ teaspoon salt, and toss to combine.

recipe creator
fruit sauces

Fruit sauces are one of the best dessert tricks around. You can make them in no time at all, and have something that will be delicious drizzled over frozen yogurt, cut-up fruit, or cake. You can use fresh fruit or frozen unsweetened. Choose from the categories below and follow these basic directions: In a food processor or blender, combine 1 FRUIT, 1 SWEETENER, 1 FLAVORING, and 1 SPICE if desired. Puree until smooth. Taste and then add 1 ACID if desired. Chill. *Makes 4 servings*

FRUITS	SWEETENERS	FLAVORINGS	SPICES*	ACIDS*
▶ Raspberries, 1 cup	▶ Honey, 2 Tbsp	▶ Vanilla extract, ½ tsp	▶ Allspice or cloves, ⅛ tsp	▶ Lemon juice, 1 Tbsp
▶ Strawberries, 1 cup	▶ Maple syrup, 2 Tbsp	▶ Almond extract, ⅛ tsp	▶ Pepper, ⅛ tsp	▶ Lime juice, 1 Tbsp
▶ Blueberries, 1 cup	▶ All-fruit spread, 2 Tbsp	▶ Orange liqueur, 1 Tbsp	▶ Cinnamon, ¼ tsp	▶ Balsamic vinegar, 1 tsp
▶ Cherries, 1 cup pitted	▶ Corn syrup, 2 Tbsp	▶ Dark rum, 1 Tbsp	▶ Ground ginger, ¼ tsp	▶ Orange juice, 3 Tbsp
▶ Pineapple, 1 cup chopped	▶ Applesauce, ⅓ cup		▶ Cardamom, ⅛ tsp	▶ Tangerine juice, 3 Tbsp
▶ Peaches, 1 cup peeled and sliced	▶ Pineapple juice concentrate, 2 Tbsp			▶ Cider vinegar, 1 tsp
▶ Mango, 1 cup sliced	▶ Apple juice concentrate, 2 Tbsp			▶ Raspberry vinegar, 1 tsp
▶ Mango, ½ cup sliced + papaya, ½ cup sliced	▶ Granulated sugar, 1 Tbsp			▶ Tarragon vinegar, 1 tsp
	▶ Brown sugar, 1 Tbsp		*optional	*optional

4 Spoon the apple mixture into a 9-inch deep-dish pie plate.

5 Preheat the oven to 425°F. On a lightly floured board, pat the chilled dough into an 8-inch circle. Gently lift the dough and place on top of the filling. Place the cobbler on a jelly-roll pan to catch any drips and bake for 15 minutes.

6 Reduce the oven to 350°F and bake for 25 minutes, or until the crust is golden brown. Transfer to a wire rack and cool 10 minutes before serving. *Makes 8 servings*

per serving: 269 calories, 5.4g total fat (2.2g saturated), 8mg cholesterol, 5g dietary fiber, 56g carbohydrate, 3g protein, 262mg sodium. good source of: fiber, selenium.

puddings & mousses

It's hard to come up with a name that encompasses all of the desserts that fall into this category. Their one unifying feature is that they have a wonderful, soothing texture. Texture is very important in a pudding and the type of thickener used determines how thick, smooth, and delicate the results are.

Cornstarch Cornstarch stirred into a flavored liquid (milk, soymilk, or fruit juice) and then heated will thicken into a pudding (*see Triple Chocolate Pudding, opposite page*). Cornstarch puddings are the type most commonly sold as storebought pudding mixes.

Other starches Any type of raw starch will thicken when it's combined with a liquid and heated (including cornstarch, of course). This accounts for two classic pudding ingredients: rice and tapioca. As these ingredients cook, they release their starch and thicken the liquid they're being cooked in (*see Almond & Apricot Rice Pudding, at right, and Mango-Tapioca Pudding, page 234*).

Eggs This is the ingredient used to thicken custards. By and large, we've found ways around using too many eggs in order to reduce the fat and cholesterol that come with them. In some puddings, we've replaced the eggs with gelatin (*see below*). Baked puddings, which are like cakes, usually require some eggs to thicken them and set them up (*see Persimmon Pudding, page 237*).

Gelatin Gelatin is a good, fat-free way to create silky, smooth-textured mousses and puddings, and is often used to replace the thickness that might have come from eggs or high-fat dairy products (*see Chocolate-Orange Latte Cotto, page 234, and Honey-Mango Mousse, page 236*).

Almond & Apricot Rice Pudding

It seems a shame to leave a canvas like rice pudding blank, so we have added shredded carrots and chopped apricots. Not only do they add spots of color, but they also add nice texture and a healthy helping of beta carotene. For an added twist, try this with an aromatic rice such as basmati.

> 2 cups water
> ¾ cup rice
> 3 cups low-fat (1%) milk
> 2 large carrots, finely shredded
> 1 teaspoon grated orange zest
> 1 teaspoon grated lime zest
> ½ cup sugar
> ½ teaspoon cinnamon
> ¼ teaspoon salt
> 1 large egg
> ⅓ cup chopped dried apricots
> 3 tablespoons slivered almonds

1 In a large saucepan, bring the water to a boil. Add the rice, cover, reduce the heat to medium-low, and cook until tender, about 20 minutes.

2 Stir in 2½ cups of the milk, the carrots, and the orange and lime zests. Uncover and cook over low heat, stirring frequently, until the milk has been absorbed, about 20 minutes.

3 Stir in the sugar, cinnamon, salt, and the remaining ½ cup milk, and cook, stirring frequently, until the rice is very tender and creamy, about 5 minutes.

4 In a small bowl, lightly beat the egg. Whisk some of the hot rice mixture into the egg to warm it, then whisk the warmed egg mixture into the saucepan. Cook, stirring constantly, for 3 minutes to cook the egg.

5 Remove from the heat and transfer to a bowl. Stir in the apricots and almonds. Chill until serving time. *Makes 6 servings*

per serving: 267 calories, 4.5g total fat (1.3g saturated), 40mg cholesterol, 2g dietary fiber, 49g carbohydrate, 8g protein, 180mg sodium. good source of: beta carotene, calcium, folate, riboflavin, selenium, thiamin, vitamin B_{12}.

Peanut Pudding with Shaved Chocolate

Though many dessert puddings get their firmness from ingredients high in saturated fat (such as cream and eggs), this satisfying combination of peanuts and chocolate is based on soymilk and gets its creamy texture from gelatin, which has no fat at all. The fat in the pudding is largely unsaturated, with only 4% of the calories coming from saturated fat. **Timing alert:** The pudding needs to chill for about 4 hours.

> 4 cups unflavored soymilk or fat-free dairy milk
>
> ½ cup packed light brown sugar
>
> 3 tablespoons creamy peanut butter
>
> ½ teaspoon dark sesame oil
>
> ¼ teaspoon salt
>
> 1 envelope plus ¾ teaspoon unflavored gelatin
>
> ¼ teaspoon almond extract
>
> ½ ounce (½ square) semisweet chocolate, grated
>
> ¼ cup dry-roasted salted peanuts, coarsely chopped

1 In a medium saucepan, combine 3 cups of the soymilk, the brown sugar, peanut butter, sesame oil, and salt. Bring to a simmer over medium heat.

2 Meanwhile, in a measuring cup, sprinkle the gelatin over the remaining 1 cup soymilk. Let stand until softened, about 2 minutes.

3 Stir the softened gelatin into the soy-peanut butter mixture and cook until the gelatin has dissolved, about 1 minute. Remove from the heat and stir in the almond extract.

4 Pour the pudding into six 6-ounce custard cups and let cool to room temperature. Refrigerate until set, about 4 hours. Just before serving, sprinkle the grated chocolate and peanuts on top. *Makes 6 servings*

per serving: 251 calories, 10g total fat (2g saturated), 0mg cholesterol, 1g dietary fiber, 31g carbohydrate, 11g protein, 253mg sodium. good source of: magnesium, potassium.

Triple Chocolate Pudding

Cocoa powder, German's sweet chocolate, and semisweet chocolate—underscored by brown sugar and cinnamon—give this pudding its rich chocolate flavor. German's chocolate is commonly (and mistakenly) referred to as German chocolate; but its name is actually the brand name, "German's," and not the chocolate's national origin.

> 3 tablespoons unsweetened cocoa powder
>
> 3 tablespoons cornstarch
>
> ⅓ cup packed dark brown sugar
>
> 3 cups low-fat (1%) milk
>
> ½ teaspoon cinnamon
>
> ¼ teaspoon salt
>
> 2 ounces German's or other sweet chocolate, coarsely chopped
>
> 2 tablespoons mini chocolate chips (1 ounce)
>
> 1 teaspoon vanilla extract

1 In a small bowl, combine the cocoa powder, cornstarch, brown sugar, and ½ cup of the milk.

2 In a medium saucepan, combine the remaining 2½ cups milk, cinnamon, and salt. Bring to a boil over medium heat. Whisk the cocoa mixture into the boiling milk and cook, whisking, just until thickened, about 4 minutes.

3 Stir in the sweet chocolate and chocolate chips. Remove from the heat, cover, and let stand until the chips have melted, about 1 minute. Stir in the vanilla extract. Spoon into 6 bowls and chill until serving time. *Makes 6 servings*

per serving: 187 calories, 5.6g total fat (3.3g saturated), 5mg cholesterol, 1g dietary fiber, 32g carbohydrate, 5g protein, 165mg sodium. good source of: calcium, riboflavin, vitamin B_{12}.

Mango-Tapioca Pudding

As the pudding cooks, the tapioca pearls swell and turn translucent, giving this dessert the appearance that earned it its affectionate nickname: fish eyes and glue. Most tapioca puddings are made with milk and eggs, but for a lighter, more tropical feeling, we've cooked the tapioca in mango nectar. You could also try this with another fruit nectar, such as apricot. **Timing alert:** Because the tapioca needs to be soaked and the cooked pudding needs to be chilled, you should start this dessert about 9 hours before you want to serve it.

> ½ cup small pearl tapioca
>
> 2 cups cold water
>
> 2 cups mango nectar
>
> ¼ cup sugar
>
> 1½ teaspoons grated lime zest
>
> ¼ cup fresh lime juice (2 to 3 limes)
>
> ½ teaspoon cinnamon
>
> ¼ teaspoon ground ginger
>
> ⅛ teaspoon salt
>
> ⅓ cup reduced-fat sour cream

1 In a large bowl, combine the tapioca and cold water, and let soak for at least 4 hours. Drain.

2 In a medium, heavy-bottomed nonaluminum saucepan, combine the mango nectar, sugar, lime zest, lime juice, cinnamon, ginger, and salt. Bring to a boil and stir in the drained tapioca. Reduce to a simmer and cook, stirring occasionally, until the tapioca "pearls" are translucent (with only the merest hint of opacity at their centers), about 25 minutes.

3 Remove from the heat and transfer the pudding to a serving bowl. Let cool to room temperature and stir in the sour cream. Cover and refrigerate until chilled, about 4 hours. *Makes 4 servings*

per serving: 222 calories, 2.5g total fat (1.5g saturated), 8mg cholesterol, 1g dietary fiber, 51g carbohydrate, 1g protein, 157mg sodium.

Chocolate-Orange Latte Cotto

This adaptation of *panna cotta* (an Italian dessert usually made with cream or a combination of milk and cream) is silky-smooth and satisfying. If you like, run a metal spatula around the edges of the dessert and invert it onto a serving plate. **Timing alert:** This dessert has to chill for at least 4 hours.

> 3 cups low-fat (1%) or fat-free milk
>
> ½ cup sugar
>
> 6 strips (½ x 2 inches) orange zest
>
> 1 envelope unflavored gelatin
>
> 3 tablespoons unsweetened cocoa powder
>
> 3 tablespoons cold water
>
> 2 tablespoons chocolate chips (1 ounce)
>
> ½ teaspoon vanilla extract
>
> ⅛ teaspoon almond extract

1 In a medium saucepan, combine 2 cups of the milk, the sugar, and orange zest. Bring to a simmer over low heat. Remove from the heat, cover, and let stand for 20 minutes for the milk to absorb the orange zest flavors. Strain and discard the zest.

2 In a small bowl, sprinkle the gelatin over the remaining 1 cup milk and let stand until softened, about 2 minutes.

3 In another small bowl, combine the cocoa and water, stirring, until the cocoa is moistened.

4 Stir the softened gelatin, moistened cocoa, and chocolate chips into the saucepan of milk. Stir over medium heat until the gelatin has dissolved and the chocolate chips have melted, about 3 minutes. Remove from the heat and stir in the vanilla and almond extracts.

5 Divide the mixture among six 6-ounce custard cups and let cool to room temperature. Refrigerate for at least 4 hours, or until set and well chilled. *Makes 6 servings*

per serving: 150 calories, 3.1g total fat (1.9g saturated), 5mg cholesterol, 1g dietary fiber, 27g carbohydrate, 6g protein, 65mg sodium. **good source of:** calcium, riboflavin, vitamin B_{12}, vitamin D.

Coeur à la Crème

Serve this creamy molded dessert with a fruit sauce (*see the "Recipe Creator" on page 231*). You can either pass the sauce at the table for diners to drizzle over their portions, or you can present the dessert sitting in a pool of the sauce. Heart-shaped ceramic molds, designed especially for this dessert, are available at specialty cookware shops. **Timing alert:** The dessert needs to drain for about 6 hours.

> 12 ounces fat-free cream cheese
>
> 4 ounces reduced-fat cream cheese (Neufchâtel)
>
> 1 cup low-fat (1%) cottage cheese
>
> ⅔ cup confectioners' sugar
>
> ½ teaspoon vanilla extract

1 In a food processor, combine the cream cheeses, cottage cheese, confectioners' sugar, and vanilla, and process to a smooth puree.

2 Line a heart-shaped ceramic coeur à la crème mold (or a 4- to 6-cup sieve set over a bowl) with a double layer of dampened cheesecloth that overhangs the mold. Spoon the cream cheese mixture into the mold, wrap the cheesecloth over, and place the mold on a plate to drain. Refrigerate for 4 to 6 hours or overnight.

3 Unfold the cheesecloth and invert the mold onto a serving plate. Remove the mold and peel off the cheesecloth. *Makes 6 servings*

per serving: 183 calories, 5.6g total fat (3.6g saturated), 20mg cholesterol, 0g dietary fiber, 18g carbohydrate, 15g protein, 538mg sodium. **good source of:** riboflavin, vitamin B$_{12}$.

Honey-Rum Semifreddo

Semifreddo in Italian means "half-cold" and it refers to any number of desserts that are almost, but not quite, frozen. Sort of soft-serve Italian style. This semifreddo has the flavors of cannoli filling. **Timing alert:** This needs about 4 hours in the freezer. If you make it the day before (in which case it will be fully frozen), it needs to sit out at room temperature for 10 to 15 minutes to soften slightly before serving.

> ½ cup golden raisins
>
> ¼ cup dark rum
>
> 2 cups low-fat (1%) cottage cheese
>
> ⅓ cup part-skim ricotta cheese
>
> ⅓ cup honey
>
> ¼ cup fat-free sour cream
>
> 1 tablespoon grated orange zest
>
> ¼ cup mini chocolate chips (2 ounces)

1 In a small bowl, stir together the raisins and rum. Set aside to soak for 10 minutes.

2 In a food processor, combine the cottage cheese, ricotta, honey, sour cream, and orange zest, and process until smooth, about 2 minutes.

3 Transfer the cheese mixture to a bowl and fold in the raisins and their soaking liquid, and the chocolate chips.

4 Line an 8½ x 4½-inch loaf pan with plastic wrap, leaving a 2-inch overhang all around. Spoon the mixture into the pan, cover with the overhang, and freeze until set but not frozen solid, about 4 hours. Unmold the semifreddo and cut into 8 slices. *Makes 8 slices*

per slice: 186 calories, 3.3g total fat (2g saturated), 6mg cholesterol, 1g dietary fiber, 28g carbohydrate, 9g protein, 250mg sodium. **good source of:** vitamin B$_{12}$.

Mochaccino Bavarian Cream

All the flavors of a mochaccino, cappuccino's chocolate-flavored cousin, come together in this chilled dessert. Because this is a dessert that's designed to be unmolded, use a decorative mold if you have one. **Timing alert:** The bavarian needs to chill for at least 4 hours.

> 1 envelope unflavored gelatin
>
> 2 cups low-fat (1%) or fat-free milk
>
> 1 large egg
>
> ¼ cup granulated sugar
>
> ¼ cup packed light brown sugar
>
> 3 tablespoons unsweetened cocoa powder
>
> 2 tablespoons instant espresso powder
>
> ½ teaspoon cinnamon
>
> ⅛ teaspoon salt
>
> ¼ teaspoon vanilla extract
>
> ⅓ cup reduced-fat sour cream

1 In a small bowl, sprinkle the gelatin over ¼ cup of the milk and let stand until softened, about 2 minutes.

2 In a medium heatproof bowl, combine the remaining 1¾ cups milk, the egg, granulated sugar, brown sugar, cocoa, espresso powder, cinnamon, and salt. Place the bowl over a saucepan of simmering water and cook, whisking, until the custard is slightly thickened, and very hot, about 5 minutes. Add the softened gelatin and cook, whisking, until the gelatin is dissolved, about 2 minutes.

3 Remove from the heat and let cool to room temperature. Stir in the vanilla. Fold in the sour cream. Pour into a small bowl or decorative mold with at least a 2½-cup capacity. Cover and refrigerate until set, at least 4 hours.

4 Run a knife or spatula around the bowl and invert the bavarian onto a serving plate. *Makes 4 servings*

per serving: 209 calories, 3.4g total fat (1.7g saturated), 60mg cholesterol, 1g dietary fiber, 38g carbohydrate, 9g protein, 176mg sodium. good source of: calcium, riboflavin, selenium, vitamin B_{12}.

Honey-Mango Mousse

For an even lighter dessert, replace all or part of the reduced-fat sour cream with plain fat-free yogurt. **Timing alert:** The mousse needs to chill for at least 2 hours.

> 2 mangoes (1½ pounds total), peeled and sliced (1½ cups)
>
> ¼ cup fresh lime juice
>
> ⅛ teaspoon salt
>
> ⅛ teaspoon allspice
>
> 1 envelope unflavored gelatin
>
> ½ cup cold water
>
> ¼ cup honey
>
> ½ cup reduced-fat sour cream

1 In a food processor, puree the mangoes with the lime juice, salt, and allspice.

2 In a small bowl, sprinkle the gelatin over ¼ cup of the water. Let the gelatin stand until softened, about 2 minutes.

3 Meanwhile, in a small saucepan, combine the honey and the remaining ¼ cup water, and bring to a boil. Stir the softened gelatin into the honey mixture and cook, stirring, until the gelatin is dissolved, about 1 minute.

4 Add the honey-gelatin mixture to the mango puree and process until well combined. Add the sour cream and process briefly just to blend.

5 Spoon into dessert bowls or glasses, cover, and refrigerate for 2 hours or until chilled and set. *Makes 4 servings*

per serving: 160 calories, 3.7g total fat (2.5g saturated), 15mg cholesterol, 1g dietary fiber, 31g carbohydrate, 3g protein, 98mg sodium. good source of: beta carotene, vitamin C.

Persimmon Pudding

Although there is a dense, plum pudding-type dessert called persimmon pudding, this is not it. This baked dessert is soft and custardy. For safety's sake, put the roasting pan with the baking dish in it on the oven rack before adding the boiling water (see step 3). **Timing alert:** This baked pudding takes 1½ hours in the oven.

    1¼ cups flour
    1 teaspoon cinnamon
    ¾ teaspoon baking powder
    ¾ teaspoon baking soda
    ½ teaspoon salt
    1¼ cups buttermilk
    ¾ cup maple syrup
    2 large eggs
    1 large egg white
    3 tablespoons extra-light olive oil
    4 very ripe and soft persimmons (about
       1¾ pounds total), peeled

1 Preheat the oven to 350°F. Spray a 7 x 11-inch glass baking dish or shallow 2-quart baking dish with nonstick cooking spray. In a large bowl, stir together the flour, cinnamon, baking powder, baking soda, and salt.

2 In a medium bowl, stir together the buttermilk, maple syrup, whole eggs, egg white, and oil. In a food processor or blender, puree the persimmons. Add the persimmon puree to the buttermilk mixture and stir until well combined.

3 Make a well in the center of the flour mixture. Add the persimmon-buttermilk mixture and stir until well combined. Pour the batter into the baking dish. Place the dish in a large roasting pan and pour boiling water to come halfway up the sides of the dish.

4 Bake for 1½ hours, or until the pudding is set, deep brown, and beginning to pull away from the sides of the dish. Serve warm or at room temperature. *Makes 8 servings*

per serving: 247 calories, 7g total fat (1.3g saturated), 55mg cholesterol, 1g dietary fiber, 42g carbohydrate, 5g protein, 375mg sodium. good source of: riboflavin, selenium, thiamin, zinc.

pies

Pie crusts get their flavor and tenderness from fat—no two ways about it. And traditionally the fat used is butter, solid vegetable shortening, or (gasp) lard. So, how do you make a pie crust worth eating without those highly saturated fats? The answer is unsaturated oils, used in two different types of crust:

Cookie crusts These crusts are made with crushed cookie crumbs, and where a typical crust recipe would have called for melted butter, we've used oil (olive, nut, or seed) instead.

Pastry crusts For the more traditional pie doughs, we've eliminated the butter (*et.al.*), and replaced it with a combination of oil and low-fat yogurt. But even with this shift away from saturated fat, the total amount of fat still needs to be high enough to make a crust worth eating. So, our solution here is to use only a top crust (*see One-Crust Apple Pie, page 239*) instead of the more usual top and bottom crusts.

---

different spins

▶ **Spiced Persimmon Pudding** Follow the directions for *Persimmon Pudding*, but add 1½ teaspoons grated orange zest, 1 teaspoon ground ginger, ¼ teaspoon ground cloves, and ⅛ teaspoon ground allspice in step 1. Substitute reduced-fat sour cream for the buttermilk.

Nectarine Cheese Pie in a Ginger Crust

Unlike most cheese pies or cheesecakes, this is made with no eggs and is not baked. Instead, homemade yogurt cheese is combined with sour cream, sugar, chopped nectarines, and gelatin and chilled until set. **Timing alert:** You will need to start the yogurt cheese a day ahead, and the filling needs about 6 hours to set.

> 3 cups plain fat-free yogurt
>
> 16 gingersnaps (4 ounces)
>
> 2 tablespoons extra-light olive oil
>
> ⅓ cup reduced-fat sour cream
>
> ¼ cup sugar
>
> 2 teaspoons grated tangerine or orange zest
>
> ½ teaspoon vanilla extract
>
> 2 teaspoons unflavored gelatin
>
> ¼ cup frozen tangerine or orange juice concentrate, thawed
>
> 1¾ cups diced nectarines (about 4)
>
> 1 cup canned juice-packed mandarin oranges, well drained

1 Set a coffee filter or a large strainer lined with cheesecloth over a bowl. Spoon in the yogurt and allow to drain, loosely covered, in the refrigerator, until the yogurt has reduced to 1¾ cups and is the consistency of soft cream cheese, about 8 hours.

2 Preheat the oven to 350°F. In a food processor, process the gingersnaps to fine crumbs. Add the oil and process briefly to combine. Spray a 9-inch pie plate with nonstick cooking spray. Press the crumb mixture into the bottom and up the sides of the plate. Bake until the crumbs are set, about 12 minutes. Transfer to a wire rack to cool.

3 In a medium bowl, beat together the yogurt cheese and sour cream until smooth. Beat in the sugar, tangerine zest, and vanilla, and set aside.

4 In a small saucepan, sprinkle the gelatin over the tangerine juice concentrate. Warm the mixture over low heat, stirring just until the gelatin is dissolved. Remove from the heat and beat the gelatin mixture into the yogurt cheese mixture.

5 Stir 1½ cups of the nectarines into the yogurt cheese mixture. Pour the filling into the prepared crust. Refrigerate until the filling is set, 6 hours or overnight.

6 Just before serving, top the pie with the remaining nectarines and the mandarin oranges. *Makes 8 wedges*

per wedge: 222 calories, 6.3g total fat (1.8g saturated), 7mg cholesterol, 1g dietary fiber, 35g carbohydrate, 7g protein, 172mg sodium. good source of: calcium, riboflavin, vitamin B_{12}, vitamin C.

Key Lime Pie

Key lime pie was created in the Florida Keys in the days when native limes were plentiful, and fresh milk was hard to come by. Canned milk (sweetened condensed, in this case) makes a rich, smooth pie filling. Now that condensed milk comes in a fat-free form, it's a real "miracle ingredient" for low saturated-fat desserts.

> Crust:
>
> 1 cup graham cracker crumbs
>
> ⅓ cup toasted wheat germ
>
> 2 tablespoons sugar
>
> 2 tablespoons extra-light olive oil
>
> 3 tablespoons water
>
> Filling:
>
> 1 large egg
>
> 2 large egg whites
>
> 1½ teaspoons grated lime zest
>
> 1 can (14 ounces) fat-free sweetened condensed milk
>
> ⅔ cup fresh lime juice (or Key lime juice)

1 Preheat the oven to 350°F.

2 Make the crust: In a medium bowl, stir together the graham cracker crumbs, wheat germ, and sugar. In a small bowl, stir together the oil and water, and mix until combined. Pour the oil mixture over the graham cracker crumb mixture and with a fork, stir to coat. Spray a 9-inch pie plate with nonstick cooking spray. Press the crumb mixture into the bottom and up the sides of the pie plate.

3 Bake the crust for 12 minutes, or until set. Leave the oven on. Cool the crust on a wire rack.

4 Make the filling: In a medium bowl, with an electric mixer, beat the whole egg, egg whites, and lime zest until fluffy. Beat in the condensed milk until combined. Beat in the lime juice until thick.

5 Pour the lime mixture into the crust. Bake for 15 minutes, or until set. Cool on a wire rack. Refrigerate and serve chilled. *Makes 8 wedges*

per wedge: 333 calories, 6.2g total fat (1g saturated), 31mg cholesterol, 1g dietary fiber, 60g carbohydrate, 10g protein, 184mg sodium. good source of: riboflavin.

One-Crust Apple Pie

The trouble with American-style fruit pies is that there's always too much crust. Too much, that is, for a health-conscious diner. Many health-oriented recipes try to solve the problem by taking the fat out of the crust, rendering it inedible. Our solution, on the other hand, is to make a single crust with lots of flavor and reasonable levels of fat (in this case all unsaturated fat from walnut oil). **Timing alert:** The dough needs to rest for 1 hour before you can roll it out.

Crust:

1 cup plus 2 tablespoons flour

2 tablespoons sugar

1 teaspoon baking powder

½ teaspoon salt

⅓ cup plain low-fat yogurt

¼ cup walnut oil or extra-light olive oil

2 tablespoons ice water

Filling:

2½ pounds apples, peeled and thinly sliced

½ cup packed light brown sugar

3 tablespoons flour

1 tablespoon fresh lemon juice

1 teaspoon cinnamon

¼ teaspoon salt

1 Make the crust: In a large bowl, combine the flour, sugar, baking powder, and salt. In a small bowl, stir together the yogurt, walnut oil, and water. Stir the yogurt mixture into the flour mix-

ture just until it forms a dough. Shape into a flat disk, wrap in plastic wrap, and refrigerate for 1 hour.

2 Preheat the oven to 450°F.

3 Make the filling: In a large bowl, toss together the apples, brown sugar, flour, lemon juice, cinnamon, and salt. Transfer to a 9-inch glass pie plate.

4 On a lightly floured surface, roll the dough out to a 13-inch round and drape over the apples. Fold the edge of the dough up to form a neat edge. With your fingers or a fork, crimp the edges of the crust. Make 4 slashes in the top of the dough for steam vents.

5 Place the pie plate on a jelly-roll pan (a baking sheet with sides) and bake for 20 minutes. Reduce the heat to 350°F and bake for 20 minutes, or until the crust is golden brown and the apples are tender. If the crust is overbrowning, tent with foil. *Makes 8 wedges*

per wedge: 275 calories, 7.5g total fat (0.7g saturated), 0mg cholesterol, 3g dietary fiber, 51g carbohydrate, 3g protein, 261mg sodium. good source of: fiber, omega-3 fatty acids, riboflavin, selenium, thiamin.

---

did you know?

Quercetin—a compound found in apples, tea, red wine, and other foods—is an important member of a large group of plant compounds called flavonoids, once thought to be vitamins. Quercetin is being intensively studied for some potential health benefits, including its ability to fight cell-damaging free radicals, help prevent heart disease, help treat or even prevent prostate cancer, and lower the risk of certain respiratory diseases. Although it is way too early to recommend quercetin as a supplement, we do think you should get as much quercetin as you can from foods. Apples, onions, raspberries, black and green tea, red wine, red grapes, citrus fruit, cherries, broccoli, and leafy greens are the way to go. And they offer lots more than just quercetin.

Spiced Blueberry Pie

The blueberry filling for this pie is made with a base mixture of blueberries cooked with spices (including black pepper) into which fresh, uncooked blueberries are stirred. The filling is poured into a prebaked gingersnap crust, made with milk and olive oil instead of butter.

> 36 gingersnaps (9 ounces)
> ⅓ cup plus 2 tablespoons sugar
> ¼ cup low-fat (1%) or fat-free milk
> 2 tablespoons extra-light olive oil
> 3 tablespoons cornstarch
> 1 teaspoon grated orange zest
> ½ teaspoon cinnamon
> ⅛ teaspoon pepper
> 6 cups fresh blueberries
> ½ cup orange juice

1 Preheat the oven to 375°F. In a food processor, process the gingersnaps and 2 tablespoons of the sugar until fine crumbs are formed. Add the milk and oil and process until evenly moistened.

2 Spray a 9-inch pie plate with nonstick cooking spray. Press the gingersnap mixture into the bottom and up the sides of the pie plate. Bake for 12 minutes to set. Cool on a wire rack.

3 Meanwhile, in a small bowl, combine the remaining ⅓ cup sugar, the cornstarch, orange zest, cinnamon, and pepper.

4 In a medium saucepan, combine 3 cups of the blueberries and the orange juice. Bring to a boil over medium heat. Stir in the sugar-cornstarch mixture, return to a boil, and cook, stirring frequently, until thickened, about 5 minutes.

5 Remove from the heat and stir in the remaining 3 cups blueberries. Spoon the blueberry mixture into the pie shell and refrigerate until serving time. *Makes 8 wedges*

per wedge: 305 calories, 9.3g total fat (1.6g saturated), 1mg cholesterol, 4g dietary fiber, 55g carbohydrate, 3g protein, 125mg sodium. **good source of:** anthocyanins.

Raspberry-Topped Lemon Tart

If you like, substitute 2½ cups of your favorite pudding for the lemon filling. **Timing alert:** The pie needs to chill for about 2 hours to set.

> 32 reduced-fat vanilla wafers (6 ounces)
> 1 tablespoon light brown sugar
> 2 teaspoons extra-light olive oil
> ¼ cup low-fat (1%) or fat-free milk
> 1 teaspoon unflavored gelatin
> ¼ cup cold water
> ¾ cup fresh lemon juice (about 3 lemons)
> 1 cup granulated sugar
> 1 large egg
> ¾ cup fat-free sour cream
> 2 tablespoons red currant jelly or seedless raspberry jam
> 1 pint raspberries

1 Preheat the oven to 350°F. In a food processor, combine the vanilla wafers and brown sugar, and process until finely ground. Add the oil and milk, and pulse until evenly moistened.

2 Spray a 9-inch tart pan with a removable bottom with nonstick cooking spray. Press the mixture into the bottom and up the sides of the pan. Bake for 12 minutes to set the crust. Let cool on a wire rack.

3 In a small bowl, sprinkle the gelatin over the water. Let stand until softened, about 2 minutes.

4 In a medium, heavy-bottomed nonaluminum saucepan, whisk together the lemon juice, granulated sugar, and egg until well combined. Cook over low heat, whisking constantly, until the mixture is hot, about 3 minutes.

5 Whisk in the softened gelatin and cook, whisking constantly, until the mixture is the consistency of thick honey and the gelatin has dissolved, about 3 minutes. Remove from the heat, transfer to a medium bowl, and let cool to room temperature.

6 Stir the sour cream into the lemon mixture. Spoon the filling into the tart shell, smoothing the top. Refrigerate until the filling is set, about 2 hours.

7 Just before serving, in a small saucepan, melt the jelly over low heat. Arrange the raspberries on the top of the tart and brush with the melted jelly. *Makes 8 wedges*

per wedge: 276 calories, 5.6g total fat (1.4g saturated), 40mg cholesterol, 3g dietary fiber, 55g carbohydrate, 4g protein, 98mg sodium. good source of: riboflavin, vitamin C.

Sweet Potato Pie in a Peanut Crust

Sweet potatoes make a delicious basis for a custard-style pie with a luscious texture. Two secret ingredients add a deep, rich flavor to the pie: Chick-peas in the pie filling and peanuts in the crust. They are botanically related (both are legumes) and have a similar nutty flavor.

1 cup graham cracker crumbs

¼ cup dry-roasted peanuts

1 tablespoon plus ¾ cup packed light brown sugar

2 tablespoons dark sesame oil

1 cup cooked sweet potato flesh (from about 8 ounces of sweet potato weighed with skin)

1 cup cooked chick-peas (page 180) or canned (rinsed and drained)

1¼ cups low-fat (2%) evaporated milk

1 large egg

2 large egg whites

2 tablespoons dark rum

1 teaspoon cinnamon

½ teaspoon ground ginger

¼ teaspoon salt

⅛ teaspoon nutmeg

1 Preheat the oven to 350°F.

2 In a food processor, combine the graham cracker crumbs, peanuts, and 1 tablespoon of the brown sugar, and pulse until the nuts are finely ground. Add the sesame oil and pulse until the mixture comes together. Don't clean the processor bowl.

3 Spray a 9-inch pie plate with nonstick cooking spray. Press the crumb mixture into the bottom and up the sides of the pie plate. Bake for 12 minutes to set the crust. Set aside while you make the filling. Leave the oven on.

4 Meanwhile, place the remaining ¾ cup brown sugar, the sweet potato, chick-peas, evaporated milk, whole egg, egg whites, rum, cinnamon, ginger, salt, and nutmeg in the food processor and process to a smooth puree.

5 Place the pie crust on a baking sheet and pour the filling mixture into the crust. Bake for 40 minutes, or until the filling is set. Serve at room temperature or chilled. *Makes 10 wedges*

per wedge: 247 calories, 7g total fat (1.4g saturated), 24mg cholesterol, 3g dietary fiber, 39g carbohydrate, 7g protein, 173mg sodium. good source of: beta carotene, calcium, folate, potassium, riboflavin.

different spins

▶**Strawberry Pie** Follow the directions for *Spiced Blueberry Pie (opposite page),* but instead of blueberries, use 6 cups of halved strawberries. Omit the black pepper and add ⅛ teaspoon allspice.

▶**Fruit-Topped Lemon Tart** Follow the directions for *Raspberry-Topped Lemon Tart (opposite page),* but substitute lemon wafers for the vanilla wafers. Instead of raspberries, top the tart with a mixture of halved straw-

berries, blueberries, and sliced kiwifruit. Instead of red currant jelly, use apricot jam that's been strained to get rid of pulp.

▶**Winter Squash Pie in a Walnut Crust** Follow the directions for *Sweet Potato Pie in a Peanut Crust,* but substitute walnuts for the peanuts, cooked and mashed winter squash for the sweet potato, and walnut oil for the sesame oil. Instead of dark rum, use amaretto or frangelico liqueur.

cakes

The major contributions that fat makes in cake baking are tenderness and moistness. We've devised a number of different strategies for baking tender, moist cakes with less fat:

Oils Whenever possible, we replace butter with an unsaturated oil. In some cases we use a toasted nut oil to maximize flavor for a minimum of fat (*see Nut-Studded Carrot Cake with Cream Cheese Frosting, page 244*).

Buttermilk Several of our cake recipes use buttermilk, which, despite its name, does not contain butter. The acid in the buttermilk gives cakes a tender crumb. Yogurt has the same effect (*see Lemon Poppyseed Cake, page 244*).

Vegetables Shredded vegetables—such as beets (yes, beets) and carrots—can provide moisture and a fair amount of sweetness (*see Chocolate Bundt Cake with Chocolate Glaze, opposite page*).

Prune butter Thick, pureed dried plums (prunes) are a good fat replacement and add moisture to dense cakes like brownies (*see Fudgy Pecan Brownies, page 247*).

angel food cakes

Angel food cakes are a rarity among cakes. They are made with no fat. They are leavened by beaten egg whites (lots of them). The resulting cake is light and airy, but only if you know the right way to cool it. As the cake bakes (in a tube pan or special angel food cake pan), the batter climbs up the tall sides and center tube. When it comes out of the oven, it needs to cool upside down so that the cake does not collapse and become dense. Some angel food cake pans have "legs" designed to suspend the pan off the counter as the cake cools. But if you use just a regular tube pan, then a good trick is to suspend the pan upside down over the neck of a bottle.

Mexican Chocolate Angel Food Cake

This cake gets its name from the combination of chocolate and spices, which is common in Mexican cooking.

> ¾ cup cake flour
>
> 1⅓ cups granulated sugar
>
> ¼ cup unsweetened cocoa powder
>
> 2 teaspoons instant espresso powder
>
> 1 teaspoon cinnamon
>
> ¼ teaspoon nutmeg
>
> ¼ teaspoon allspice
>
> 12 large egg whites, at room temperature
>
> 1 teaspoon cream of tartar
>
> ¼ teaspoon salt
>
> 1½ teaspoons vanilla extract
>
> ¼ teaspoon almond extract
>
> ¼ cup mini chocolate chips (2 ounces)
>
> 1 tablespoon confectioners' sugar (optional)

1 Preheat the oven to 350°F. If your angel food cake pan doesn't have "legs," have a long-necked bottle ready to hang the cake on as it cools.

2 On a sheet of wax paper, sift together the flour, ⅓ cup of the granulated sugar, the cocoa powder, espresso powder, cinnamon, nutmeg, and allspice. Set aside.

3 In a large bowl, with an electric mixer, beat the egg whites, cream of tartar, and salt until soft peaks form. Gradually beat in the remaining 1 cup granulated sugar, 1 tablespoon at a time, until very stiff peaks form. Beat in the vanilla and almond extracts until well combined.

4 Sift the flour-cocoa mixture over the egg whites and sprinkle the chocolate chips lightly over the top. Fold into the egg whites.

5 Pour the batter into an ungreased 10-inch angel food cake pan or tube pan and bake for 1 hour, or until the cake is set and pulls away from the sides of the pan. Invert the cake pan over the neck of the bottle and allow the cake to cool upside down.

6 With a small metal spatula, loosen the sides of the cake and invert onto a cake plate. Dust with the confectioners' sugar, if desired, before serving. *Makes 10 slices*

per slice: 190 calories, 1.7g total fat (1g saturated), 0mg cholesterol, 1g dietary fiber, 39g carbohydrate, 6g protein, 126mg sodium. good source of: riboflavin, selenium.

Chocolate Bundt Cake with Chocolate Glaze

The secret ingredient in this cake is beets, which add fiber and the B vitamin folate, two nutrients not commonly found in chocolate cake. In addition to the nutritional bonus, the beets contribute a hint of sweetness, a dark chocolate-like color, and moisture.

    3 ounces (3 squares) unsweetened
       chocolate
    1 can (14½ ounces) sliced beets with their
       liquid
    2¾ cups flour
    ⅔ cup plus 4 teaspoons unsweetened
       cocoa powder
    1½ teaspoons baking powder
    ¾ teaspoon baking soda
    ¾ teaspoon salt
    2 large eggs
    2 large egg whites
    2 cups granulated sugar
    1¾ cups buttermilk
    ⅓ cup extra-light olive oil
    1 cup confectioners' sugar
    2 tablespoons low-fat (1%) or fat-free milk
    ½ teaspoon vanilla extract

1 Preheat the oven to 350°F. Spray a bundt pan with nonstick cooking spray. Dust with flour, shaking off the excess.

2 In the top of a double boiler, melt the chocolate. Let cool to room temperature. In a food processor, puree the beets and their liquid. Set the beet puree aside.

3 In a medium bowl, combine the flour, ⅔ cup of the cocoa, the baking powder, baking soda, and salt.

4 In a large bowl, with an electric mixer, beat the whole eggs, egg whites, and granulated sugar until light and lemon-colored. Beat in the melted chocolate, the beet puree, buttermilk, and oil. Fold in the flour mixture.

5 Pour the batter into the bundt pan. Bake for 1 hour and 5 minutes, or until a toothpick inserted in the center comes out clean and the cake has begun to pull away from the sides of the pan. Cool the cake in the pan for 30 minutes, then turn out onto a wire rack to cool completely.

6 Meanwhile, in a small bowl, stir together the remaining 4 teaspoons cocoa, the confectioners' sugar, milk, and vanilla, stirring until smooth. Drizzle the glaze onto the top and down the sides of the cooled cake. *Makes 12 slices*

per slice: 286 calories, 12g total fat (4g saturated), 37mg cholesterol, 4g dietary fiber, 41g carbohydrate, 8g protein, 395mg sodium. good source of: fiber, folate, riboflavin, selenium, thiamin.

did you know?
A bundt pan is a fluted cake pan with a tube in the center, and bears a resemblance to such other cake molds as kugelhopfs or turk's heads. The bundt pan was introduced (and trademarked) in this country in the 1950s by an American manufacturer of Scandinavian bakeware. The name has since come to mean any similar fluted tube pan for baking. The cakes that are baked in bundt pans have a fine crumb and a dense texture, which is what allows them to unmold properly.

Nut-Studded Carrot Cake with Cream Cheese Frosting

A light cream cheese frosting turns this one-layer cake into a party-worthy dessert, perfect for decorating. If you are making this cake in advance and freezing it, freeze it unfrosted; thaw at room temperature, then decorate the cake shortly before serving.

2 cups flour

½ cup toasted wheat germ

1½ teaspoons baking powder

1 teaspoon baking soda

1½ teaspoons cinnamon

½ teaspoon cardamom

½ teaspoon salt

2 large eggs

1⅓ cups granulated sugar

1¼ cups buttermilk

3 tablespoons extra-light olive oil

3 cups coarsely grated carrots

⅓ cup dried currants

¼ cup shelled pistachios, coarsely chopped

4 ounces reduced-fat cream cheese (Neufchâtel)

4 ounces fat-free cream cheese

¼ cup confectioners' sugar

½ teaspoon vanilla extract

1 Preheat the oven to 350°F. Spray a 9 x 13-inch baking pan with nonstick cooking spray. Dust with flour, shaking out the excess.

2 In a medium bowl, combine the flour, wheat germ, baking powder, baking soda, cinnamon, cardamom, and salt.

3 In a large bowl, with an electric mixer, beat the eggs and granulated sugar until light and lemon-colored. Beat in the buttermilk and oil.

4 Fold in the flour mixture. Stir in the carrots, currants, and pistachios.

5 Spread the batter evenly in the prepared pan. Bake for 30 to 35 minutes, or until a toothpick inserted in the center comes out clean and the cake has begun to pull away from the sides of the pan. Let the cake cool in the pan on a rack for 10 minutes before turning out onto the rack to cool completely.

6 Meanwhile, in a small bowl, beat the cream cheeses, confectioners' sugar, and vanilla together. When the cake is cool, frost the top and sides with the cream cheese frosting. *Makes 16 pieces*

per piece: 226 calories, 5.1g total fat (1g saturated), 29mg cholesterol, 2g dietary fiber, 39g carbohydrate, 7g protein, 238mg sodium. good source of: beta carotene, selenium, thiamin.

Lemon Poppyseed Cake

This update on a classic cake is low in fat without sacrificing flavor. Buttermilk makes the cake especially tender.

3 tablespoons poppy seeds

2½ cups cake flour

1½ teaspoons baking powder

½ teaspoon baking soda

¼ teaspoon salt

2 large eggs

1 large egg white

4 tablespoons unsalted butter

2 tablespoons extra-light olive oil

1 tablespoon grated lemon zest

1¾ cups sugar

1½ cups buttermilk

¼ cup fresh lemon juice

1 Preheat the oven to 350°F. Spray a 10-inch tube pan with nonstick cooking spray. Dust with flour, shaking off the excess. Place the poppy seeds in a baking pan and cook until lightly toasted, about 4 minutes.

2 On a sheet of wax paper, combine the flour, baking powder, baking soda, salt, and poppy seeds. In a small bowl, whisk together the whole eggs and egg white.

3 In a large bowl, with an electric mixer, beat the butter, oil, and lemon zest until creamy. Gradually beat in 1½ cups of the sugar until light and fluffy. Add the egg mixture, 1 teaspoon at a time, until light in texture.

4 With a rubber spatula, alternately fold in the flour mixture and the buttermilk, beginning and ending with the flour mixture, until just blended.

5 Scrape the batter into the tube pan, smoothing the top. Bake for 35 minutes, or until a toothpick inserted in the center of the cake comes out clean. Transfer the pan to a wire rack to cool. Once cool turn out onto a cake plate.

6 In a small saucepan, stir together the remaining ¼ cup sugar and the lemon juice. Bring to a boil over medium heat and cook, stirring, until the sugar dissolves, about 2 minutes. With a fork, prick holes in the top of the cake and pour the hot syrup over the cake. *Makes 16 slices*

per slice: 231 calories, 6.1g total fat (2.3g saturated), 35mg cholesterol, 1g dietary fiber, 41g carbohydrate, 4g protein, 134mg sodium. **good source of:** thiamin.

Pumpkin Cheesecake in a Ginger Crust

If you've got leftover cooked sweet potato or winter squash on hand, substitute 1¾ cups mashed for the pumpkin puree. **Timing alert:** The cheesecake needs to chill for at least 4 hours.

- *36 gingersnaps (9 ounces)*
- *1 tablespoon extra-light olive oil*
- *1 tablespoon granulated sugar*
- *2 packages (8 ounces each) reduced-fat cream cheese (Neufchâtel)*
- *1 package (8 ounces) fat-free cream cheese*
- *⅔ cup packed light brown sugar*
- *1 can (15 ounces) unsweetened pumpkin puree*
- *½ cup plain fat-free yogurt*
- *2 tablespoons dark rum*
- *1½ teaspoons cinnamon*
- *½ teaspoon ground ginger*
- *¼ teaspoon nutmeg*
- *¼ teaspoon salt*
- *2 large eggs*
- *4 large egg whites*

1 Preheat the oven to 300°F. Spray a 9-inch springform pan with nonstick cooking spray.

2 In a food processor, combine the gingersnaps, oil, and granulated sugar. Process until the crumbs are evenly moistened. Press the crumb mixture into the bottom of the prepared pan. Set aside.

3 In a medium bowl, with an electric mixer, beat the cream cheeses and brown sugar until well combined. Beat in the pumpkin, yogurt, rum, cinnamon, ginger, nutmeg, and salt. Beat in the whole eggs and egg whites, one at a time, beating well after each addition.

4 Pour the batter into the crust and bake for 1 hour and 30 minutes, or until set. Turn the oven off and let the cheesecake stand in the oven for 30 minutes. Transfer to a wire rack to cool. Refrigerate until well chilled, about 4 hours. *Makes 12 wedges*

per wedge: 276 calories, 9.2g total fat (4.1g saturated), 53mg cholesterol, 2g dietary fiber, 36g carbohydrate, 12g protein, 512mg sodium. **good source of:** beta carotene, riboflavin, selenium, vitamin B$_{12}$.

different spins

▶**Pumpkin Cheesecake in a Vanilla-Walnut Crust** Follow the directions for *Pumpkin Cheesecake in a Ginger Crust,* but substitute vanilla wafers for the gingersnaps and walnut oil for the olive oil. Substitute fat-free vanilla yogurt for the plain yogurt.

▶**Pumpkin Cheesecake in a Lemon Crust** Follow the directions for *Pumpkin Cheesecake in a Ginger Crust,* but substitute lemon wafers for the gingersnaps and fat-free lemon yogurt for the plain yogurt.

Chocolate Cheesecake

Silken tofu and low-fat cottage cheese make a surprisingly rich-tasting cheesecake. Although silken tofu has the smoothest texture, you could also make this with regular tofu. **Timing alert:** The cheesecake needs to chill for at least 4 hours.

24 chocolate wafer cookies (5 ounces)

1 tablespoon extra-light olive oil

1 tablespoon water

¼ cup unsweetened cocoa powder

2 tablespoons hazelnut liqueur or amaretto

1 pound firm silken tofu

1 cup low-fat (1%) cottage cheese

¼ cup mini chocolate chips (2 ounces), melted

¾ cup packed dark brown sugar

2 tablespoons flour

1 large egg

2 large egg whites

1 teaspoon vanilla extract

1 Preheat the oven to 375°F. In a food processor, process the cookies until finely ground. Add the oil and water, and process until combined.

2 Spray a 9-inch springform pan with nonstick cooking spray. Press the crumb mixture into the bottom and partway up the sides of the pan. Bake for 10 minutes to set the crust. Let cool on a wire rack. Reduce the oven temperature to 350°F.

3 In a small bowl, combine the cocoa and liqueur until well moistened. In a food processor, combine the cocoa mixture, tofu, cottage cheese, chocolate chips, brown sugar, flour, whole egg, egg whites, and vanilla, and process until very smooth.

4 Pour the batter into the prepared crust and bake for 40 minutes.

5 Reduce the oven temperature to 250°F and bake for 10 minutes, or until the cheesecake is just set. Cool to room temperature, then refrigerate until chilled, about 4 hours. *Makes 12 wedges*

per wedge: 191 calories, 5.2g total fat (2g saturated), 19mg cholesterol, 1g dietary fiber, 29g carbohydrate, 7g protein, 214mg sodium. **good source of:** isoflavones.

cookies

Butter makes cookies crisp and rich, and there are some cookie recipes where you just can't avoid it—in butter cookies, for example. There's really no point in trying to make low-fat versions of such cookies, and so we haven't. But certain cookies work well with less fat, such as Italian biscotti, which are crisped by being twice-baked (*see Carrot-Pistachio Biscotti, page 249*). And some cookies naturally have no fat, such as macaroons, which are made with egg whites (*see Apricot-Pumpkin Seed Macaroons, page 249*). For cakey cookies, like brownies, we've applied the same rules as for baking cakes.

Fig Squares with a Walnut Crust

Fig paste on top of a buttery-tasting crust makes a satisfying bar cookie. The crust can be baked several hours or up to a day ahead, and without the topping makes a delicious shortbread.

½ cup walnuts

1 cup flour

⅓ cup cup confectioners' sugar

1½ teaspoons grated orange zest

⅛ teaspoon salt

¼ cup walnut oil

1 cup dried figs (8 ounces), stemmed and coarsely chopped

⅔ cup port wine

¼ cup orange juice

2 tablespoons honey

½ teaspoon cardamom

1 Preheat the oven to 350°F. On a baking sheet, toast the walnuts for 7 minutes, or until crisp and fragrant. Leave the oven on.

2 Transfer the walnuts to a food processor. Add the flour, confectioners' sugar, orange zest, and salt, and process until finely ground. Add the walnut oil and process until evenly moistened.

3 Press the mixture into an 8-inch square metal baking pan. With the tines of a fork, prick the dough all over. Bake for 20 minutes, or until the crust is crisp. Cool the crust on a wire rack, but leave the oven on.

4 Meanwhile, in a small saucepan, combine the figs, port, orange juice, honey, and cardamom. Bring to a simmer. Cover and cook until the figs are soft and most of the liquid has been absorbed, about 20 minutes.

5 Transfer the mixture to a food processor and process to a smooth paste. Spread the fig paste over the cooled crust and put back in the oven and bake for 20 minutes to set the topping. Cool in the pan on a wire rack before cutting into 16 squares. *Makes 16 squares*

per square: 145 calories, 5.7g total fat (0.5g saturated), 0mg cholesterol, 2g dietary fiber, 21g carbohydrate, 2g protein, 39mg sodium. good source of: omega-3 fatty acids.

Peanut Butter Blondies

Here's a blondie that does not have a killer amount of fat.

> 1 cup flour
> ½ teaspoon baking powder
> ½ teaspoon baking soda
> ¼ teaspoon salt
> ⅓ cup chunky peanut butter
> 2 tablespoons extra-light olive oil
> ⅔ cup packed light brown sugar
> 2 tablespoons light corn syrup
> ½ cup prune butter (lekvar)
> 2 large egg whites
> 1 teaspoon vanilla extract

1 Preheat the oven to 350°F. Spray an 8-inch square baking pan with nonstick cooking spray. In a small bowl, whisk together the flour, baking powder, baking soda, and salt.

2 In a large bowl, with an electric mixe[r] peanut butter, oil, brown sugar, and [...] until creamy. Beat in the prune butte[r] combined. Beat in the egg whites and [...] well combined. Fold in the flour mixt[ure.]

3 Spoon the batter into the pan. Bake for 25 minutes, or until a toothpick inserted in the center comes out clean. Cool the cake in the pan on a rack. *Makes 16 blondies*

per blondie: 138 calories, 4.4g total fat (0.8g saturated), 0mg cholesterol, 1g dietary fiber, 23g carbohydrate, 3g protein, 122mg sodium.

Fudgy Pecan Brownies

Prune butter (pureed dried plums) helps to make these brownies especially fudgy. Look for prune butter (also called lekvar) in the jams and jelly aisle of the supermarket.

> ⅓ cup pecans
> ⅔ cup flour
> ⅓ cup unsweetened cocoa powder
> 2 tablespoons cornstarch
> 1 teaspoon baking powder
> ¼ teaspoon baking soda
> ¼ teaspoon salt
> 1 cup packed light brown sugar

continued on page 248

did you know?

Don't avoid commercial peanut butter because of rumors that it contains trans fats. According to a new analysis by a USDA researcher, most peanut butters contain very small amounts of trans fats (trans fats, created when vegetable oil is hydrogenated, act like saturated fats in the body and thus increase the risk of heart disease). And although peanut butter is high in fat, this is highly monounsaturated and does not boost blood cholesterol. In fact, studies show that a diet rich in peanuts and peanut butter may help reduce blood cholesterol.

continued from page 247

⅓ cup prune butter (lekvar)

2 tablespoons extra-light olive oil

2 large egg whites

1 tablespoon water

¼ cup dried cherries, coarsely chopped

¼ cup mini chocolate chips

1 Preheat the oven to 350°F. Spray an 8-inch square baking pan with nonstick cooking spray.

2 In a small baking pan, toast the pecans in the oven until crisp and fragrant, about 7 minutes. Coarsely chop.

3 In a medium bowl, stir together the flour, cocoa powder, cornstarch, baking powder, baking soda, and salt.

4 In a large bowl, with an electric mixer, beat the brown sugar, prune butter, oil, egg whites, and water until thick and well combined. Stir in the flour mixture until just combined. Gently fold in the pecans, cherries, and chocolate chips.

5 Scrape the batter into the prepared pan. Bake for 15 to 18 minutes, or until a toothpick inserted in the center comes out slightly wet and the sides of the brownies begin to pull away from the pan. Cool the brownies in the pan on a wire rack. *Makes 12 brownies*

per brownie: 166 calories, 5.8g total fat (1.3g saturated), 0mg cholesterol, 2g dietary fiber, 28g carbohydrate, 2g protein, 106mg sodium.

---

different spins

▶**Almond-Ginger Biscotti** Follow the directions for *Carrot-Pistachio Biscotti (opposite page)*, but substitute coarsely chopped almonds for the pistachios. Substitute 3 tablespoons chopped crystallized ginger for the apricots.

▶**Cranberry-Sunflower Macaroons** Follow the directions for *Apricot-Pumpkin Seed Macaroons (opposite page)*, but substitute 3 tablespoons of roasted sunflower seeds for the pumpkin seeds, and substitute dried cranberries for the apricots. Add ¼ cup mini chocolate chips.

Toasted Oatmeal Cookies with Cranberries

Toasted oats and flaxseeds contribute a slightly nutty flavor to these cookies, while adding heart-healthy soluble fiber and omega-3 fatty acids.

1¼ cups old-fashioned rolled oats

¼ cup flaxseeds

¾ cup flour

½ teaspoon baking soda

½ teaspoon salt

3 tablespoons extra-light olive oil

2 tablespoons butter, at room temperature

½ cup packed light brown sugar

¼ cup granulated sugar

1 large egg

½ teaspoon vanilla extract

1 cup dried cranberries

1 Preheat the oven to 350°F. Spread the oats on a jelly-roll pan and bake for 10 minutes, stirring midway, until light golden. Remove from the oven and let cool slightly. Leave the oven on.

2 In a spice mill or coffee grinder, grind the flaxseeds until they're the texture of cornmeal. In a large bowl, stir together the ground flaxseeds, toasted oats, flour, baking soda, and salt.

3 In a large bowl, with an electric mixer, beat the oil, butter, brown sugar, and granulated sugar until light and fluffy. Add the egg and beat until well combined. Beat in the vanilla. Stir in the flour mixture. Stir in the dried cranberries.

4 Spray 2 large baking sheets with nonstick cooking spray. Drop the dough by tablespoons, 2 inches apart, on the baking sheets. Bake for 10 to 12 minutes, or until set and lightly golden. Midway through the baking, reverse the baking sheets from front to back and top to bottom for more even cooking. Cool the cookies on a wire rack. *Makes 3½ dozen*

per cookie: 60 calories, 2.2g total fat (0.6g saturated), 7mg cholesterol, 1g dietary fiber, 9g carbohydrate, 1g protein, 46mg sodium. good source of: fiber, omega-3 fatty acids.

Carrot-Pistachio Biscotti

Biscotti (which means "twice cooked" in Italian) are crisp cookies intended for dunking into coffee or tea (and sometimes wine). To make biscotti, a log of cookie dough is baked once, then cut into slices that are baked again to make them crunchy. The carrots and carrot juice add a faint sweetness, a nice golden color, and beta carotene.

> 1¼ cups flour
> ½ cup sugar
> 2 tablespoons yellow cornmeal
> 1½ teaspoons grated lemon zest
> ¾ teaspoon cinnamon
> ½ teaspoon baking powder
> ¼ teaspoon salt
> 1 large carrot, finely shredded
> ¼ cup coarsely chopped pistachio nuts
> 3 tablespoons finely chopped dried apricots
> ½ cup carrot juice

1 Preheat the oven to 350°F. Spray a large baking sheet with nonstick cooking spray.

2 In a large mixing bowl, whisk together the flour, sugar, cornmeal, lemon zest, cinnamon, baking powder, and salt. Stir in the shredded carrot, pistachios, and apricots. Add the carrot juice and stir until a firm dough forms.

3 Shape the dough into a log 15 inches long by 3 inches wide by ½ inch high. Place on the baking sheet and bake for 30 minutes, or until firmly set and golden brown.

4 Remove the baking sheet from the oven, but leave the oven on. Let the log cool slightly, then slice crosswise but on the diagonal into ½-inch-thick cookies. Return the cookies to the oven and bake for 20 minutes, turning them over after 10 minutes, until they are lightly colored and crisp.
Makes 2½ dozen

per cookie: 45 calories, 5g total fat (0.1g saturated), 0mg cholesterol, 1g dietary fiber, 9g carbohydrate, 1g protein, 25mg sodium.

Apricot-Pumpkin Seed Macaroons

Macaroons are cookies that are made by binding the ingredients with egg whites instead of a flour-and-fat dough. Classic macaroons are made with either almonds or coconut. Our version improves the nutrition profile by using oats, pumpkin seeds, and dried apricots.

> 2 cups old-fashioned rolled oats
> ¼ cup hulled pumpkin seeds (pepitas)
> ½ cup chopped dried apricots
> ¾ cup sugar
> ¼ teaspoon salt
> 3 large egg whites
> 1 teaspoon vanilla extract

1 Preheat the oven to 350°F. Spray 2 large baking sheets with nonstick cooking spray.

2 In a baking pan, combine the oats and pumpkin seeds, and toast in the oven for 7 minutes, or until the oats are lightly browned, crisp, and fragrant. Transfer the oats and seeds to a large bowl and let cool to room temperature.

3 Add the apricots, sugar, and salt to the bowl and toss to combine. Stir in the egg whites and vanilla until well combined.

4 Drop the batter by rounded tablespoons, 1 inch apart, onto the baking sheets. Bake for 8 minutes, then reverse the baking sheets from front to back and top to bottom for more even cooking. Bake for 9 minutes, or until golden brown and slightly firm, but not hard.

5 Cool the cookies for 5 minutes on the pans, then transfer to a wire rack to cool completely.
Makes 2 dozen

per cookie: 67 calories, 1.1g total fat (0.2g saturated), 0mg cholesterol, 1g dietary fiber, 13g carbohydrate, 2g protein, 32mg sodium.

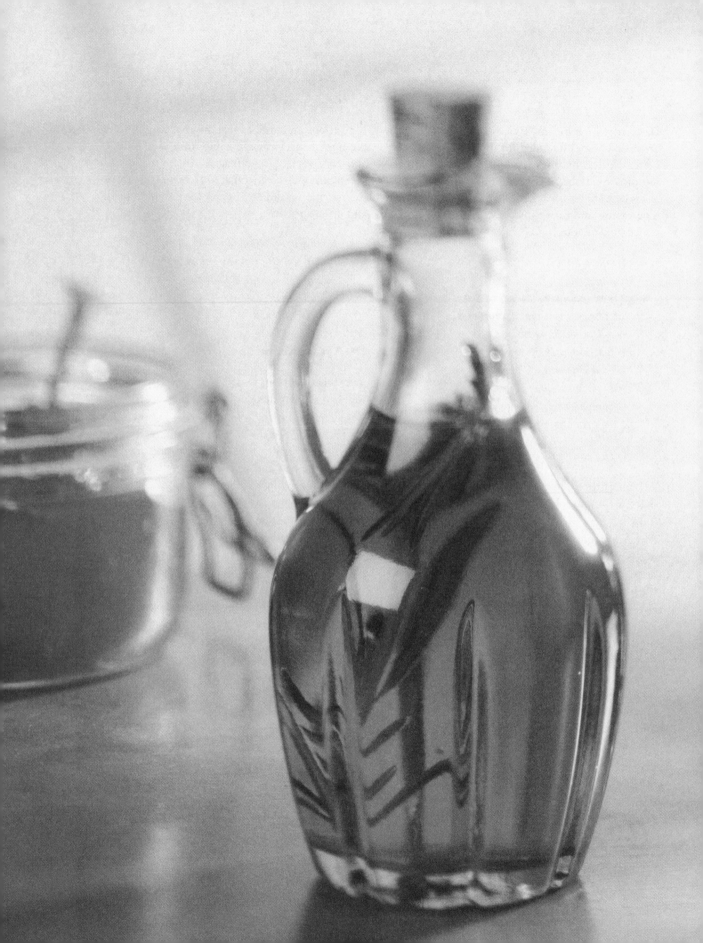

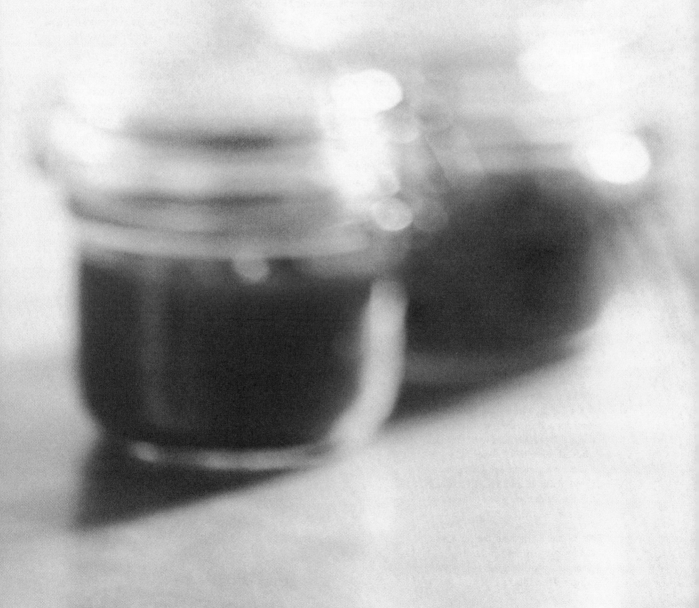

the pantry

Mushroom-Onion Broth

Use this anywhere that you would ordinarily use chicken broth.

MAKES 8 CUPS

½ cup dried mushrooms

1 cup boiling water

2 pounds white mushrooms, quartered

1 pound onions, thickly sliced

1 large carrot, thickly sliced

8 cloves garlic, unpeeled

2 teaspoons olive oil

2 tablespoons tomato paste

½ teaspoon thyme

½ teaspoon salt

¼ teaspoon pepper

10 cups water

1 In a small heatproof bowl, combine the dried mushrooms and the boiling water, and let stand for 20 minutes, or until softened. Reserving the soaking liquid, scoop out the dried mushrooms. Strain the soaking liquid through a coffee filter or a paper towel-lined sieve.

2 Meanwhile, preheat the oven to 400°F. In a large roasting pan, combine the mushroom soaking liquid, the reconstituted dried mushrooms, the white mushrooms, onions, carrot, garlic, and oil. Cover with foil and roast for 15 minutes, or until the mushrooms have begun to soften.

3 Roast, uncovered, for 50 minutes, or until the onions are browned.

4 Transfer to a large soup pot or stockpot and add the tomato paste, thyme, salt, pepper, and water. Bring to a boil. Reduce to a simmer and cook, uncovered, until the broth is richly flavored, about 45 minutes. Strain. Cool to room temperature and refrigerate or freeze.

PER ½ CUP: 39 CALORIES, 0.8G TOTAL FAT (0.1G SATURATED), 0MG CHOLESTEROL, 0G DIETARY FIBER, 7G CARBOHYDRATE, 0G PROTEIN, 91MG SODIUM.

Homemade Chicken Broth

This basic broth is easy to make and infinitely more healthful than store-bought. It is much lower in sodium and there are good amounts of beta carotene and lycopene from the vegetable juices. If chicken legs are on sale, you can certainly use them in place of the whole chickens.

MAKES 8 CUPS

2 whole chickens (about 3 pounds each), cut up

8½ cups water

4 cups carrot juice

1 cup low-sodium tomato-vegetable juice

2 large onions, unpeeled and halved

2 large carrots, thickly sliced

1 large leek, thinly sliced

2 stalks celery, thinly sliced

8 cloves garlic, unpeeled

¾ teaspoon rosemary

¾ teaspoon thyme

10 sprigs of parsley

2 bay leaves

1 Preheat the oven to 450°F. Spread the chicken in a large roasting pan and roast for 30 minutes, or until browned and crisp.

2 With tongs or a slotted spoon, transfer the chicken to a large stockpot. Pour off and discard all the fat from the roasting pan. Pour ½ cup of the water into the roasting pan, scraping up any browned bits clinging to the bottom and sides. Add these juices to the stockpot along with the chicken.

3 Add the remaining 8 cups water, the carrot juice, and tomato-vegetable juice, and bring to a boil over high heat, skimming off the foam as it rises to the surface. Continue skimming until no foam remains.

4 Add the onions, carrots, leek, celery, garlic, rosemary, thyme, parsley, and bay leaves. Return to a boil, continuing to skim any foam that rises. Reduce the heat to low and simmer until the broth is rich and flavorful, about 2 hours.

5 Strain the broth and discard the solids. Refrigerate and remove the fat that solidifies on the surface. Refrigerate for up to 3 days or freeze.

PER ½ CUP: 56 CALORIES, 2.5G TOTAL FAT (0.6G SATURATED), 3MG CHOLESTEROL, 1G DIETARY FIBER, 7G CARBOHYDRATE, 1G PROTEIN, 46MG SODIUM. **GOOD SOURCE OF:** BETA CAROTENE, LYCOPENE.

Seasoned Olive Oil

No point in buying expensive flavored olive oils when it's so easy to make your own. Below are a few suggestions for flavorings, but use them as a guideline to create your own.

MAKES 2 CUPS

Seasonings (*see below*)
2 cups mild-flavored olive oil

1 In a sterilized (and cooled) 1-quart jar, combine the seasonings (*see below*) and the olive oil. Close tightly and let sit at room temperature for 1 to 2 days. (Shake the jar and taste the oil after 1 day.)
2 Strain the oil into a clean bottle. Discard the solids. Store the oil in the refrigerator.

PER TABLESPOON: 119 CALORIES, 14G TOTAL FAT (1.8G SATURATED), 0MG CHOLESTEROL, 0G DIETARY FIBER, 0G CARBOHYDRATE, 0G PROTEIN, 0MG SODIUM.

Lemon-Pepper Olive Oil ¼ cup strips of lemon zest and 1 tablespoon of cracked black peppercorns.
Orange-Chili Olive Oil ¼ cup strips of orange zest and 2 fresh red chili peppers (split).
Vanilla-Cinnamon Oil 2 split vanilla beans and 2 cinnamon sticks. This unusual combination would be good in baked goods or for cooking pancakes.
Herbed Olive Oil In a small pot of boiling water, blanch 1 cup of leaves and stems of either basil, mint, cilantro, or parsley for 15 seconds. Rinse under cold running water; drain and dry well. Transfer to a food processor and add the oil. Coarsely puree.
Shallot & Ginger Olive Oil In a small pot of boiling water, blanch 3 shallots for 2 minutes. Drain. Cool and coarsely chop. Combine with 2 tablespoons chopped fresh ginger.
Rosemary-Garlic Olive Oil In a small pot of boiling water, blanch 3 cloves garlic for 2 minutes. Drain. Cool and coarsely chop. Combine with ⅓ cup minced fresh rosemary.

Dill-Caper Dressing

Silken tofu makes a wonderful salad dressing. The rich creaminess of the tofu is accented in this dressing by spicy Dijon mustard, chopped capers, and fresh dill. In addition to using this as a salad dressing, it would make a tasty sauce for fish or chicken.

MAKES 1½ CUPS

1 cup (8 ounces) firm low-fat silken tofu
¼ cup cider vinegar
2 tablespoons Dijon mustard
½ teaspoon salt
½ teaspoon pepper
¼ cup capers, drained and minced
¼ cup chopped fresh dill

In a food processor or blender, combine the tofu, vinegar, mustard, salt, and pepper, and puree until smooth. Stir in the capers and dill. Store the dressing in the refrigerator.

PER ¼ CUP: 11 CALORIES, 0.4G TOTAL FAT (0G SATURATED), 0MG CHOLESTEROL, 0G DIETARY FIBER, 1G CARBOHYDRATE, 1G PROTEIN, 281MG SODIUM. GOOD SOURCE OF: ISOFLAVONES.

Creamy Roasted Garlic Dressing

This rich and creamy dressing works well in any situation where you might use a ranch-style dressing.

MAKES 1¼ CUPS

1 head of garlic (about 3½ ounces)
15 ounces firm low-fat silken tofu
1½ teaspoons grated lemon zest
¼ cup fresh lemon juice
1 tablespoon flaxseed oil or dark sesame oil
¾ teaspoon salt

1 Preheat the oven to 400°F. Wrap the garlic in foil, place on a baking sheet, and bake until the foil package feels soft to the touch, about 30 minutes.
2 When cool enough to handle, unwrap, slice off one end of the garlic head, and squeeze the garlic pulp into a blender or food processor.
3 Add the tofu, lemon zest, lemon juice, flaxseed oil, and salt, and process until smooth. Store the dressing in the refrigerator.

PER 2 TABLESPOONS: 42 CALORIES, 1.7G TOTAL FAT (0.2G SATURATED), 0MG CHOLESTEROL, 0G DIETARY FIBER, 4G CARBOHYDRATE, 3G PROTEIN, 212MG SODIUM. GOOD SOURCE OF: ISOFLAVONES, OMEGA-3 FATTY ACIDS.

Orange-Balsamic Dressing

If you haven't got honey mustard on hand, substitute 1 tablespoon of mustard and ½ teaspoon of honey.

MAKES ½ CUP

⅓ cup orange juice

2 tablespoons balsamic vinegar

1 tablespoon honey mustard

2 teaspoons olive oil

¼ teaspoon salt

¼ teaspoon pepper

1 shallot, minced

In a screw-top jar, combine the orange juice, vinegar, mustard, olive oil, salt, and pepper. Close and shake to combine. Stir in the shallot. Store the dressing in the refrigerator.

PER TABLESPOON: 24 CALORIES, 1.5G TOTAL FAT (0.2G SATURATED), 0MG CHOLESTEROL, 0G DIETARY FIBER, 3G CARBOHYDRATE, 0G PROTEIN, 79MG SODIUM.

Fresh Ginger & Lime Dressing

When shopping for fresh ginger, look for pieces that are smooth and plump, avoiding those that are dry or withered, as they won't yield much juice. If you'd rather not grate and squeeze fresh ginger, look for bottled ginger juice and substitute 2 tablespoons for the fresh squeezed.

MAKES ½ CUP

2 tablespoons fresh ginger juice (from about ⅓ cup grated fresh ginger)

1 teaspoon grated lime zest

¼ cup fresh lime juice

2 tablespoons honey

2 teaspoons olive oil

¼ teaspoon salt

1 Place the grated ginger in a small fine-mesh sieve set over a small bowl. Press the ginger to extract the juice. Discard the ginger solids.

2 Whisk in the lime zest, lime juice, honey, oil, and salt. Store the dressing in the refrigerator.

PER TABLESPOON: 31 CALORIES, 1.2G TOTAL FAT (0.2G SATURATED), 0MG CHOLESTEROL, 0G DIETARY FIBER, 6G CARBOHYDRATE, 0G PROTEIN, 73MG SODIUM.

Blue Cheese Dressing

A little bit of blue cheese goes a long way in this creamy dressing. If you prefer your dressing thinner, add a little water or fat-free (skim) milk.

MAKES 1 CUP

¾ cup plain fat-free yogurt

1 ounce blue cheese

1 tablespoon white wine vinegar

1 tablespoon fresh lemon juice

½ teaspoon pepper

⅛ teaspoon salt

2 tablespoons minced chives or scallion greens

In a food processor or blender, combine the yogurt, blue cheese, vinegar, lemon juice, pepper, and salt. Process until smooth. Transfer to a bowl and stir in the chives. Store the dressing in the refrigerator.

PER 2 TABLESPOONS: 27 CALORIES, 1.1G TOTAL FAT (0.7G SATURATED), 3MG CHOLESTEROL, 0G DIETARY FIBER, 2G CARBOHYDRATE, 2G PROTEIN, 104MG SODIUM.

Creamy Carrot Dressing

This is equally at home as a dressing for tossed salad or stirred into cooked rice.

MAKES ¾ CUP

⅓ cup carrot juice

⅓ cup plain fat-free yogurt

1 tablespoon fresh lemon juice

1 large shallot, quartered

1 teaspoon cumin

½ teaspoon ground ginger

½ teaspoon pepper

¼ teaspoon salt

In a food processor or blender, combine the carrot juice, yogurt, lemon juice, shallot, cumin, ginger, pepper and salt. Puree until smooth. Store the dressing in the refrigerator.

PER 2 TABLESPOONS: 18 CALORIES, 0.1G TOTAL FAT (0G SATURATED), 0MG CHOLES- TEROL, 0G DIETARY FIBER, 3G CARBOHY- DRATE, 1G PROTEIN, 112MG SODIUM.

Shallot, Mustard & Flaxseed Oil Dressing

Flaxseed oil is more ordinarily thought of in connection with health-food supplements than with cooking. Yet this rich source of alpha-linolenic acid (a type of omega-3 fatty acid) has a deep, nutty flavor that is delicious in a salad dressing. If you don't have flax- seed oil, you can still make a reasonable facsimile of this dressing by using 5 teaspoons extra-virgin olive oil and 1 teaspoon dark sesame oil. Keep this dressing on hand for tossing with steamed vegetables, drizzling on toma- toes, or for any occasion when you would use a vinaigrette.

MAKES ½ CUP

¼ cup balsamic vinegar

2 tablespoons flaxseed oil

2 teaspoons Dijon mustard

1 teaspoon light brown sugar

1 shallot, minced, or 2 tablespoons minced red onion

1 clove garlic, minced

¼ teaspoon salt

In a screw-top jar, combine the vine- gar, flaxseed oil, mustard, brown sugar, shallot, garlic, and salt. Close and shake to blend. Store the dressing in the refrigerator.

PER TABLESPOON: 41 CALORIES, 3.5G TOTAL FAT (0.3G SATURATED), 0MG CHOLESTEROL, 0G DIETARY FIBER, 2G CARBOHYDRATE, 0G PROTEIN, 107MG SODIUM. **GOOD SOURCE OF:** OMEGA-3 FATTY ACIDS.

Sweet & Sour Peanut Sauce

Use this sauce to dress noodles or steamed vegetables.

MAKES 1¼ CUPS

2 cloves garlic, peeled

½ cup creamy peanut butter

⅔ cup cilantro

½ cup water

2 tablespoons rice vinegar or cider vinegar

1 tablespoon plus 1 teaspoon reduced-sodium soy sauce

2 teaspoons honey

¾ teaspoon hot pepper sauce

¼ teaspoon salt

1 In a small saucepan of boiling water, cook the garlic for 2 minutes to blanch. Drain.

2 Transfer the garlic to a blender or food processor. Add the peanut butter, cilantro, water, vinegar, soy sauce, honey, hot sauce, and salt, and process until smooth. Store the sauce in the refrigerator.

PER 2 TABLESPOONS: 84 CALORIES, 6.6G TOTAL FAT (1.3G SATURATED), 0MG CHOLES- TEROL, 1G DIETARY FIBER, 5G CARBOHY- DRATE, 3G PROTEIN, 200MG SODIUM. **GOOD SOURCE OF:** NIACIN, VITAMIN E.

Tofu-Lemon Pepper Dipping Sauce

This is a good dipping sauce for artichokes or steamed asparagus. It's also a flavorful stand-in for mayonnaise in salad dressings or as a sandwich spread.

MAKES 2 CUPS

12 ounces extra-firm low-fat silken tofu

1 teaspoon grated lemon zest

3 tablespoons fresh lemon juice

2 teaspoons Dijon mustard

½ teaspoon pepper

¼ teaspoon salt

In a blender or food processor, combine the tofu, lemon zest, lemon juice, mustard, pepper, and salt, and process to a smooth puree. Store the sauce in the refrigerator.

PER 2 TABLESPOONS: 13 CALORIES, 0.3G TOTAL FAT (0G SATURATED), 0MG CHOLESTEROL, 0G DIETARY FIBER, 1G CARBOHYDRATE, 2G PROTEIN, 98MG SODIUM.

Pesto Sauce

This traditional basil-garlic sauce from Genoa is normally made with a substantial amount of oil (in addition to a lot of cheese and nuts). We've trimmed the cheese and nuts a bit, but the oil has been cut from ½ cup to 1 tablespoon, allowing the other flavors to shine. This sauce makes enough to coat 1 pound of pasta. When ready to serve, toss the pesto with the cooked pasta and ½ cup of the pasta cooking water. Using the hot pasta cooking water helps to melt the Parmesan in the pesto so that it nicely coats the pasta.

MAKES 1 CUP

2 cups packed basil leaves

2 cloves garlic, peeled

⅓ cup grated Parmesan cheese

¼ cup walnuts

⅓ cup water

1 tablespoon olive oil

¾ teaspoon salt

In a food processor, combine the basil, garlic, Parmesan, walnuts, water, oil, and salt. Process until finely ground. Store the sauce in the refrigerator.

PER 2 TABLESPOONS: 58 CALORIES, 4.9G TOTAL FAT (1.2G SATURATED), 3MG CHOLESTEROL, 1G DIETARY FIBER, 1G CARBOHYDRATE, 3G PROTEIN, 296MG SODIUM.

Hot & Spicy Cocktail Sauce

This sauce gets its heat from a smoky chipotle pepper and a healthy amount of cayenne. Chipotle peppers packed in adobo can be found at Mexican markets and many supermarkets. If you can't find chipotles, substitute a canned or bottled jalapeño and increase the chili powder to 2½ teaspoons.

MAKES 1¼ CUPS

1 cup ketchup

2 tablespoons fresh lime juice

2 teaspoons chili powder

1 teaspoon coriander

¼ teaspoon cayenne pepper

¼ teaspoon salt

1 chipotle pepper packed in adobo, minced

In a medium bowl, whisk together the ketchup, lime juice, chili powder, coriander, cayenne, and salt. Stir in the chipotle pepper. Store the sauce in the refrigerator.

PER 2 TABLESPOONS: 29 CALORIES, 0.2G TOTAL FAT (0G SATURATED), 0MG CHOLESTEROL, 1G DIETARY FIBER, 7G CARBOHYDRATE, 0G PROTEIN, 360MG SODIUM.
GOOD SOURCE OF: LYCOPENE.

Romesco Sauce

This flavorful Spanish sauce is typically served with grilled meat, poultry, or fish. You could also toss it with cooked pasta, or stir it into rice. Blanching the garlic for 2 minutes takes away its sharp bite without sacrificing flavor.

MAKES 1⅓ CUPS

2 red bell peppers, roasted (*page 190*)

3 garlic cloves, peeled

¼ cup orange juice

2 tablespoons tomato paste

2 tablespoons coarsely chopped unblanched almonds

2 teaspoons olive oil

½ teaspoon Louisiana-style hot pepper sauce

¼ teaspoon salt

1 Preheat the broiler. Roast the peppers. When they are cool enough to handle, peel them.

2 Meanwhile, in a small saucepan of boiling water, blanch the garlic for 2 minutes. Drain.

3 In a food processor, combine the roasted peppers, garlic, orange juice, tomato paste, almonds, oil, hot sauce, and salt. Process to a smooth puree. Store the sauce in the refrigerator.

PER ⅓ CUP: 71 CALORIES, 3.6G TOTAL FAT (0.4G SATURATED), 0MG CHOLESTEROL, 2G DIETARY FIBER, 9G CARBOHYDRATE, 1.7G PROTEIN, 212MG SODIUM. **GOOD SOURCE OF:** BETA CAROTENE, VITAMIN B$_6$, VITAMIN C, VITAMIN E.

Red Pepper Harissa

Harissa is the fiery hot condiment that normally accompanies the North African stew called couscous. Our version is tempered by the addition of roasted bell peppers, but it's still on the spicy side. (Those with a taste for spice should add up to ¼ teaspoon additional cayenne.) Stir this condiment into soups or stews, spread on sandwiches, or mix with low-fat yogurt as a dip for vegetables.

MAKES 1 CUP

2 red bell peppers, roasted (*page 190*)

3 garlic cloves, peeled

½ teaspoon caraway seeds, lightly crushed

2 teaspoons olive oil

1 teaspoon ground cumin

½ teaspoon coriander

½ teaspoon cayenne pepper

¼ teaspoon salt

1 Preheat the broiler. Roast the peppers. When they are cool enough to handle, peel them.

2 Meanwhile, in a small saucepan of boiling water, blanch the garlic for 2 minutes. Drain.

3 In a food processor, combine the roasted pepper, garlic, caraway seeds, oil, cumin, coriander, cayenne, and salt. Process to a smooth puree. Store the harissa in the refrigerator.

PER TABLESPOON: 13 CALORIES, 0.7G TOTAL FAT (0.1G SATURATED), 0MG CHOLESTEROL, 1G DIETARY FIBER, 2G CARBOHYDRATE, 0G PROTEIN, 37MG SODIUM. **GOOD SOURCE OF:** VITAMIN C.

Green Curry Paste

Thai cooks make up batches of curry paste that they then use as seasonings for various curry dishes. Curry pastes come in many colors and flavors, including green curry paste, which is herbal and usually not very spicy. You can use the curry paste as the flavoring base for soups, stews, stir-fries, and (of course) curries, as well as a topping for grilled poultry or fish.

MAKES ¾ CUP

½ cup packed cilantro leaves and stems

2 scallions, cut into large pieces

2 tablespoons fresh lime juice

1 canned or bottled jalapeño pepper

1½ teaspoons ground coriander

½ teaspoon salt

½ teaspoon black pepper

¼ cup water

½ teaspoon coconut extract

In a food processor or blender, combine the cilantro, scallions, lime juice, jalapeño, coriander, salt, and black pepper. Add the water and coconut extract, and process to a smooth paste, about 30 seconds. Store the curry paste in the refrigerator.

PER 2 TABLESPOONS: 7 CALORIES, 0.1G TOTAL FAT (0G SATURATED), 0MG CHOLESTEROL, 1G DIETARY FIBER, 1G CARBOHYDRATE, 0G PROTEIN, 207MG SODIUM.

Chimichurri Sauce

Argentina's answer to ketchup, this bright green sauce is good on just about anything—from grilled poultry or meat, to fish and vegetables.

MAKES ¾ CUP

1 cup packed parsley leaves

1 cup packed cilantro leaves

4 cloves garlic, peeled

3 tablespoons red wine vinegar

2 tablespoons fresh lime juice

4 teaspoons olive oil

¼ teaspoon salt

¼ teaspoon cayenne pepper

In a food processor, combine the parsley, cilantro, garlic, vinegar, lime juice, oil, salt, and cayenne, and puree until smooth. Store the sauce in the refrigerator.

PER TABLESPOON: 21 CALORIES, 1.6G TOTAL FAT (0.2G SATURATED), 0MG CHOLESTEROL, 0G DIETARY FIBER, 1G CARBOHYDRATE, 0G PROTEIN, 54MG SODIUM. **GOOD SOURCE OF:** VITAMIN C.

Agliata Sauce

This Italian garlic-based sauce dates back to Roman times. It's similar to a pesto but uses stale breadcrumbs for body instead of cheese. Toss with hot cooked pasta; this make enough to coat 10 ounces of pasta for 4 servings.

MAKES 1⅓ CUPS

2 slices (1 ounce each) stale whole-grain bread

6 cloves garlic, peeled

½ cup parsley leaves

2 tablespoons walnuts

2 teaspoons olive oil

¾ teaspoon salt

¼ teaspoon red pepper flakes

In a food processor, combine the bread, garlic, parsley, walnuts, oil, salt, and red pepper flakes. Process until finely ground. Store the sauce in the refrigerator.

PER ⅓ CUP: 85 CALORIES, 4.9G TOTAL FAT (0.6G SATURATED), 0MG CHOLESTEROL, 1G DIETARY FIBER, 9G CARBOHYDRATE, 2G PROTEIN, 219MG SODIUM. **GOOD SOURCE OF:** OMEGA-3 FATTY ACIDS, VITAMIN C.

Salsa Verde

A wide range of green sauces are used in Hispanic cooking, and the exact ingredients vary with the region—and the cook. New World sauces tend toward the spicy, and Old World tend toward the herbal. This one is an amalgam. Serve it over broiled fish, chicken, or vegetables.

MAKES 1¼ CUPS

1 large green bell pepper, roasted (*page 190*)

⅓ cup parsley leaves

⅓ cup cilantro leaves and stems

1 canned or bottled jalapeño

¼ cup water

2 tablespoons fresh lime juice

1 tablespoon olive oil

½ teaspoon salt

1 Preheat the broiler. Roast the bell pepper. When it's cool enough to handle, peel.

2 In a food processor, combine the parsley, cilantro, jalapeño, water, lime juice, oil, and salt, and pulse on and off until finely chopped. Add the roasted pepper and pulse until well combined. Store the sauce in the refrigerator.

PER 2 TABLESPOONS: 18 CALORIES, 1.4G TOTAL FAT (0.2G SATURATED), 0MG CHOLESTEROL, 0G DIETARY FIBER, 2G CARBOHYDRATE, 0G PROTEIN, 124MG SODIUM. **GOOD SOURCE OF:** VITAMIN C.

Charmoula

Charmoula is a traditional Moroccan sauce made by blending garlic with lemon juice, parsley (and/or cilantro), and other seasonings. In North Africa, it's often served as a dipping sauce. But it would also be good spooned over steamed vegetables, stirred into rice, or served with grilled meats or fish. It also makes a good marinade for fish and poultry.

MAKES 1⅓ CUPS

1 tablespoon cumin

¾ cup canned diced tomatoes

2 cloves garlic, minced

3 tablespoons fresh lemon juice

4 teaspoons olive oil

1½ teaspoons paprika

¼ teaspoon salt

¼ teaspoon cayenne pepper

½ cup chopped cilantro

½ cup chopped parsley

1 In a small, heavy-bottomed saucepan, toast the cumin over low heat until lightly browned and very fragrant, about 2 minutes.
2 Add the tomatoes and garlic, and cook until slightly thickened, about 5 minutes. Transfer to a medium bowl.
3 Stir in the lemon juice, oil, paprika, salt, and cayenne. Stir in the cilantro and parsley. Store the sauce in the refrigerator.

PER 4 TEASPOONS: 33 CALORIES, 2.6G TOTAL FAT (0.3G SATURATED), 0MG CHOLESTEROL, 1G DIETARY FIBER, 3G CARBOHYDRATE, 1G PROTEIN, 110MG SODIUM. **GOOD SOURCE OF:** VITAMIN C.

Spicy Cranberry Sauce

This interesting twist on traditional cranberry sauce is spiked with hot spices: ground ginger, cloves, and black pepper.

MAKES 4 CUPS

1½ cups orange juice

1¼ cups sugar

2 packages (12 ounces each) cranberries, fresh or frozen

1 lime, finely chopped with skin, any seeds discarded

1 teaspoon ground ginger

¼ teaspoon ground cloves

¼ teaspoon pepper

¼ teaspoon salt

1 In a large nonaluminum saucepan, bring the orange juice and sugar to a boil over medium heat. Boil until the sugar has dissolved, about 3 minutes.
2 Add the cranberries, lime, ginger, cloves, pepper, and salt. Bring to a boil over medium heat, reduce to a simmer, and cook, stirring frequently, until the berries have popped and the mixture has thickened, about 15 minutes.
3 Let cool to room temperature. Store the sauce in the refrigerator.

PER ½ CUP: 187 CALORIES, 0.3G TOTAL FAT (0G SATURATED), 0MG CHOLESTEROL, 4G DIETARY FIBER, 48G CARBOHYDRATE, 1G PROTEIN, 75MG SODIUM. **GOOD SOURCE OF:** ANTHOCYANINS, FIBER, VITAMIN C.

Curried Fruit Sauce

Mango gives this sauce its silky texture and rich flavor. Delicious with fish, meat, or poultry, this would also work well as a topping for frozen yogurt. If you'd rather not grate and squeeze fresh ginger, look for bottled ginger juice and substitute 1 tablespoon for the fresh-squeezed.

MAKES 1 CUP

¼ cup grated fresh ginger

1 large mango, peeled, pitted, and coarsely chopped

¼ cup apricot or mango nectar

¼ cup packed fresh mint leaves

2 teaspoons curry powder

2 tablespoons fresh lime juice

¼ teaspoon salt

1 Place the grated ginger in a small fine-mesh sieve set over a small bowl. Press the ginger to extract the juice. Discard the ginger solids.
2 In a food processor or blender, combine the ginger juice, chopped mango, apricot nectar, mint, curry powder, lime juice, and salt. Process to a smooth puree. Store the sauce in the refrigerator. Use within 3 days as the flavor will dissipate with time.

PER ¼ CUP: 52 CALORIES, 0.4G TOTAL FAT (0.1G SATURATED), 0MG CHOLESTEROL, 2G DIETARY FIBER, 13G CARBOHYDRATE, 1G PROTEIN, 149MG SODIUM. **GOOD SOURCE OF:** BETA CAROTENE, VITAMIN C.

Cranberry-Tomato Barbecue Sauce

Use this sweet and tangy barbecue sauce as you would any other, brushing it on during the final few minutes of cooking. For a spicier sauce, increase the cayenne.

MAKES 2 CUPS

1 tablespoon olive oil

1 medium onion, finely chopped

2 cloves garlic, minced

1 package (12 ounces) cranberries, fresh or frozen

½ cup maple syrup

2 tablespoons molasses

3 tablespoons tomato paste

2 tablespoons balsamic vinegar

1½ teaspoons Worcestershire sauce

½ teaspoon cumin

¼ teaspoon salt

¼ teaspoon cayenne pepper

1 In a large saucepan, heat the oil over medium heat. Add the onion and garlic, and cook, stirring frequently, until the onion is soft, about 7 minutes.
2 Add the cranberries, maple syrup, and molasses, and cook, stirring frequently, until most of the cranberries have popped, about 7 minutes.
3 Stir in the tomato paste, vinegar, Worcestershire sauce, cumin, salt, and cayenne, and cook until the sauce has a ketchup-like consistency, about 5 minutes. Cool to room temperature and store the sauce in the refrigerator.

PER ¼ CUP: 116 CALORIES, 1.9G TOTAL FAT (0.3G SATURATED), 0MG CHOLESTEROL, 2G DIETARY FIBER, 26G CARBOHYDRATE, 1G PROTEIN, 136MG SODIUM. GOOD SOURCE OF: VITAMIN C.

Smoky Tomato Barbecue Sauce

Cans of smoky chipotle peppers (in adobo sauce) can be found at Latin American grocery stores and many supermarkets. You can add more or less chipotle depending upon how hot you like your barbecue. The amount of chipotle used here makes a moderately hot sauce.

MAKES 1½ CUPS

2 teaspoons olive oil

1 small onion, finely chopped

3 cloves garlic, minced

1¾ cups canned crushed tomatoes

3 chipotle peppers in adobo, minced (1 tablespoon)

1½ teaspoons honey

½ teaspoon coriander

¼ teaspoon cumin

¼ teaspoon salt

⅛ teaspoon cinnamon

1 In a medium nonstick saucepan, heat the oil over medium heat. Add the onion and garlic, and cook, stirring frequently, until the onion is soft, about 5 minutes.
2 Add the tomatoes, chipotle, honey, coriander, cumin, salt, and cinnamon, and bring to a boil. Reduce to a simmer, cover, and cook until thick, about 5 minutes. Cool to room temperature and store the sauce in the refrigerator.

PER ¼ CUP: 37 CALORIES, 1.7G TOTAL FAT (0.2G SATURATED), 0MG CHOLESTEROL, 1G DIETARY FIBER, 5.6G CARBOHYDRATE, 0.8G PROTEIN, 192MG SODIUM. GOOD SOURCE OF: LYCOPENE.

Cilantro-Garlic Barbecue Sauce

If you like, make a double batch of this sauce and use it to toss with pasta or to spoon over grilled vegetables.

MAKES 1 CUP

2 heads of garlic (3½ ounces each)

3 cups cilantro leaves and stems

1 cup flat-leaf parsley leaves

½ cup fresh lemon juice

2 tablespoons olive oil

1 teaspoon salt

1 Preheat the oven to 400°F. Wrap the garlic in foil, place on a baking sheet, and bake until the packet is soft to the touch, about 30 minutes. When cool enough to handle, squeeze the garlic into a food processor bowl.
2 Add the cilantro, parsley, lemon juice, oil, and salt, and process to a smooth puree. Store the sauce in the refrigerator.

PER ¼ CUP: 77 CALORIES, 3.6G TOTAL FAT (0.5G SATURATED), 0MG CHOLESTEROL, 1G DIETARY FIBER, 11G CARBOHYDRATE, 2.2G PROTEIN, 309MG SODIUM. GOOD SOURCE OF: VITAMIN C.

Big-Batch Chili Marinara

There aren't very many reasons to make your own pasta sauce these days. Commercial brands come not only in low-fat, low-sodium versions, but also with just about any flavor you can think of, from red wine to roasted garlic. However, this homemade marinara has them all beat on the health front: Hidden underneath the spicy tomato sauce are cabbage, carrots, and bell peppers, adding fiber, beta carotene, vitamin B_6, and indoles to the sauce.

MAKES 6 QUARTS

4 teaspoons olive oil

2 large onions, finely chopped

3 carrots, finely chopped

8 cloves garlic, minced

3 red bell peppers, diced

2 green bell peppers, diced

3 cups finely chopped green cabbage

1 Granny Smith apple, peeled and finely chopped

¼ cup unsweetened cocoa powder

4 cans (28 ounces each) crushed tomatoes

3 cans (14½ ounces) no-salt-added diced tomatoes

1 can (6 ounces) no-salt-added tomato paste

¼ cup chipotle peppers in adobo, finely chopped

4 teaspoons chili powder

1¾ teaspoons oregano

1½ teaspoons salt

1 In an 8-quart Dutch oven, heat the oil over medium-low heat. Add the onions and cook, stirring frequently, until tender, about 10 minutes.
2 Stir in the carrots and garlic, and cook, stirring frequently, until the carrots are crisp-tender, about 5 minutes.
3 Stir in the bell peppers, cabbage, apple, and cocoa, and cook, stirring frequently, until the peppers are tender, about 7 minutes.
4 Stir in the crushed tomatoes, diced tomatoes and their juice, tomato paste, chipotle peppers, chili powder, oregano, and salt, and bring to a simmer. Simmer, uncovered, until the sauce is richly flavored and slightly thickened, about 20 minutes.
5 Cool the sauce to room temperature and transfer to quart containers. Refrigerate or freeze.

PER CUP: 97 CALORIES, 1.5G TOTAL FAT (0.3G SATURATED), 0MG CHOLESTEROL, 6G DIETARY FIBER, 21G CARBOHYDRATE, 4G PROTEIN, 358MG SODIUM. **GOOD SOURCE OF:** BETA CAROTENE, FIBER, INDOLES, LYCOPENE, MAGNESIUM, NIACIN, POTASSIUM, SULFORAPHANE, THIAMIN, VITAMIN B_6, VITAMIN C, VITAMIN E.

Tomatillo Salsa

Tomatillos look like small green tomatoes covered in a tan, papery husk. If you can't find fresh tomatillos, substitute 2 cups of canned tomatillos, but omit step 2 and blanch 3 cloves of garlic in a small saucepan of water, then add to the food processor in step 3 along with the canned tomatillos. Serve the salsa with grilled meats, chicken, vegetables, or chips.

MAKES 3 CUPS

2 pounds fresh tomatillos

3 cloves garlic, peeled

1 large red bell pepper, roasted (*page 190*)

½ cup cilantro, finely chopped

2 scallions, thinly sliced

3 tablespoons fresh lime juice

½ teaspoon cumin

½ teaspoon salt

1 Remove the papery husks covering the tomatillos. Wash the tomatillos.
2 In a large saucepan, combine the tomatillos, garlic, and cold water to cover by 1 inch. Bring to a boil and boil for 2 minutes. Drain, rinse under cold water, and drain again.
3 Cut the tomatillos into large pieces, then transfer to a food processor along with the garlic. Pulse until the tomatillos are finely chopped. Transfer to a large bowl.
4 Meanwhile, preheat the broiler. Roast the pepper. When it's cool enough to handle, peel and coarsely dice.
5 Add the pepper to the tomatillos along with the cilantro, scallions, lime juice, cumin, and salt, and stir to combine. Store the salsa in the refrigerator.

PER ¼ CUP: 30 CALORIES, 0.8G TOTAL FAT (0.1G SATURATED), 0MG CHOLESTEROL, 2G DIETARY FIBER, 6G CARBOHYDRATE, 1G PROTEIN, 99MG SODIUM. **GOOD SOURCE OF:** VITAMIN C.

recipe creator
fruit salsas

Tart and spicy fruit salsas are a cross between a condiment and a fruit salad. They are quick to make and are a wonderful complement to savory dishes like broiled poultry, fish, and meat. Choose from the categories listed below and follow these basic instructions: In a medium bowl, combine 2 cups of FRUIT (all one type or a combination), 1 CRUNCHY vegetable, 1 SAVORY vegetable, 1 FRESH HERB, and 1 ACID. Add ½ teaspoon salt and ⅛ teaspoon cayenne (you can omit the cayenne if you don't like spiciness, or increase the cayenne if you do). *Makes about 3 cups*

FRUITS	CRUNCHY	SAVORY	FRESH HERBS	ACIDS
▶ Mango, diced	▶ Jícama, ½ cup diced	▶ Red onion, ¼ cup minced	▶ Cilantro, ¼ cup chopped	▶ Lemon juice, 1 Tbsp
▶ Pineapple, diced	▶ Cucumber, ½ cup diced	▶ Plum tomatoes, 2, diced	▶ Fresh basil, ¼ cup chopped	▶ Lime juice, 1 Tbsp
▶ Banana, diced	▶ Red bell pepper, ⅓ cup diced	▶ Scallions, 2, thinly sliced	▶ Fresh mint, 2 Tbsp chopped	▶ Cider vinegar, 1 Tbsp
▶ Strawberries, halved	▶ Water chestnuts, ¼ cup diced	▶ Grape tomatoes, ½ cup halved	▶ Parsley, ¼ cup chopped	▶ Rice vinegar, 1 Tbsp
▶ Grapes, red or green seedless, halved	▶ Fresh fennel, ⅓ cup diced	▶ Corn kernels, ½ cup		▶ White vinegar, 1 Tbsp
▶ Cherries, halved and pitted	▶ Celery, ⅓ cup diced			▶ Balsamic vinegar, 1 Tbsp
▶ Plums, diced	▶ Daikon radish, ¼ cup diced			▶ Pomegranate molasses, 1 Tbsp
▶ Oranges or grapefruits, seeded and diced				▶ Passionfruit juice (unsweetened), 1 Tbsp
▶ Nectarines, diced				
▶ Peaches, peeled and diced				
▶ Cantaloupe, diced				

Grilled Pepper & Tomato Salsa

If you don't have a grill, you can broil the peppers and tomatoes. The timing should be approximately the same, depending on how close you can get your broiler pan to the heat.

MAKES 4 CUPS

2 yellow bell peppers, halved lengthwise and seeded

2 jalapeño peppers, halved lengthwise and seeded

2 pounds plum tomatoes

1 small red onion, finely chopped

⅓ cup chopped fresh mint

3 tablespoons red wine vinegar

1 teaspoon olive oil

½ teaspoon oregano

½ teaspoon salt

1 Spray a grill topper with nonstick cooking spray. Preheat the grill to medium. Grill the bell peppers and the jalapeños on the grill topper, cut-sides up, covered, for 10 minutes, or until the skin is charred. Remove from the grill and set aside. When cool enough to handle, peel and coarsely chop.
2 Place the tomatoes on the grill topper. Grill, covered, until they char and soften, about 7 minutes; turn them once or twice as they grill. Remove from the grill and set aside. Do not peel the tomatoes, but coarsely chop.
3 In a large bowl, combine the chopped bell peppers, jalapeños, and tomatoes (with their skins). Add the red onion, mint, vinegar, oil, oregano, and salt. Serve at room temperature. Store the salsa in the refrigerator.

PER ¼ CUP: 53 CALORIES, 1.2G TOTAL FAT (0.2G SATURATED), 0MG CHOLESTEROL, 2G DIETARY FIBER, 11G CARBOHYDRATE, 2G PROTEIN, 160MG SODIUM. **GOOD SOURCE OF:** POTASSIUM, VITAMIN B_6, VITAMIN C.

Tomato-Melon Salsa

Serve this mildly spiced salsa with grilled duck, chicken, or pork. You could use another type of tomato in this salsa, but the advantage to plum tomatoes is that they're meaty, without a lot of extra liquid.

MAKES 3 CUPS

2 tablespoons red currant jelly

4 teaspoons balsamic vinegar

2 teaspoons Dijon mustard

¼ teaspoon salt

3 cups cubed (½ inch) cantaloupe

1 small cucumber, peeled, seeded, and cut into ½-inch cubes (¾ cup)

½ cup cubed (½ inch) plum tomato

⅓ cup minced red onion

1 In a medium bowl, whisk together the currant jelly, vinegar, mustard, and salt until well combined.
2 Add the cantaloupe, cucumber, tomato, and red onion, and toss to combine. Refrigerate for up to 1 day; after that the salsa will be too watery.

PER ½ CUP: 61 CALORIES, 0.5G TOTAL FAT (0.1G SATURATED), 0MG CHOLESTEROL, 1G DIETARY FIBER, 14G CARBOHYDRATE, 1G PROTEIN, 152MG SODIUM. **GOOD SOURCE OF:** BETA CAROTENE, POTASSIUM, VITAMIN C.

Papaya-Corn Salsa

The papayas that most frequently appear on the market are the Solo varieties from Hawaii. These fruits are pear-shaped, about 6 inches long, and weigh from 1 to 2 pounds each.

MAKES 3 CUPS

1 small papaya (12 ounces) or 2 medium mangoes, peeled, pitted, and diced

1 large red bell pepper, diced

½ cup corn kernels, thawed frozen or fresh (from 2 ears)

¼ cup minced cilantro

2 tablespoons fresh lime juice

¼ teaspoon chili powder

In a medium bowl, stir together the papaya, bell pepper, corn, cilantro, lime juice, and chili powder. Refrigerate until ready to use. This will keep for up to 1 day; after that the fruit will be too watery.

PER ½ CUP: 33 CALORIES, 0.2G TOTAL FAT (0G SATURATED), 0MG CHOLESTEROL, 2G DIETARY FIBER, 8G CARBOHYDRATE, 1G PROTEIN, 4MG SODIUM. **GOOD SOURCE OF:** VITAMIN C.

Spicy Pear & Pepper Salsa

This chunky salsa would be good with roast pork or turkey.

MAKES 3 CUPS

3 tablespoons red wine vinegar

2 tablespoons honey

1 teaspoon Louisiana-style hot pepper sauce

¼ teaspoon salt

¼ teaspoon black pepper

¾ pound Bosc or Bartlett pears, peeled and cut into ½-inch chunks

1 red bell pepper, cut into ½-inch squares

⅓ cup finely chopped red onion

In a medium bowl, stir together the vinegar, honey, hot sauce, salt, and black pepper. Add the pears, bell pepper, and onion, and toss to combine. Store the salsa in the refrigerator.

PER ½ CUP: 66 CALORIES, 0.3G TOTAL FAT (0G SATURATED), 0MG CHOLESTEROL, 2G DIETARY FIBER, 17G CARBOHYDRATE, 1G PROTEIN, 119MG SODIUM. **GOOD SOURCE OF:** VITAMIN C.

Red Onion Marmalade

In the past decade or so, restaurant chefs decided to adopt the term marmalade (technically a fruit preserve with pieces of fruit suspended in a clear jelly) and apply it to onion relishes such as this. Maybe it's because the sweetness of onions makes them a natural partner of meat and poultry, much like certain fruit sauces (think duck à l'orange). This sweet-and-sour onion marmalade can be made a week in advance and refrigerated until serving time.

MAKES 2 CUPS

1 tablespoon olive oil

1¼ pounds red onions (about 4 medium), finely chopped

3 tablespoons balsamic vinegar

1 tablespoon light brown sugar

½ teaspoon grated orange zest

2 tablespoons orange juice

½ teaspoon salt

1 In a large skillet, heat the oil over low heat. Add the onions and cook, stirring frequently, until soft, about 15 minutes.

2 Stir in the vinegar, brown sugar, orange zest, orange juice, and salt. Cook, stirring frequently, until glossy, about 15 minutes. Serve warm, at room temperature, or chilled. Store the marmalade in the refrigerator.

PER ¼ CUP: 54 CALORIES, 1.8G TOTAL FAT (0.3G SATURATED), 0MG CHOLESTEROL, 1G DIETARY FIBER, 9G CARBOHYDRATE, 1G PROTEIN, 150MG SODIUM. **GOOD SOURCE OF:** QUERCETIN.

Corn Relish

Serve alongside grilled meats, poultry, or fish.

MAKES 4 CUPS

½ cup cider vinegar

¼ cup raisins

2 tablespoons sugar

2 teaspoons chili powder

½ teaspoon salt

¼ teaspoon cayenne pepper

1 green bell pepper, diced

3 cups frozen corn kernels

3 scallions, thinly sliced

1 In a large nonaluminum saucepan, combine the vinegar, raisins, sugar, chili powder, salt, and cayenne. Bring to a boil over medium-high heat. Boil for 2 minutes.

2 Add the bell pepper and cook until the pepper is crisp-tender, about 3 minutes.

3 Remove from the heat and stir in the corn and scallions. Cool to room temperature. Store the relish in the refrigerator.

PER ¼ CUP: 46 CALORIES, 0.3G TOTAL FAT (0.1G SATURATED), 0MG CHOLESTEROL, 1G DIETARY FIBER, 11G CARBOHYDRATE, 1G PROTEIN, 78MG SODIUM. **GOOD SOURCE OF:** LUTEIN, VITAMIN C.

Fresh Vidalia Onion Relish

Vidalia onions are sweet and mild. If they aren't in season you may be able to find another sweet onion such as a Walla Walla or a Texas 1020. If not, substitute a red onion.

MAKES 1 CUP

1 medium Vidalia onion, diced

1 yellow bell pepper, diced

¼ cup pitted green olives (about 6), coarsely chopped

3 tablespoons chopped fresh mint

3 tablespoons fresh lemon juice

4 teaspoons honey

1 tablespoon balsamic vinegar

¼ teaspoon salt

¼ teaspoon pepper

In a medium bowl, combine the onion, bell pepper, olives, mint, lemon juice, honey, vinegar, salt, and pepper. Cover and refrigerate for at least 1 hour before using. Store the relish in the refrigerator.

PER ¼ CUP: 79 CALORIES, 1G TOTAL FAT (0.1G SATURATED), 0MG CHOLESTEROL, 2G DIETARY FIBER, 18G CARBOHYDRATE, 2G PROTEIN, 292MG SODIUM. **GOOD SOURCE OF:** VITAMIN B$_6$, VITAMIN C.

Fresh Pineapple-Jícama Relish

This sweet-tart sandwich relish goes well with smoked poultry or ham. Or serve it as a condiment with broiled chicken or salmon. Try to make the relish as close to serving time as possible, since the enzymes in the pineapple and kiwifruit will turn the other ingredients mushy if they sit too long.

MAKES 3 CUPS

2 cups finely diced fresh pineapple

2 kiwifruit, peeled and finely diced

½ cup finely diced jícama or tart, crisp apple

2 tablespoons honey

2 tablespoons chopped cilantro

1 tablespoon fresh lime juice

In a large bowl, stir together the pineapple, kiwifruit, jícama, honey, cilantro, and lime juice. Refrigerate for up to 2 hours.

PER ⅓ CUP: 45 CALORIES, 0.2G TOTAL FAT (0G SATURATED), 0MG CHOLESTEROL, 1G DIETARY FIBER, 11G CARBOHYDRATE, 0G PROTEIN, 2MG SODIUM. **GOOD SOURCE OF:** VITAMIN C.

Banana Chutney

This spicy banana chutney would work well as an accompaniment to simple grilled poultry or pork, or with any curried main dish. If you like chutney extra hot, add a finely chopped canned or bottled jalapeño.

MAKES 2¼ CUPS

4 cloves garlic, peeled

2 tablespoons coarsely chopped fresh ginger

¾ cup red wine vinegar

1 cup packed light brown sugar

½ teaspoon salt

1 medium red onion, cut into ½-inch chunks

½ teaspoon pepper

1½ pounds ripe bananas (about 5 medium), thickly sliced

⅓ cup raisins

1 In a blender or food processor, process the garlic, ginger, and ¼ cup of the vinegar until smooth.

2 In a medium saucepan, stir together the brown sugar, salt, remaining ½ cup vinegar, and the garlic mixture. Stir in the onion and pepper. Bring to a boil over medium heat. Cook until the onion is glossy and tender, about 20 minutes.

3 Stir in the bananas and raisins, and cook until the chutney is thick and the bananas have lost their shape, about 15 minutes. Cool to room temperature. Store the chutney in the refrigerator.

PER **3** TABLESPOONS: 134 CALORIES, 0.3G TOTAL FAT (0.1G SATURATED), 0MG CHOLESTEROL, 2G DIETARY FIBER, 34G CARBOHYDRATE, 1G PROTEIN, 107MG SODIUM. **GOOD SOURCE OF:** POTASSIUM, VITAMIN B$_6$.

Fresh Rhubarb Chutney

Serve this spicy sauce alongside grilled chicken or pork. If fresh rhubarb is not available, substitute an equal amount of frozen rhubarb.

MAKES 3 CUPS

4 cups sliced rhubarb (from 1¼ pounds rhubarb)

1 cup diced onion

1 large McIntosh apple, cut into ½-inch chunks

1 red bell pepper, diced

⅓ cup honey

¼ cup dried currants

2 tablespoons balsamic vinegar

2 tablespoons minced fresh ginger

1 teaspoon yellow mustard seeds

½ teaspoon black pepper

½ teaspoon salt

1 In a large saucepan, stir together the rhubarb, onion, apple, bell pepper, honey, currants, vinegar, ginger, mustard seeds, black pepper, and salt. Bring to a boil, reduce to a simmer, cover, and cook until the mixture is thick, about 20 minutes.

2 Cool to room temperature. Store the chutney in the refrigerator.

PER ⅓ CUP: 93 CALORIES, 0.4G TOTAL FAT (0.1G SATURATED), 0MG CHOLESTEROL, 3G DIETARY FIBER, 23G CARBOHYDRATE, 1G PROTEIN, 134MG SODIUM. GOOD SOURCE OF: FIBER, POTASSIUM, VITAMIN C.

Nectarine-Pineapple Chutney

This fresh fruit chutney is delicious served just after cooking, but it will keep well in the refrigerator.

MAKES 2 CUPS

1 can (20 ounces) juice-packed crushed pineapple, drained

2 large nectarines, coarsely chopped

8 scallions, coarsely chopped

⅓ cup diced dried apricots

⅓ cup cider vinegar

6 tablespoons dark brown sugar

2 cloves garlic, chopped

½ teaspoon ground ginger

¼ teaspoon cinnamon

¼ teaspoon red pepper flakes

½ cup diced red bell pepper

1 In a large nonaluminum saucepan, stir together the pineapple, nectarines, scallions, apricots, vinegar, brown sugar, garlic, ginger, cinnamon, and pepper flakes. Bring to a boil over medium-high heat, reduce the heat to medium, and cook, stirring frequently, until the nectarines begin to soften, about 8 minutes.

2 Remove the mixture from the heat and stir in the bell pepper. Serve at room temperature or chilled. Store the chutney in the refrigerator.

PER ⅓ CUP: 140 CALORIES, 0.5G TOTAL FAT (0G SATURATED), 0MG CHOLESTEROL, 3G DIETARY FIBER, 36G CARBOHYDRATE, 2G PROTEIN, 10MG SODIUM. GOOD SOURCE OF: FIBER, POTASSIUM, THIAMIN, VITAMIN C.

Mixed Fruit Chutney

There are packages of already diced mixed dried fruit, some of them with a tropical theme, but you could also make your own mixture. For example, a diced dried pear and cranberry chutney would be nice. Or try diced dried peaches and cherries.

MAKES 1 CUP

⅔ cup distilled white vinegar

⅓ cup packed brown sugar

1 green bell pepper, diced

1 small red onion, finely chopped

1 cup mixed diced dried fruit

½ cup canned crushed tomatoes

1 clove garlic, minced

1 teaspoon coriander

1 teaspoon chili powder

½ teaspoon salt

1 In a 3-quart nonaluminum saucepan, stir together the vinegar, brown sugar, bell pepper, onion, mixed fruit, tomatoes, garlic, coriander, chili powder, and salt.

2 Bring to a boil, reduce the heat to a simmer, cover, and cook, stirring frequently, until the pepper and onion are tender and the chutney is slightly thickened, about 20 minutes. Cool to room temperature. Store the chutney in the refrigerator.

PER 2 TABLESPOONS: 84 CALORIES, 0.2G TOTAL FAT (0G SATURATED), 0MG CHOLESTEROL, 2G DIETARY FIBER, 22G CARBOHYDRATE, 1G PROTEIN, 164MG SODIUM. GOOD SOURCE OF: VITAMIN C.

Butternut Squash & Fruit Chutney

Much like salsas, chutneys can be made of all sorts of things, though the most familiar type is mango chutney. The flavor of mango is present here, but the star ingredient is butternut squash, which is rich in beta carotene. If you like, you can use frozen butternut squash cubes, but add them when you add the apple (step 3), because they are softer than fresh squash. Serve as a condiment with meat or poultry.

MAKES 4 CUPS

¾ cup mango or apricot nectar

3 tablespoons apricot all-fruit spread

1 tablespoon cider vinegar

1½ teaspoons curry powder

½ teaspoon salt

2 cups diced butternut squash

½ cup dried apricots, coarsely chopped

1 Granny Smith apple, cut into ½-inch chunks

⅓ cup finely chopped red onion

1 In a medium saucepan, bring the mango nectar, fruit spread, vinegar, curry powder, and salt to a boil over medium heat.
2 Add the squash and apricots, and reduce the heat to low. Cover and cook until the squash is firm-tender, about 10 minutes.
3 Stir in the apple and red onion. Cover and cook until the apple and squash are tender, about 5 minutes. Cool to room temperature. Store the chutney in the refrigerator.

PER ½ CUP: 79 CALORIES, 0.2G TOTAL FAT (0G SATURATED), 0MG CHOLESTEROL, 3G DIETARY FIBER, 21G CARBOHYDRATE, 1G PROTEIN, 152MG SODIUM. GOOD SOURCE OF: BETA CAROTENE, FIBER, POTASSIUM, VITAMIN C.

Lime-Raisin Chutney

This sweet-tart puree was inspired by a southern Indian condiment made from tamarind. Sweet raisins and tart lime juice mimic the flavors of tamarind, an ingredient available mostly at Indian markets. Serve this chutney with any curried dish, or use it as a sauce to serve over simple broiled chicken or pork.

MAKES 1⅓ CUPS

⅔ cup water

½ cup fresh lime juice

1 tablespoon sugar

1 teaspoon yellow mustard

½ teaspoon turmeric

¼ teaspoon salt

2 cups dark or golden raisins

1 In a medium saucepan, combine the water, lime juice, sugar, mustard, turmeric, and salt. Bring to a boil over medium heat.
2 Add the raisins and reduce to a simmer. Cover and cook, stirring occasionally, until the raisins are very soft, about 40 minutes.
3 Transfer the mixture to a food processor or blender and process to a smooth puree. Cool to room temperature. Store the chutney in the refrigerator.

PER TABLESPOON: 109 CALORIES, 0.2G TOTAL FAT (0.1G SATURATED), 0MG CHOLESTEROL, 1G DIETARY FIBER, 29G CARBOHYDRATE, 1G PROTEIN, 80MG SODIUM.

Tomato-Orange Chutney

Grated orange and lemon zests add fresh citrusy flavors to this thick tomato chutney. Serve with grilled chicken or fish, or use as a burger and sandwich topping.

MAKES 1 CUP

1 can (14½ ounces) stewed tomatoes, chopped with their juice

2 tablespoons sugar

2½ teaspoons grated orange zest

1 teaspoon grated lemon zest

1 tablespoon distilled white vinegar

1½ teaspoons coriander

¼ teaspoon salt

¼ teaspoon pepper

1 In a medium nonaluminum saucepan, combine the tomatoes and their juice, sugar, orange zest, lemon zest, vinegar, coriander, salt, and pepper. Bring to a boil over medium heat.
2 Reduce to a simmer and cook, uncovered, stirring occasionally, until the chutney is the consistency of jam, about 15 minutes.
3 Cool to room temperature. Store the chutney in the refrigerator.

PER ¼ CUP: 58 CALORIES, 0.3G TOTAL FAT (0G SATURATED), 0MG CHOLESTEROL, 2G DIETARY FIBER, 14G CARBOHYDRATE, 1G PROTEIN, 373MG SODIUM. GOOD SOURCE OF: LYCOPENE, VITAMIN C.

Double-Pineapple Sauce

This sauce can be served with either sweet or savory dishes. It's equally delicious over frozen yogurt or alongside grilled chicken or pork.

MAKES 2⅔ CUPS

1 cup pineapple juice
3 tablespoons honey
½ teaspoon cinnamon
½ teaspoon chili powder
⅛ teaspoon ground cloves
1 fresh pineapple (about 3 pounds), peeled, cored, and coarsely chopped

1 In a large nonreactive skillet, stir together the pineapple juice, honey, cinnamon, chili powder, and cloves. Bring to a boil and cook, stirring frequently, until reduced by half, about 7 minutes.
2 Stir in half of the chopped pineapple and cook, stirring frequently, until thickened, about 5 minutes.
3 Remove from the heat and let cool to room temperature. Stir in the remaining chopped pineapple. Serve at room temperature or chilled. Store the sauce in the refrigerator.

PER ⅔ CUP: 115 CALORIES, 0.6G TOTAL FAT (0.1G SATURATED), 0MG CHOLESTEROL, 2G DIETARY FIBER, 29G CARBOHYDRATE, 1G PROTEIN, 7MG SODIUM. **GOOD SOURCE OF**: THIAMIN, VITAMIN C.

Refrigerator Peach-Ginger Jam

This quick, fresh jam (made without added pectin) gets thicker the longer you cook it. Test it by spooning some out of the pot and then dropping it back in—it should stick to the spoon and fall off slowly in a thick mound.

MAKES 6 CUPS

3½ pounds ripe peaches
3½ cups sugar
1 tablespoon grated lemon zest
2 tablespoons fresh lemon juice
⅓ cup finely chopped crystallized ginger

1 In a large pot of boiling water, working in batches, blanch the peaches for 1 minute to loosen their skin. Run the peaches under cold water to cool them down. Peel, halve, and pit the peaches. Then cut into wedges.
2 Transfer the peach wedges to a large nonaluminum saucepan. Add the sugar, lemon zest, and lemon juice, and bring to a full boil over high heat. Reduce to a simmer and cook, stirring frequently, for 15 minutes. Mash the peaches with a potato masher or a fork.
3 Stir in the crystallized ginger and cook until the jam is thick enough to remain on a spoon once it's been lifted out of the pot, 10 to 20 minutes.
4 Let cool to room temperature. Store the jam in the refrigerator.

PER TABLESPOON: 36 CALORIES, 0G TOTAL FAT (0G SATURATED), 0MG CHOLESTEROL, 0G DIETARY FIBER, 9G CARBOHYDRATE, 0G PROTEIN, 0MG SODIUM.

Fresh Blueberry Jam

A small amount of cardamom and ginger gives this jam a slightly spicy note.

MAKES 1½ CUPS

3 cups blueberries
1 cup sugar
4 strips (2 x ¼-inch) lime zest
2 tablespoons fresh lime juice
¾ teaspoon cinnamon
½ teaspoon ground ginger
¼ teaspoon cardamom
⅛ teaspoon salt
⅛ teaspoon pepper

1 In a medium saucepan, combine the blueberries, sugar, lime zest, lime juice, cinnamon, ginger, cardamom, salt, and pepper. Cook over medium heat, stirring frequently, until thick, about 20 minutes.
2 Remove from the heat. Discard the zest. Let cool to room temperature. Store the jam in the refrigerator.

PER TABLESPOON: 43 CALORIES, 0.1G TOTAL FAT (0G SATURATED), 0MG CHOLESTEROL, 1G DIETARY FIBER, 11G CARBOHYDRATE, 0G PROTEIN, 13MG SODIUM. **GOOD SOURCE OF**: ANTHOCYANINS.

Apple Butter

If you'd like to store the apple butter for a longer period, sterilize a 1-quart canning jar (or 3 half-pint jars). Transfer the apple butter to the hot jar. Place the screw lid on top and seal. Place the jar in a boiling water bath, and process for 10 minutes after the water returns to a boil. **Timing alert:** This apple butter needs to be tended on stovetop for about 1½ hours.

MAKES 2½ CUPS

4 pounds apples (use a mix of types), peeled and cut into eighths

¼ cup apple cider or apple juice

6 strips (2 x ½-inch) lemon zest

¾ cup sugar

1½ teaspoons cinnamon

½ teaspoon ground ginger

¼ teaspoon grated nutmeg

1 In a large saucepan, combine the apples, apple cider, and lemon zest. Bring to a boil over medium heat. Reduce to a simmer. Cook, stirring often, until the apples are very tender and falling apart, about 20 minutes.

2 Stir in the sugar, cinnamon, ginger, and nutmeg, and cook over low heat, stirring frequently, until the mixture is very thick, about 1 hour. Test the apple butter by placing a spoonful on a plate. If it doesn't weep any liquid and doesn't spread out, it's ready.

3 Store the apple butter in the refrigerator.

PER 2 TABLESPOONS: 83 CALORIES, 0.3G TOTAL FAT (0.1G SATURATED), 0MG CHOLESTEROL, 2G DIETARY FIBER, 22G CARBOHYDRATE, 0G PROTEIN, 1MG SODIUM.

Pumpkin Butter

Serve this thick spread as you would jam or preserves. For longer storage, sterilize 5 half-pint canning jars. Transfer the pumpkin butter to the hot jars. Place the screw lids on top and seal. Place the jars in a boiling water bath, and process for 10 minutes after the water returns to a boil. Once processed, the pumpkin butter will keep for several months. **Timing alert:** This pumpkin butter needs to be tended on stovetop for about 1½ hours.

MAKES 4 CUPS

3 cans (15 ounces each) unsweetened pumpkin puree

½ cup packed brown sugar

½ cup granulated sugar

¼ cup orange juice

1 teaspoon cinnamon

¾ teaspoon ground ginger

¼ teaspoon allspice

⅛ teaspoon ground cloves

⅛ teaspoon salt

1 In a large heavy saucepan, combine the pumpkin puree, brown sugar, granulated sugar, orange juice, cinnamon, ginger, allspice, cloves, and salt. Bring to a boil.

2 Reduce to a simmer and cook, uncovered, stirring frequently, until the mixture is very thick, about 1½ hours. Store the pumpkin butter in the refrigerator.

PER 2 TABLESPOONS: 40 CALORIES, 0.2G TOTAL FAT (0G SATURATED), 14MG CHOLESTEROL, 2G DIETARY FIBER, 10G CARBOHYDRATE, 1G PROTEIN, 12MG SODIUM. **GOOD SOURCE OF:** BETA CAROTENE.

Fresh Kim Chee

Kim chee, Korean pickled vegetables, can be mildly hot to extremely hot. This recipe makes a moderately hot kim chee, so if you like very spicy dishes, increase the cayenne accordingly. Serve the kim chee alongside meat or poultry. **Timing alert:** A true Korean kim chee would be set aside for months to ferment (like sauerkraut), but this fresh kim chee still takes 2 days to "pickle."

MAKES 4 CUPS

1 head napa cabbage (about 3 pounds), halved lengthwise and cut crosswise into 2-inch-wide pieces

3 tablespoons coarse (kosher) salt

3 tablespoons hot water

2 tablespoons soy sauce

2 tablespoons distilled white vinegar

2 teaspoons anchovy paste

¾ teaspoon cayenne pepper

3 cloves garlic, thinly sliced

1 tablespoon matchstick strips of fresh ginger

6 scallions, thinly sliced

1¼ cups matchstick strips of daikon radish

1 In a large bowl, combine the cabbage and salt, and toss well. Let stand for 3 hours. Rinse the cabbage under cold water and squeeze well to get rid of any excess liquid.

2 In a large bowl, stir together the hot water, soy sauce, vinegar, anchovy paste, and cayenne. Add the cabbage, garlic, ginger, scallions, and daikon, and toss well. Cover and let stand at room temperature, turning the cabbage occasionally in the sauce, for 2 days. Store the kim chee in the refrigerator.

PER ½ CUP: 37 CALORIES, 0.4G TOTAL FAT (0.1G SATURATED), 0MG CHOLESTEROL, 5G DIETARY FIBER, 7G CARBOHYDRATE, 3G PROTEIN, 359MG SODIUM. **GOOD SOURCE OF:** BETA CAROTENE, CALCIUM, FIBER, FOLATE, INDOLES, POTASSIUM, VITAMIN B₆, VITAMIN C.

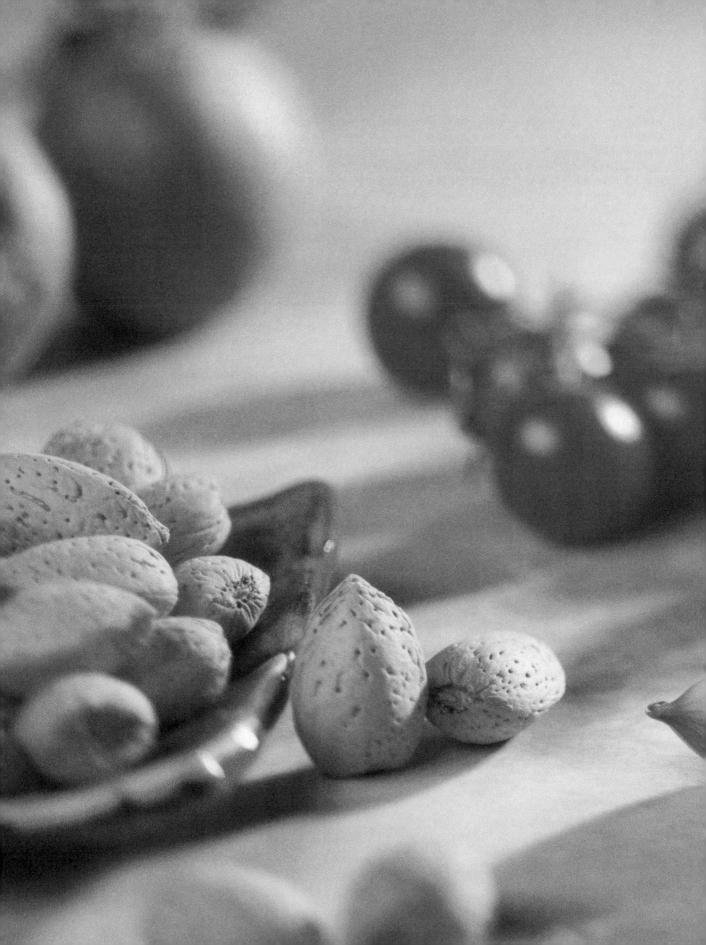

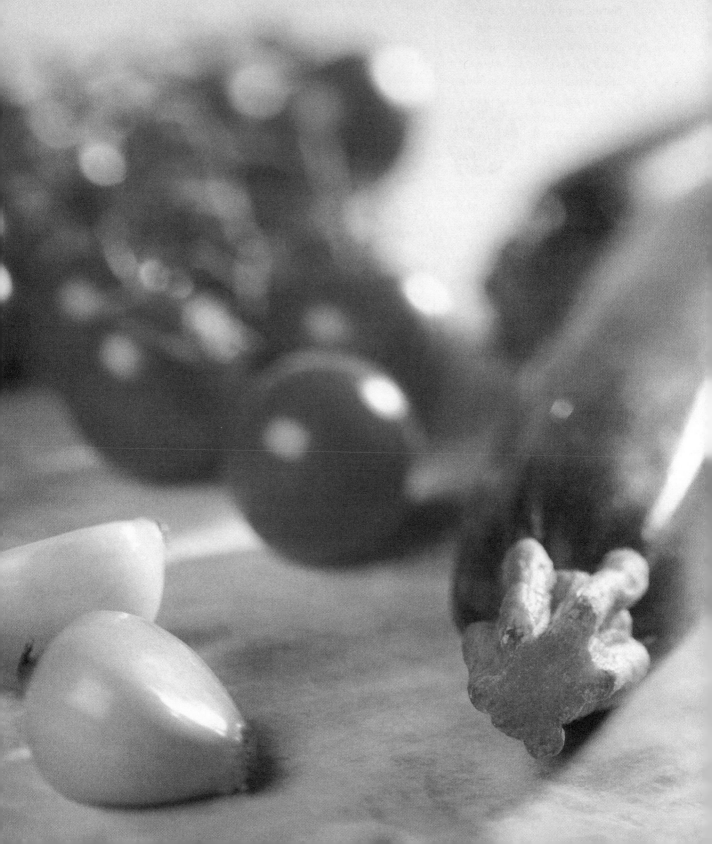

foods a to z

acorn squash

Nutrition profile Acorn squash is rich in carotenoid pigments (such as beta carotene, alpha carotene, and lutein) that lend vivid autumn color to its flesh. In addition, 1 cup of cooked mashed acorn squash will give you 11 g of fiber, 25% of the RDA for magnesium, 28% of the RDA for vitamin B_6, and 29% of the RDA for vitamin C. Acorn squash also has good amounts of thiamin, potassium, and iron.

Maximizing nutrients The carotenoids in acorn squash are made more bioavailable when the squash is cooked, and when it's cooked or served with a small amount of unsaturated fat, such as olive oil. Because acorn squash is deeply ridged and therefore difficult to peel, it is most often cooked as unpeeled halves. Most people do not eat the skin (it has a neutral flavor, but is on the tough side), but its dark color indicates that is has lots of plant pigments, some of which may have health benefits.

almonds

Nutrition profile Almonds, like many nuts, are nutrient-dense, which means that relative to the number of calories in a serving, you'll get a lot of valuable nutrients. For example, for 1 ounce (about 23 almonds) you get over 3 g of dietary fiber, 6 g of protein, 20% of the RDA for mag-nesium, and 46% of the RDA for the antioxidant vitamin E. In addition, almonds provide riboflavin, iron, and fiber, as well as plant sterols. And although that same ounce of almonds brings 15 g of fat, the fat is mostly monounsaturated fat, a beneficial, heart-healthy fat. Studies show that nuts, when replacing saturated fat, offer heart health benefits by reducing levels of artery-damaging LDL (low-density lipoprotein), the "bad" cholesterol. Don't go overboard with almonds, though, because (like other nuts) they are high in calories.

Maximizing nutrients Cooking does not adversely affect the nutrients in almonds, but proper storage (in the refrigerator or freezer) is important to help prevent their oils from going rancid.

amaranth

Nutrition profile Amaranth leaves (also called callaloo, Indian spinach, or Chinese spinach) are rich in beta carotene, folate, potassium, and calcium; and 1 cup of cooked amaranth leaves will also give you a good amount of vitamin C (60% of the RDA). The same plant also provides a tiny seed packed with powerful nutritional value. Compared with other grains, amaranth seeds are high in protein (7 g per ¼ cup), and aren't deficient in the essential amino acids lysine and methionine. In addition ¼ cup of amaranth seeds has 31% of the RDA for magnesium, good amounts of iron and zinc, and over 7 g of dietary fiber.

Maximizing nutrients Cooking amaranth leaves will enhance the availability of their beta carotene, but it should be cooked in little or no water to limit the loss of its water-soluble nutrients such as folate (and other B vitamins) and vitamin C. Eating the leaves uncooked, in a salad, will give you more vitamin C, which is heat-sensitive. Cooking amaranth grain (seeds) will not adversely affect their mineral, fiber, or protein content, but eating the grain with a food high in vitamin C will improve the body's ability to absorb the non-heme iron.

apples

Nutrition profile Apples provide a good amount of both insoluble and soluble fiber, including a type of soluble fiber called pectin. Studies show that pectin and other types of soluble fiber help to lower blood cholesterol. In addition, apples contain phytochemicals such as quercetin, and red apples supply natural pigments in their skin called anthocyanins.

Maximizing nutrients A good percentage of the fiber in an apple is in the skin or just under it, so unpeeled apples will give you the most fiber. And the bioavailability of the soluble fiber pectin will be somewhat increased when the apples are cooked.

apricots

Nutrition profile Fragrant and delicate, fresh apricots supply beta carotene, vitamin C, fiber, and potassium. Dried apricots are a concentrated source of the nutrients in fresh apricots, though their vitamin C is destroyed by the drying process. Dried apricots are also a fairly good source of iron.

Maximizing nutrients Although eating fresh apricots is the way to get the most vitamin C, other substances—such as beta carotene and the soluble fiber pectin—are actually made more available to the body when the apricots (either fresh or dried) are cooked.

artichokes

Nutrition profile Artichokes are a good source of potassium, magnesium, and folate. They are also very rich in fiber: A 2-ounce serving (the heart of one big artichoke) has 3 g of fiber, which is over 10% of the minimum amount of fiber recommended daily.

Maximizing nutrients Although frozen and canned "hearts" are the most available market form of artichokes, it's best to cook and eat fresh, whole artichokes as often as possible to take advantage of the nutrients found in the leaves. To preserve as much of the water-soluble folate as possible, steam rather than boil artichokes.

arugula

Nutrition profile Along with its pleasant, peppery taste, arugula also provides folate, beta carotene, and potassium.

Maximizing nutrients Arugula is most often served uncooked in salads. But if you like its pungent and assertive taste, then try sautéing it with garlic and a small amount of olive oil; the cooking and the addition of the oil will make the beta carotene more bioavailable.

asparagus

Nutrition profile Asparagus is a member of the lily family and thus closely related to garlic, onions, and leeks. Low in fat and calories, and high in fiber, asparagus provides an impressive array of nutrients such as iron, beta carotene, vitamin C, and a wealth of B vitamins—most exceptionally folate: 1 cup of cooked asparagus yields 263 mcg of folate, which is 66% of the RDA.

Maximizing nutrients To retain more of the water-soluble B vitamins, steam or microwave asparagus instead of boiling it.

avocados

Nutrition profile Avocados are nutritious; they are rich in B vitamins, especially folate (which, along with vitamin B_6, may help to lower the risk for heart disease): One Hass avocado provides 57 mcg of folate, which is about 14% of the RDA. And though avocados are high in fat, their fat is mostly beneficial monounsaturated fat that, when substituted for saturated fat, helps to lower LDL cholesterol levels.

bananas

Nutrition profile Bananas provide significant amounts of potassium, a mineral that may protect against high blood pressure. One banana contains 467 mg of potassium, which is about 16% of the daily recommended intake. Bananas are also an excellent source of heart-healthy soluble fiber pectin and vitamin B_6.

barley

Nutrition profile A versatile grain with a nutlike flavor, barley is a rich source of complex carbohydrates, thiamin, niacin, vitamin B_6, iron, and zinc. It also provides ample amounts of fiber, particularly beta glucan, a soluble fiber that helps to lower LDL cholesterol. In addition, 1 cup of cooked pearl barley will supply 55 mcg (about 25% of the RDA)

b

of the antioxidant mineral selenium. Hulled barley, the form of the grain in which the bran is left intact, has even more vitamins and minerals than the more common pearl (or pearled) barley; look for it in health-food stores. Whole-grain barley also has the phytochemicals called saponins.

Maximizing nutrients When barley is cooked in water and then drained, it loses some portion of its water-soluble B vitamins. Therefore, one of the most nutritious ways to cook barley is in a soup, where the cooking water is consumed, too. And eating barley with a food high in vitamin C will improve the body's ability to absorb the grain's nonheme iron.

beans, dried

Nutrition profile A nourishing, low-fat source of plant protein, dried beans are high in complex carbohydrates, fiber, B vitamins (especially folate), and minerals, such as potassium, magnesium, and selenium. Beans are particularly rich in cholesterol-lowering soluble fiber as well as plant sterols. And the insoluble fiber in dried beans helps to improve regularity by speeding the passage of food through the intestine. The ample fiber content of dried beans also bolsters weight-control efforts by contributing to a feeling of fullness.

Maximizing nutrients Cooking beans is most efficiently done in

a fair amount of water, which means that some of the water-soluble folate will be lost to the cooking water. However, ½ cup of most cooked beans still has handsome amounts of folate. It's always best to cook your own beans (*see page 180*), but canned beans are a good solution if you're pressed for time. Canned beans do have substantial amounts of sodium in the packing liquid, however; so be sure to rinse them well before using. The gas-causing culprits in beans are carbohydrates called oligosaccharides. Some research suggests that presoaking beans, and then discarding the soaking water before cooking the beans, will get rid of some of their oligosaccharides.

beans, fresh

Nutrition profile The carotenoids beta carotene, lutein, zeaxanthin, as well as folate and vitamin C are found in most fresh edible-pod beans (such as snap beans). Fresh beans are also low in calories and rich in fiber. Shell beans—fresh beans out of the pod, such as lima beans—are considerably higher in calories and carbohydrates, though they are still very low in fat (with the exception of soybeans, which have quite a bit of fat).

Maximizing nutrients Edible-pod beans eaten uncooked will have the most vitamin C (which is found largely in the pod, not the beans), but cooking increases the bioavailability of the carotenoids. The best cooking methods are

steaming or microwaving—as opposed to boiling—which help preserve the water-soluble B vitamins.

beef

Nutrition profile Beef can fit into a healthful diet if you select lean cuts, trim all visible fat before cooking, and eat small portions (3 ounces, cooked). At only 183 calories, a 3-ounce serving of cooked sirloin will give you 26 g of protein as well as 99% of the RDA for vitamin B_{12}, 48% of the RDA for zinc, and 34% of the RDA for iron.

Maximizing nutrients The levels of these nutrients are approximately the same for lean or fatty beef, and trimming the fat from beef will not remove any of the meat's nutrients. For information on healthful ways to cook beef, see page 91.

beet greens

Nutrition profile Although beets are generally known for their deep red roots (*see Beets, opposite page*), their leaves are actually the most nutritious part of the plant. Not only are the large, long-stemmed, tender young beet leaves among the mildest cooking greens of all, but they are also rich in beta carotene and vitamin C (40% of the RDA in 1 cup cooked). And though they have good calcium levels, the greens contain substances called oxalates, which interfere with the absorption of this mineral.

Maximizing nutrients To preserve vitamin C content, cook beet greens with a quick, low-moisture method (such as steaming, microwaving, or stir-frying), and serve or cook with a small amount of unsaturated oil (such as olive oil or canola oil) to enhance the bioavailability of the beta carotene.

beets

Nutrition profile Beets are a rich source of fiber, potassium, and folate. Notable for their sweet, earthy flavor, beets have the highest sugar content of any vegetable, while remaining very low in calories (1 cup of cooked beets has only 75 calories). And unlike many other vegetables, their full flavor is retained whether they are fresh or canned (which is the way most beets are sold in the United States). Fresh beets, though, have a characteristic earthy-sweet flavor and a crisp texture that you don't find in canned versions; and some of the B vitamins and plant pigments in canned beets leach out into the packing liquid.

Maximizing nutrients The best way to cook beets is to microwave or roast them whole, with their skins on and their stem and root ends untrimmed. The reason for this is that if you peel beets, or cut into them at all, their deep purple color (which derives in part from natural plant

pigments called betacyanins) will leach out as they cook.

belgian endive

Nutrition profile Pale Belgian endive has minimal nutritional value, but adds a satisfying, slightly bitter flavor to dishes.

blackberries

Nutrition profile Plump, juicy, and slightly tart, the blackberry is not only generous in flavor and texture but is high in fiber (over 7 g per cup), low in calories, and rich in vitamin C and folate. In addition, blackberries get their purplish-black color from anthocyanin pigments. Ellagic acid is another phytochemical found in blackberries.

Maximizing nutrients Cooking will destroy some of the folate and vitamin C in blackberries, so to get the benefit of these vitamins, eat fresh berries. The fiber and pigments, on the other hand, are not affected by heat.

blueberries

Nutrition profile Blueberries are low in calories (1 cup has 81 calories) and rich in flavor. Blueberries also contain significant amounts of vitamin C, as well as pectin, a soluble fiber that helps lower cholesterol levels.

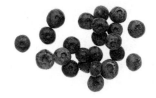

Blueberries have also been studied for their antioxidant properties; and they contain anthocyanins—a group of phytochemical pigments that put the "blue" in blueberry.

Maximizing nutrients Fresh, uncooked blueberries will have the most vitamin C, which is partly destroyed by heat. The soluble fiber pectin, on the other hand, will be more bioavailable in cooked blueberries. One solution to this is to always use a mix of cooked and fresh blueberries. This technique has many culinary virtues as well: The contrast between the rich, soft cooked blueberries and the firm, fresh berries is very satisfying (*see Spiced Blueberry Pie, page 240*).

bok choy

Nutrition profile One cup of cooked bok choy will give you 24% of the recommended daily intake for beta carotene, 17% of the RDA for vitamin B_6, and almost half of the RDA for vitamin C. Bok choy also offers folate, calcium, fiber, and potassium. What bok choy will *not* give you is a lot of calories: 1 cup has only 20 calories. And because bok choy is a cruciferous vegetable, it contains phytochemicals called isothiocyanates and indoles.

b

Maximizing nutrients Bok choy is ideally suited to stir-fries not only because of its Asian origins, but also because by cooking the bok choy in a small amount of oil, the beta carotene content of the vegetable becomes more available to the body. This quick-cooking method also helps preserve the B vitamin content, since these vitamins are water-soluble and would be reduced if you cooked the bok choy in water. The phytochemicals in bok choy are heat stable and are not significantly lost in the cooking process; in fact, the indole content will be improved by cooking.

brazil nuts

Nutrition profile In relation to their size, Brazil nuts contain a large assortment of nutrients including protein, fiber, vitamin E, thiamin, iron, magnesium, and zinc. Their most notable nutritional attribute, however, is their exceptional selenium content: A single Brazil nut can supply more than twice the RDA for selenium (a large nut has 140 mcg, or 254% of the RDA). Brazil nuts are also a rich source of heart-healthy plant sterols and monounsaturated fatty acids.

Maximizing nutrients Brazil nuts are uncommon cooking ingredients, perhaps because they are difficult to shell and are rarely sold in a convenient form. They are most often sold in the shell, to be eaten as is. Like other nuts, because of their high fat content they should be stored in the refrigerator or freezer.

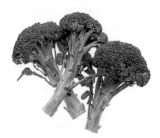

broccoli

Nutrition profile A high-fiber, nutrient-dense food, broccoli is a good source of folate, riboflavin, vitamin B_6, vitamin C, and potassium, as well as the carotenoids, beta carotene and lutein. Noted for its wealth of phytochemicals, broccoli (and especially broccoli sprouts) is a leading source of sulforaphane, indoles, and isothiocyanates.

Maximizing nutrients Raw broccoli will have more vitamin C and B vitamins than cooked broccoli, but its carotenoid bioavailability will be improved by cooking. Unfortunately, raw broccoli is not to everyone's taste, and most people eat it cooked. To conserve broccoli's heat-sensitive and water-soluble nutrients, cook it as briefly as possible and not in a lot of water. Try a low-moisture, quick-cooking method such as steaming, microwaving, or stir-frying. And if possible, include the leaves—most people throw them away, but they contain a lot of the plant's beta carotene—and

the peels on the stalks; or if you do peel the stalks, try not to peel too deeply. The phytochemicals in broccoli and broccoli sprouts are heat stable and are not significantly lost in the cooking process; in fact, there is research that indicates that the bioactivity of indoles may actually be increased by cooking.

broccoli rabe

Nutrition profile Resembling thin broccoli stalks with small clusters of tiny buds and large leaves, broccoli rabe (also known as rapini) is a good source of vitamin C and beta carotene. In addition, like all cruciferous vegetables, broccoli rabe is rich in certain phytochemicals, including sulforaphane and indoles. The seeds of the broccoli rabe plant are used to make rapeseed oil, also known as canola.

Maximizing nutrients Broccoli rabe should be cooked much the same way as broccoli (*at left*), the only difference being that broccoli rabe is generally too bitter to be eaten uncooked.

brussels sprouts

Nutrition profile Along with their savory flavor and satisfying texture, Brussels sprouts offer vitamin C, fiber, folate, and other B vitamins, as well as the carotenoids lutein and zeaxanthin. In addition, because they are cruciferous vegetables, Brussels sprouts also contain the phytochemicals indoles, isothiocyanates, and sulforaphane.

Maximizing nutrients Like other cruciferous vegetables, Brussels sprouts are on the bitter side and many people are not up to eating them uncooked. However, shredded raw Brussels sprouts make a very interesting slaw that is higher in vitamin C and B vitamins than cooked sprouts. Nonetheless, cooked sprouts are by far the norm, and the best way to cook them is quickly and in minimal liquid, such as steaming, microwaving, sautéing, or stir-frying. If you cook or serve Brussels sprouts with a little bit of unsaturated oil, it improves the absorption of their carotenoids, which are fat-soluble. In addition, cooking will enhance the availability of the indoles.

buckwheat

Nutrition profile The "wheat" in the name buckwheat is misleading, as it isn't related to wheat at all. In fact, buckwheat isn't a true grain, but rather the fruit of a leafy plant belonging to the rhubarb family. Robust and nutlike in flavor, buckwheat provides good-quality plant protein and is also a respectable source of niacin and fiber. The protein in buckwheat is of high quality because it contains all eight essential amino acids in good proportions, including significant amounts of lysine, the amino acid in which true grains, such as wheat, are most deficient. One

cup of buckwheat gives you 20% of the RDA for magnesium. In addition, buckwheat contains a type of flavonoid phytochemical called rutin.

Maximizing nutrients Cook buckwheat in a small amount of water (as you would cook rice) to get the most nutrients.

bulgur

Nutrition profile Just one cup of cooked bulgur will give you a generous amount of fiber (8.2 g) as well as a good amount of iron, magnesium, and niacin. Like other whole grains, bulgur also has various phytochemicals, such as lignans and saponins.

Maximizing nutrients Bulgur, which is parcooked and cracked, is one of the easiest forms of whole wheat to cook, requiring nothing more than steeping (soaking) in boiling water. It should be steeped in the minimum of water required to soften it, thus retaining maximum nutrients.

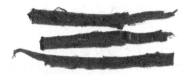

burdock

Nutrition profile A good source of magnesium and potassium, burdock is a root vegetable that has an earthy, sweet flavor. Burdock contains inulin (a nondigestible fiber), which is a prebiotic—something that may

help promote the growth of "good" bacteria in the colon. Some people may experience an allergic reaction to inulin.

Maximizing nutrients The minerals and fiber in burdock are not significantly affected by heat, though if cooked in too much water, some of the minerals will leach out.

butternut squash

Nutrition profile The deep orange flesh of butternut squash indicates the presence of carotenoids: In fact, 1 cup of cooked, mashed butternut squash provides 93% of the recommended daily intake for the carotenoid beta carotene. Rich in complex carbohydrates, butternut squash is also a good source of fiber, vitamin C, magnesium, and potassium.

Maximizing nutrients The carotenoids in butternut squash are made more bioavailable when it's cooked and/or served with a small amount of unsaturated fat, such as olive oil.

cabbage

Nutrition profile Along with its distinctive flavor, cabbage has good amounts of vitamin C, folate, and fiber (1 cup of cooked cabbage provides 6.6 g of fiber, and uncooked has 7.6 g). It also contains phytochemicals called

C

indoles, isothiocyanate and sulforaphane. Other phytochemicals called anthocyanins give red cabbage its color.

Maximizing nutrients Raw cabbage is a good source of vitamin C, but don't cut the cabbage up until fairly close to serving time: Cutting activates an enzyme that destroys vitamin C. Cooked cabbage will lose some of its folate and vitamin C, so it's best to use quick, minimum-liquid methods, such as steaming, microwaving, or stir-frying. The indole content, on the other hand, will be enhanced by cooking.

cantaloupe

Nutrition profile Low in calories and rich in potassium, vitamin B_6, and vitamin C, cantaloupe is an excellent source of the antioxidant beta carotene, providing more of this carotenoid than any other melon.

Maximizing nutrients Be sure to wash the rinds of cantaloupe (as well as other melons); they are susceptible to bacterial contamination because they grow on the ground. To preserve their vitamin C content, buy whole cantaloupes rather than pre-cut halves or cubes: This vitamin is diminished when the melon is cut and/or exposed to air.

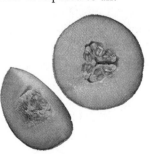

carrots

Nutrition profile Carrots are an exceptional source of plant pigments called carotenoids, which are so named because they were first identified in carrots. Carrots are the leading source in the American diet of beta carotene. Along with beta carotene, carrots also supply alpha carotene and lutein, other carotenoids that have antioxidant properties. The carrots with the deepest color contain the most carotenoids. Carrots are also a good source of vitamin B_6 and fiber.

Maximizing nutrients Because carotenoids are fat-soluble nutrients, cooking carrots with a little bit of fat (preferably monounsaturated fat, such as canola or olive oil), or eating them with other sources of fat, makes the beta carotene more available for absorption by the body. Cooking also makes the soluble fiber in the carrots more bioavailable; heat breaks down the cellulose walls and makes the soluble fiber within more available (this is the same process that tenderizes the carrots as they cook).

cashews

Nutrition profile Cashews provide magnesium, zinc, and vitamin E. They also are a rich source of plant sterols and monounsaturated fats, both of which are linked with heart health. Like most other nuts, cashews are high in calories (163 calories per ounce) and should be eaten in moderation.

Maximizing nutrients Cooking does not adversely affect the nutrients in cashews, but the proper storage (in the refrigerator or freezer) is important to help prevent their oils from going rancid.

cauliflower

Nutrition profile Vitamin C-rich cauliflower is a good source of the B vitamins folate and vitamin B_6. It is also exceptionally low in calories: You could eat 3 cups of cauliflower florets and still be getting under 100 calories. Like broccoli, cabbage, and its other cruciferous relatives, cauliflower is a reservoir of phytochemicals, such as isothiocyanates and indoles.

Maximizing nutrients Raw cauliflower will have more vitamin C than cooked, but as with all vegetables that contain vitamin C, cutting into the vegetable activates an enzyme that destroys the vitamin. So it's best to prepare cauliflower as close to serving time as possible. Because most of the vitamin C and the B vitamins in cauliflower can be lost if the vegetable is cooked in too much water or for too long, it is best to steam or microwave it quickly, or else use the cooking water for soup. On the other hand, cooking enhances the availability of the indoles in cauliflower.

celeriac (celery root)

Nutrition profile Closely related to celery, celeriac is low in calories and has modest amounts of vitamin C and potassium. However, what celeriac lacks in nutritional power it makes up for with its intense celery flavor.

Maximizing nutrients Celeriac can be eaten both raw and cooked. Raw celeriac (good in salads) will have the most vitamin C. The potassium content will not be affected by heat, but if cooked in too much water the potassium will leach out; steaming or braising are best for mineral retention.

celery

Nutrition profile Celery is mostly water, with little or no sugar, so it is very low in calories (about 6 per stalk). It has 35 mg of sodium—not much, but more than most vegetables. A large stalk also has small amounts of potassium, vitamin C, folate, fiber, and the carotenoid lutein.

Maximizing nutrients If possible, include the celery leaves when cooking. They contain a higher concentration of nutrients than the stalks.

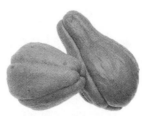

chayote

Nutrition profile Chayote (pronounced chy-OH-tay) is a summer squash, but unlike most other summer squashes, it is a rich source of fiber (4.5 g for 1 cup cooked). It is also a good source of vitamins C and B_6.

Maximizing nutrients To preserve their vitamin B_6 content, chayotes should be cooked in a minimum of water: Steaming, microwaving, and stir-frying are good choices. Or use it in a soup, where the liquid it's cooked in is also consumed.

cheese

Nutrition profile Rich in protein and an excellent source of the bone-building mineral calcium, cheese provides vitamin A, vitamin B_{12}, riboflavin, and zinc. The downside to cheese, however, is fat and calories: In fact, just an ounce (an average slice) of cheese contains 100 calories and more fat—most of it saturated—than a typical serving of ice cream. Some cheeses are already lower in fat (such as cottage cheese, part-skim mozzarella, and ricotta), but for other cheeses, there is a range of fat levels available: reduced-fat (25% or less fat per serving than regular, full-fat cheese), low-fat (no more than 3

g of fat per serving), and nonfat (less than 0.5 g fat per serving). In addition, sodium is a problem with most cheeses—almost all contain about 300 mg per ounce.

Maximizing nutrients Two things that fat brings to cheese are flavor and an ability to melt. So using reduced-fat cheeses can be a challenge on both fronts. For example, if reduced-fat cheeses (including low-fat and nonfat types) are exposed to high heat or are heated for too long, they go past "melted" and on to "rubber." However, if you add these cheeses toward the end of the cooking time, they will melt and not bind. The lower the fat content of the cheese, the more this is a delicate maneuver: Nonfat cheeses, for example, are best used in recipes where little to no heat is involved. As to the flavor issue, you might be better off using a small amount of a highly flavored full-fat cheese, such as Parmesan. This way you can significantly reduce the amount of saturated fat in the dish and still get cheese flavor (which is really what you're after anyway).

cherries

Nutrition profile Low in calories (½ cup has only 52) and abundant in flavor, cherries contain soluble fiber and vitamin C as well as phytochemicals such as quercetin (a flavonoid) and phenolic com-

C

pounds. In addition, cherries contain anthocyanins, which give a reddish-blue color to foods. Proponents of a folk remedy for gout believe that drinking cherry juice can help relieve pain and inflammation linked to gout, though there is no scientific evidence to support this belief.

Maximizing nutrients Uncooked cherries are best for preserving heat-sensitive vitamin C, and cooked cherries are best for increasing the availability of soluble fiber. Anthocyanin pigments will leach out when cherries are cooked in a liquid, but the liquid usually remains part of the dish (as in a cherry pie or sauce).

chestnuts

Nutrition profile Chestnuts provide potassium, protein, and B vitamins: 6 roasted chestnuts will supply 10% of the RDA for thiamin and 15% for vitamin B_6. Unlike most other nuts, chestnuts also furnish a respectable amount of vitamin C, and are very low in fat.

Maximizing nutrients Most chestnuts are cooked first (by roasting or boiling) in order to be added to another dish, such as a stuffing, and then cooked again. A second cooking will further diminish the vitamin C and vitamin B_6, since both can be destroyed by heat. Plain roasted chestnuts are probably the most nutritious form of this low-fat nut.

chick-peas

Nutrition profile Like most legumes, chick-peas (or garbanzo beans) are highly nutritious. Rich in complex carbohydrates, folate, iron, and zinc, chick-peas are an excellent source of both soluble and insoluble fiber. And ½ cup of cooked chick-peas supplies 7 g of protein and only 2 g of fat.

Maximizing nutrients Cooking beans is most efficiently done in a fair amount of water, which means that some of the water-soluble folate will be lost to the cooking water. However, ½ cup of cooked chick-peas still has 35% of the RDA for folate. It's always best to cook your own beans (*see page 180*): Not only can you control the sodium levels, but canned beans tend to be a little mushy. However, canned chick-peas retain their flavor and shape better than most other canned beans. They still have substantial amounts of sodium in the packing liquid, however; so be sure to rinse them well before using.

chicken

Nutrition profile Chicken (without the skin) supplies low-fat protein and is a rich source of vitamins and minerals. Chicken is a very good source of a number of B vitamins (riboflavin, niacin, B_6, and B_{12}) as well as the minerals iron, selenium, and zinc. Although dark-meat chicken, such as the thigh, is higher in fat than white meat (3 to 5 times

higher, depending on the bird), it also brings with it a higher concentration of minerals.

Maximizing nutrients For information on healthful ways to cook chicken, see page 104.

chicory

Nutrition profile An array of vitamins and minerals is found in the dark-green leaves of this salad green: beta carotene, riboflavin, vitamin C, vitamin E, and potassium, calcium, iron, and magnesium. Chicory provides a particularly impressive amount of folate (100% of the RDA in 2 cups).

chili peppers

Nutrition profile Noted for their hot, pungent bite, chili peppers are distinguished from sweet peppers by their burning flavor, which comes from a volatile substance called capsaicin. Producing a sudden sensation of heat (and often pain) in the mouth by targeting and stimulating pain receptors in the skin and mucous membranes, capsaicin can cause discomfort, sweating, watery eyes, and exhilaration. The amount of capsaicin varies considerably from one type of chili pepper to another. All chili peppers are a good source of vitamin C—though you would have to eat 1 tablespoon of them to get 25% of the RDA (not impossible for real chili lovers). And red chili peppers contain far more beta carotene than their green counterparts.

Maximizing nutrients The vitamin C in chili peppers is diminished by both chopping and cooking, but since the amount of chilies you have to eat to get the vitamin C is sizable, its nutritional contribution to a meal is really not the issue. The heat of chili peppers for many people acts as a flavor enhancer, often helping those on sodium-restricted diets.

chocolate

Nutrition profile Chocolate provides not only sensory satisfaction and luscious flavor, but also magnesium, copper, iron, zinc, and small amounts of protein. Ounce for ounce, the most minerals are found in unsweetened

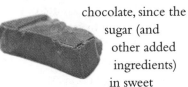

chocolate, since the sugar (and other added ingredients) in sweet chocolates displace some of the nutrients. The fat in chocolate is comprised almost equally of oleic acid (a monounsaturated fat also found in olive oil) and stearic and palmitic acids (both saturated fats). Recent studies indicate that dark chocolate contains phytochemicals called catechins (flavonoids also found in tea). And contrary to common belief, chocolate doesn't have a lot of caffeine; for exam-

ple, 1 ounce of semisweet chocolate has 5 to 10 mg of caffeine compared with a 6-ounce cup of coffee, which has 100 to 150 mg. Note that white chocolate isn't regarded by the FDA as real chocolate because it is made without cocoa solids, rather, it is derived from cocoa butter, sugar, milk, and added flavorings.

clams

Nutrition profile Clams are teeming with iron, and they also supply selenium and zinc, B vitamins, and are an exceptional source of vitamin B_{12}: A half dozen cooked clams has only 166 calories but provides about 40 times the required daily amount of vitamin B_{12}. And don't shun clams because shellfish have a reputation for being high in cholesterol: Clams are actually slightly lower in cholesterol per ounce than chicken or beef.

Maximizing nutrients The danger of contamination has made it quite risky to eat raw clams: Raw shellfish may harbor various kinds of bacteria and other potentially harmful organisms and should be cooked to avoid food poisoning. For healthful ways to cook clams, see page 65.

collard greens

Nutrition profile Collard greens supply a pleasant, piquant flavor as well as beta carotene, calcium, vitamin C, folate, and fiber. Like other cruciferous vegetables, collards provide phytochemicals,

including sulforaphane and indoles.

Maximizing nutrients The carotenoids, fiber, and indoles will all be more bioavailable when the collards are cooked. And cooking (or eating) the collards with a bit of unsaturated oil (such as olive or canola) will enhance the absorption of the beta carotene. The folate, on the other hand, will be diminished if the collards are cooked in a lot of water, so either use minimum-moisture cooking techniques, such as steaming or stir-frying, or be sure that the cooking water is part of the dish.

corn

Nutrition profile One of America's more popular foods, corn provides fiber, thiamin, folate, potassium, iron, and magnesium, and is a good source of complex carbohydrates. Only yellow corn, however, contains the carotenoids beta carotene, lutein and zeaxanthin.

Maximizing nutrients To preserve more of the water-soluble B vitamins (folate and thiamin) in corn, it's best to steam rather than boil it. If this isn't practical (since people often cook at least a dozen ears of corn), cook for no longer than 5 minutes in rapidly boiling water to minimize nutrient loss.

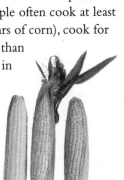

C

crab

Nutrition profile Low in fat and calories, crabmeat is a good source of protein, niacin, folate, zinc, iron, and provides an ample amount of the antioxidant mineral selenium. The notable nutrient in crabmeat, though, is vitamin B$_{12}$, with 3 ounces of cooked crabmeat supplying over 250% of the RDA. When you eat crab, you'll also benefit from their heart-healthy omega-3 fatty acids, which studies show may help to prevent fatal heart attacks. And although crabmeat is high in cholesterol, it is low in saturated fat, which may be more of a risk factor for heart disease than dietary cholesterol.

Maximizing nutrients For information on healthful ways to cook crab, see page 64.

cranberries

Nutrition profile Low in calories and high in vitamin C and fiber, fresh cranberries are more than a colorful holiday garnish. The pigments in cranberries are anthocyanins, similar to those in red grapes, blueberries, and many other red/blue/purple fruits and vegetables. In addition, other phytochemicals called procyanidins are found in cranberries and cranberry juice.

Maximizing nutrients The only way to eat cranberries is cooked (or dried), which forfeits their vitamin C content. However, their fiber is not compromised by cooking; and although their anthocyanin pigments will leach out into the cooking liquid, cranberries are generally eaten with this liquid (as in a cranberry sauce).

cucumbers

Nutrition profile Although the cucumber belongs to the same vegetable family as pumpkin, watermelon, and other squash, it doesn't offer the same nutritional value as its relatives, though it does have some potassium. The skin of cucumbers also contains the carotenoid lutein.

dandelion greens

Nutrition profile Dark leafy greens are among the most nutritious and adaptable of foods, and that well-known lawn pest and harbinger of spring, the dandelion, is no exception. Dandelion greens are rich in beta carotene, calcium, potassium, and fiber, along with some vitamin C and iron, but minimal calories. But be cautious: If you use pesticides, herbicides, or lawn fertilizers on your grass or nearby, stick with storebought dandelion greens. Don't pick dandelions by the roadside, either. If pets have access to your lawn, that's another reason to buy the greens at the store.

Maximizing nutrients Young dandelion greens are eaten fresh in salads, thus providing the most vitamin C. But you can also braise them in a small amount of liquid with a bit of oil to enhance the bioavailability of their beta carotene.

dates

Nutrition profile Low in fat and rich in potassium and fiber, dried dates are among the sweetest of fruits (up to 70% sugar by weight). A small amount of dates (only 2 ounces) has over 150 calories, but over 4 g of fiber.

duck

Nutrition profile Duck, like other types of poultry, is a good source of protein, B vitamins, iron (twice the amount found in turkey, and four times that in chicken), and selenium. And although most people think of duck as too fatty to eat, duck meat (the breast in particular) is actually leaner than chicken. A 3-ounce serving of skinless cooked duck breast has 30% less fat than the same amount of skinless chicken breast.

Maximizing nutrients For healthful ways to cook duck, see page 136.

eggplant

Nutrition profile High in fiber and low in fat, eggplant has a full flavor and a substantial, "meaty" texture that makes it an ideal food for vegetarians.

Maximizing nutrients Eggplant can act as a sponge for fats, so steaming, broiling/grilling, or baking are all good low-fat cooking options. Eggplant can also be successfully stir-fried and sautéed when it's cooked with a minimum of oil and other ingredients that provide some moisture. Many recipes call for salting eggplant before cooking it. This step draws out some of the moisture and produces a denser-textured flesh, which means the eggplant will exude less water and absorb less fat in cooking. Rinsing the eggplant thoroughly after salting will remove most of the salt; however, if you are following a sodium-restricted diet, you should not use this method.

eggs

Nutrition profile Eggs are a rich source of vitamin B$_{12}$, riboflavin, and selenium. The yolks contain the carotenoids, lutein and zeaxanthin and vitamin A, and are one of the few foods that naturally contain vitamin D. Egg whites are an excellent source of high-quality protein, considered nearly perfect because of its exemplary balance of amino acids.

With the increased awareness that dietary cholesterol is not the criminal it was once thought to

be, the per capita consumption of eggs in the U.S. has been steadily increasing. Nonetheless, people with high cholesterol would still be wise to limit egg consumption.

Maximizing nutrients It is possible to trim cholesterol and fat from egg recipes by cooking with fewer yolks than whites. You can substitute two whites for one whole egg for up to half the eggs in scrambled eggs or omelets. In other recipes, try substituting two egg whites plus 1 teaspoon of olive oil for each whole egg; this significantly reduces the cholesterol and saturated fat content of the dish, but drops the total fat content by only about 1 gram per egg. Sometimes you can simply substitute two egg whites for each whole egg called for, but only experimenting with your favorite recipes will tell which of them can be adapted this way: Eggs do perform very specific functions, especially in baking and sauce-making, and sometimes there is just no workable substitute or modification.

escarole

Nutrition profile A member of the chicory family, escarole is a bitter salad green with a good amount of folate, as well as some fiber (3 g per 2 cups), beta carotene, and potassium.

Maximizing nutrients Escarole can be served both uncooked in salad, and braised. Cooking the escarole in a minimum of liquid

and with a little bit of unsaturated fat will keep the loss of water-soluble folate to a minimum and maximize the availability of fat-soluble beta carotene.

fennel

Nutrition profile Although the pale green stalks of the fennel plant look like celery, there is no mistaking fennel's sweet licoricelike flavor. Like celery, though, fennel is low in calories, making it an ideal food for anyone who is watching his/her weight. Fennel also provides some vitamin C and potassium.

Maximizing nutrients Fennel is delicious both raw and cooked, though heat will diminish its vitamin C content.

figs

Nutrition profile Both fresh and dried figs are nutritious, with dried figs ounce for ounce being more nutrient-dense (as well as higher in calories) than the fresh form. Figs also provide some potassium and, because of their multitudes of tiny seeds, very good amount of fiber, including heart-healthy soluble fiber. Figs also contain plant sterols.

Maximizing nutrients Fresh figs are generally eaten uncooked, but dried figs are often stewed to soften them, making their soluble fiber more available.

fish

Nutrition profile While there are so many different types of fish, for practical purposes—both from a health standpoint and a cooking standpoint—it is easiest to divide fish into two main categories: lean or fatty. Lean fish are less than 5% fat by weight; and conversely, fatty fish are more than 5% fat by weight, though only a few so-called fatty fish are truly high in fat, with more than 10 g of fat per 3 ounces cooked.

All fish—both lean and fatty—are admirable sources of high-quality protein minus the artery-clogging saturated fat present in other high-protein foods. And fish contain the form of iron ("heme" iron) that is most readily and easily absorbed by our bodies. Most fish also contain notable amounts of B vitamins, especially thiamin, niacin, vitamin B_6, and vitamin B_{12}.

Fatty fish—which include mackerel, salmon, herring, and sardines—are very rich in the polyunsaturated fatty acids called omega-3s, which are important for heart health. And because this is one instance where fat may help protect the heart, the American Heart Association advises eating at least two servings of fish a week, especially fatty fish.

Salmon, sardines, and mackerel are also important sources of bone-strengthening vitamin D. And canned fish that include the bones provide good amounts of calcium: A 3-ounce serving of canned sardines with bones contains over 25% of a day's requirement for this mineral.

Maximizing nutrients For healthful ways to cook fish, see page 44.

flaxseeds

Nutrition profile Flaxseed is an ancient seed that is undergoing a resurgence of popularity. The health benefits of this tiny seed are linked to a wide range of nutrients, including alpha-linolenic acid (ALA), one of the fatty acids essential for human growth and development. The body converts ALA into the same type of heart-healthy omega-3 fatty acids found in fish. Flaxseed is also high in potassium and phytochemicals called lignans.

Generous quantities of both soluble and insoluble fiber are also present in flaxseed. The insoluble fiber helps to promote bowel regularity by preventing constipation. A considerable amount of the soluble fiber in flaxseed is mucilage, a thick, sticky substance that may help to lower LDL cholesterol. The oil pressed from flaxseeds also contains

ALA, but the fiber and lignans found in the whole seeds are lost during processing.

Maximizing nutrients Because flaxseeds are tiny and have a hard outer coating, they must be ground or thoroughly chewed; otherwise they can pass through the body undigested. Use a coffee grinder or spice grinder to grind them before adding them to a recipe. To preserve the oil's ALA and prevent it from going rancid, store flaxseed oil in the refrigerator and use it mostly in uncooked dishes such as salads.

flour, wheat

Nutrition profile Most of the wheat flour we eat is white flour, which has been stripped of the bran and germ of the wheat kernel, and thus also most of its fiber and many of its nutrients. For that reason, white flour is usually enriched with iron, niacin, riboflavin, thiamin, and folate and, sometimes even with fiber. Whole-wheat flour is made from the entire wheat kernel-bran, germ, and endosperm. Because all of the healthful parts of the grain are used, vitamins, minerals, fiber, and phytochemicals are plentiful in whole-wheat flour.

garlic

Nutrition profile Garlic contains a sulfur compound called allicin, released only when the clove is crushed or cut and allowed to stand for 10 minutes. This (and the compounds it converts into) is what gives these vegetables their strong taste and smell, and is what's thought to be beneficial. Since the amount of garlic used in most recipes is relatively small, it cannot confer any appreciable health benefit.

ginger

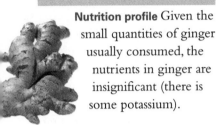

Nutrition profile Given the small quantities of ginger usually consumed, the nutrients in ginger are insignificant (there is some potassium).

grapefruit

Nutrition profile Ounce for ounce, red, pink, and white grapefruits have the same number of calories and amount of vitamin C, but the red and pink varieties have more than 40 times more beta carotene, plus some lycopene, another important carotenoid. When shopping for grapefruit and grapefruit juice, pink is better, but red is best. The redder the pulp, the more lycopene. Whatever its color, grapefruit is also rich in vitamin C, potassium, and pectin (the soluble fiber that helps to lower cholesterol levels). In addition, citrus flavonoids are also present in grapefruit. Grapefruit juice is also highly nutritious, though it lacks the fiber present in the whole fruit.

Maximizing nutrients Don't remove all of the pith, which is the white spongy layer between the zest and the pulp, because it contains a good amount of the fruit's fiber.

grapes

Nutrition profile While table grapes have modest amounts of vitamins and minerals, some varieties are good sources of vitamin C. The skins of red and purple grapes (as well as red and purple grape juice and red wine) contain a phytochemical called resveratrol. Grapes also contain the flavonoid phytochemical called quercetin.

guava

Nutrition profile An excellent source of vitamin C (a single guava provides more than twice the RDA), guava also supplies fiber (including heart-healthy pectin) and small amounts of the carotenoid lycopene, a red plant pigment.

Maximizing nutrients It's rare to find fresh guava outside Asian or Hispanic neighborhoods. Its more widely available form tends to be guava nectar, guava jelly, or cooked down guava paste. None of these forms has much vitamin C left (it's diminished by the processing), but the lycopene and pectin will be fine; in fact, they will be concentrated in the guava paste (along with a substantial amount of sugar).

hazelnuts

Nutrition profile Hazelnuts are a good source of thiamin, vitamin B_6, iron, and magnesium; and, compared with other nuts, they have a high vitamin E profile. If consumed in moderation (all nuts are calorie-dense), hazelnuts may yield cardiovascular benefits: they are high in monounsaturated fats, which are believed to lower LDL ("bad") cholesterol levels. They are a source of plant sterols, substances thought to reduce the risk of heart disease. And they have small amounts of alpha-linolenic acid (ALA), an omega-3 fatty acid related to those in fish. Studies indicate that even small amounts of this fat may help to prevent fatal heart attacks.

Maximizing nutrients Cooking does not adversely affect the nutrients in hazelnuts, but the proper storage (in the refrigerator or freezer) is important in preventing their oils from going rancid.

honeydew melon

Nutrition profile This sweet and juicy, white-green fleshed melon is a good source of the carotenoid, zeaxanthin. One cup of honeydew provides a mere 62 calories, as well as potassium, thiamin, and 49% of the RDA for the antioxidant vitamin C.

Maximizing nutrients Cutting the melon as close to serving time as possible will preserve more of its vitamin C.

h

jerusalem artichokes

Nutrition profile Jerusalem artichokes (also called sunchokes) contain quite a lot of iron (almost 30% of the RDA in 1 cup), potassium, B vitamins, and inulin (a nondigestible fiber), which is a prebiotic—something that may assist in the growth of "good" bacteria in the colon. Some people experience an allergic reaction to inulin.

Maximizing nutrients Serve cooked jerusalem artichokes with citrus juice or other vitamin-C rich food to enhance the absorption of their nonheme iron.

jícama

Nutrition profile Jícama, a tuber with a crisp apple-like flesh, provides vitamin C and fiber.

Maximizing nutrients Jícama is best eaten uncooked to retain its crunchy texture and vitamin C content.

kale

Nutrition profile One of the top sources of the carotenoid lutein, kale is low in calories and rich in vitamin B$_6$ and vitamin C. Other carotenoids found in kale are zeaxanthin and beta

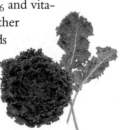

carotene. Because kale is a cruciferous vegetable, it is endowed with phytochemicals called sulforaphane and indoles.

Maximizing nutrients Cook kale to enhance its indole content, and with a small amount of unsaturated oil (such as canola or olive oil) to enhance the bioavailability of the carotenoids beta carotene, lutein, and zeaxanthin. Though cooking diminishes kale's vitamin C content, 1 cup of cooked kale still has a respectable amount: a little over 50% of the RDA.

kiwifruit

Nutrition profile Kiwifruit provides a rich assortment of nutrients, such as vitamin C, fiber, potassium, folate, and magnesium. Particularly noteworthy is its abundance of the carotenoid lutein. Furthermore, kiwifruit contains the antioxidant vitamin E—and unlike most other sources of vitamin E (such as vegetable oils and nuts), kiwifruit is low in fat and calories.

Maximizing nutrients To preserve the vitamin C content in kiwifruit, it is best to eat the fruit uncooked. If you combine kiwifruit with meat, poultry, or fish (in a salad, for example), don't let the mixture sit too long before serving; kiwi's enzyme, actinidin, will begin to "tenderize" the animal protein and turn it mushy.

kohlrabi

Nutrition profile Kohlrabi is a member of the cabbage family and provides a hefty amount of potassium as well as fiber, vitamin B$_6$, an impressive supply of vitamin C (1 cup cooked will give you almost 100% of the RDA), and a good deal of potassium. In addition, this crisp, sweet-tasting vegetable is a rich source of vitamin E, which is unusual considering that vitamin E is mostly found in high-fat foods: 1 cup will give you about 18% of this antioxidant vitamin. And because it is a cruciferous vegetable, you will also be getting phytochemicals such as indoles, sulforaphane, and isothiocyanates.

Maximizing nutrients Uncooked kohlrabi will have the most vitamin C, but cooking will enhance it's indole availability. To best preserve kohlrabi's water-soluble vitamin C and vitamin B, use a quick-cooking, minimum-liquid method such as steaming, microwaving, or stir-frying.

lamb

Nutrition profile Cut for cut, lamb contains approximately the same amount of internal fat as beef, and offers similarly significant levels of riboflavin, vitamin B$_{12}$, niacin, iron, and zinc.

Maximizing nutrients For healthful ways to cook lamb, see page 97.

leeks

Nutrition profile Highly versatile, with a delicate flavor, leeks are low in calories (only about 32 calories per cup cooked) and a good source of fiber and iron. And because they are members of the *Allium* family (onions, shallots), they contain a phytochemical called diallyl sulfide.

Maximizing nutrients While many recipes call for only the white part of leeks, you should consider using the dark green leaves as well, since they are a good source of nutrients.

lemons

Nutrition profile Beyond their tart, intense, refreshing flavor, lemons also supply potassium and a wealth of vitamin C (2 tablespoons of lemon juice provides more than 15% of the RDA). Whole lemons also offer fiber. Phytochemicals called limonenes are in lemon peels.

Maximizing nutrients Since vitamin C is destroyed by exposure to heat, light, and oxygen, squeeze lemons to make juice as close as possible to when you plan on using it. Also, the vitamin C content will be the highest when the juice is added to uncooked dishes. To get the most limonenes, grate the zest (the colored outer layer of the peel) of the lemons and use it in the dish, too.

lentils

Nutrition profile An inexpensive source of high-quality protein, lentils provide an excellent amount of fiber and the B vitamin folate. For example, a mere ½-cup serving of lentils will supply almost half of the RDA for folate and 30% of the recommended daily intake for fiber. Lentils also have other B vitamins (vitamin B_6 and thiamin), as well as potassium, iron, and zinc.

Maximizing nutrients To protect the water-soluble vitamins folate and vitamin B_6, don't cook lentils in too much water; and if any cooking liquid needs to be drained off, try to use it in the recipe or save for soups or other dishes. The soluble fiber in lentils is made more bioavailable as the lentils cook and the fiber dissolves. Eat foods high in vitamin C along with lentils to enhance nonheme iron absorption.

lettuce

Nutrition profile Most lettuce will provide vitamin C and the B vitamin folate, and some will also supply beta carotene. However, compared with many other leafy green vegetables, lettuce offers minimal nutritional value. There are many different types of lettuce, with the darker varieties generally offering a greater number of nutrients. For example, a darker leaf lettuce such as romaine contains far more folate, iron, and potassium than do the types of lettuce with pale leaves such as iceberg lettuce.

Maximizing nutrients Because cutting vegetables activates an enzyme that destroys vitamin C, whole lettuce leaves would have the most vitamin C. However, since eating whole leaves is impractical with large lettuces, it does suggest that there is a nutritional benefit to eating baby lettuces (as in mesclun) that do not need to be cut up. For large-leaf lettuce, cut it or tear it into bite-size pieces close to serving time.

lima beans

Nutrition profile Lima beans are a good source of B vitamins (vitamin B_6, niacin, folate), protein (including the important amino acid lysine), fiber (especially soluble fiber in the form of pectin), iron, potassium, and magnesium; and they have very little fat.

Maximizing nutrients Lima beans come fresh (rare), frozen, and dried. For fresh and frozen, cook the beans with a minimum of water (steaming or microwaving) to preserve as much of their water-soluble B vitamins as possible. For dried limas, in which a good deal of water is required to cook them, try to incorporate the cooking water into the dish. Cooking limas in soup is a good solution.

limes

Nutrition profile Fragrant and tangy, the lime is an excellent seasoning as well as a good source of vitamin C, with 2 tablespoons of lime juice providing about 10% of the RDA for this indispensable antioxidant vitamin. The whole fruit contains fiber. And as with lemons, limes contain phytochemicals called limonenes.

Maximizing nutrients Since vitamin C is destroyed by exposure to heat, light, and oxygen, squeeze limes to make juice as close to cooking time as possible. Also, the vitamin C content will be the highest when the juice is added to uncooked dishes. To get the most limonenes, grate the zest (the colored outer layer of the peel) of the limes and use it in the dish, too.

lobster

Nutrition profile Lobster provides huge amounts of vitamin B_{12} and the antioxidant mineral selenium, as well as some zinc. In spite of its cholesterol content, which is high compared with other shellfish (61 mg for a 3-ounce serving), its fat is largely healthful unsaturated fats, including some omega-3s.

Maximizing nutrients For healthful ways to cook lobster, see page 64.

mackerel

Nutrition profile All types of mackerel are high-fat fish, which means that they contain omega-3s, beneficial fats that may protect against fatal heart attacks. In fact, mackerel is among the leading sources for these heart-healthy fats. Highly nourishing, mackerel is a good source of protein, riboflavin, niacin, vitamin B_6, vitamin E, iron, magnesium, and it also provides a hefty amount of vitamin B_{12} (almost 675% of the RDA for this important vitamin) and about 80% of the RDA for the antioxidant mineral selenium.

Maximizing nutrients To retain the maximum amount of its water-soluble B vitamins, mackerel are best cooked by dry-heat methods such as grilling, baking, or roasting.

mangoes

Nutrition profile Mangoes are not only delicious tropical fruits with a lush texture and beautiful color, they are also rich in nutrients. Mangoes have good amounts of soluble fiber, vitamin C, and vitamin E. Their orange flesh also indicates the presence of beta carotene as well as small amounts of another carotenoid, beta cryptoxanthin.

Maximizing nutrients Eating a mango with a small amount of unsaturated oil (as in a salad or a salsa) will improve the body's ability to absorb the carotenoids in the fruit.

milk

Nutrition profile In relation to its calories, milk provides an abundance of nutrients, which makes it an important, nutrient-dense food. It offers high-quality protein, and is also the leading source of the bone-nourishing mineral calcium in the American diet. Milk is a rich source of potassium, vitamins A and D, riboflavin, and vitamin B_{12}. Fat-free and low-fat (1%) milks contain all the nutrients of whole milk without the extra fat.

Maximizing nutrients You can substitute low-fat (1%) milk for whole milk in many baking, pudding, sauce, and soup recipes. The result will be a somewhat less rich dish, but saturated fat levels will be considerably lower. To add richness to low-fat milk, without adding any fat, stir 2 tablespoons of nonfat dry milk powder into 1 cup liquid milk.

millet

Nutrition profile Millet is an ancient grain that deserves to be rediscovered. Low in fat and a good source of plant protein and fiber, millet supplies an impressive assortment of essential nutrients. For example, ½ cup of cooked millet will give you 8 g of protein and over 15% of the RDA for the following: thiamin (21%), riboflavin (15%), niacin (20%), vitamin B_6 (15%), iron (19%), magnesium (a whopping 25%), and zinc (20%).... not bad for only ½ cup.

Maximizing nutrients To get the most out of millet's wealth of water-soluble B vitamins, cook it in a minimum of water that doesn't get drained off (as you would cook rice).

mushrooms

Nutrition profile Mushrooms are more than just wonderful flavor enhancers: They provide riboflavin, niacin, vitamin B_6, and a type of soluble fiber called beta glucan. And as a boon to those watching their calorie intake, mushrooms have a complex, satisfying flavor and texture for almost no calories (2 whole cups of raw mushrooms have about 40 calories).

Maximizing nutrients Fresh mushrooms are sponges, so when sautéing or stir-frying, try to use as little fat as possible. There are two ways to accomplish this: You can start sautéing the mushrooms with a combination of water or broth plus a small amount of olive oil. Or, you can start the mushrooms with a small amount of oil over very low heat, in a covered pan. In a short time, the mushrooms will give off enough liquid to provide their own "broth" for cooking

in. For dried mushrooms, when you soak them to reconstitute them, use the soaking water in the recipe. This not only adds flavor to the dish, but also uses whatever B vitamins might have leached into the soaking water.

mussels

Nutrition profile Mussels are low in fat and rich in nutrients, including heart-healthy omega-3 fatty acids. Sweet and delicate in flavor, mussels offer a good supply of protein, and an extraordinary quantity of vitamin B_{12} (3 ounces cooked will give you 851% of the RDA for this important B vitamin). In addition, just 3 ounces of cooked mussels, at only 146 calories, will give you substantial amounts of thiamin, riboflavin, niacin, folate, iron, zinc, and a hefty 139% of the RDA for the antioxidant mineral selenium.

Maximizing nutrients For healthful ways of cooking mussels, see page 65.

mustard greens

Nutrition profile The piquant and nutritious leafy part of the plant from which we get mustard seed, mustard greens are rich in beta carotene, vitamin C, and folate. In addition, because they are a cruciferous vegetable, mustard greens provide phytochemicals called indoles and isothiocyanates.

Maximizing nutrients To preserve its folate and enhance the beta

carotene availability, cook mustard greens in a small amount of liquid with a bit of monounsaturated fat (such as olive or canola oil). Cooking will also enhance the availability of indoles.

napa cabbage

Nutrition profile Napa cabbage (also called Chinese cabbage) is a rich source of folate, with 1 cup cooked supplying 12% of the RDA for this B vitamin. In addition, 1 cup will also give you 37% of the RDA for zinc.

Maximizing nutrients Napa cabbage is good both uncooked (in salads) and cooked, usually in stir-fries, soups, or stews. Although heat will destroy some of the folate, any that leaches into the cooking liquid will be consumed along with the dish.

n

nectarines

Nutrition profile Sweeter and darker-fleshed than peaches, nectarines are low in calories and are a good source of potassium and fiber. Two antioxidant carotenoids, beta carotene and beta cryptoxanthin, bestow a vivid golden-yellow hue to nectarine flesh. In addition, rosey-skinned nectarines contain natural plant pigments called anthocyanins.

Maximizing nutrients Nectarines can be eaten (cooked or uncooked) with their skin, which in brightly colored specimens will contribute healthful carotenoids and other pigments.

nut oils

Nutrition profile With the exception of fiber, nut oils generally provide the same minerals, vitamins, and beneficial monounsaturated fats found in the nuts themselves. Like the nuts from which they're pressed, nut oils are very low in saturated fats. Almond, hazelnut, macadamia, pecan, and pistachio oils are rich sources of monounsaturated fats, which help to lower blood cholesterol; walnut oil also supplies heart-healthy alpha-linolenic acid (ALA); and almond and hazelnut oils are notable sources of vitamin E.

Maximizing nutrients Store nut oils in the refrigerator to prevent them from becoming rancid. Overheating will diminish the flavor of nut oils, so either add them at the end of the cooking time, or use the oils unheated in salad dressings.

okra

Nutrition profile Cooked sliced okra exudes a slimy juice that is a combination of tongue-twisting chemical substances (acetylated acidic polysaccharide and galacturonic acid). It is this mucilaginous quality that makes some people avoid okra, but causes others to seek it out, especially for its ability to add a thickness to stews like gumbo. This unusual vegetable has much to offer nutritionally. It is a good source of B vitamins, vitamin C, magnesium, potassium, and fiber, as well as the carotenoids lutein and zeaxanthin. It is particularly rich in soluble fiber, which may help to lower LDL ("bad") cholesterol levels.

Maximizing nutrients For a stand-alone vegetable side dish, briefly cooking whole okra in a low-moisture method (steaming or microwaving) preserves more of its water-soluble B vitamins, keeps the vegetable crisp, and keeps its thickening juices contained. When okra's thickening capability is desirable, the pods can be sliced and cooked along with the other ingredients in the soup or stew.

olive oil

Nutrition profile An excellent source of the monounsaturated fatty acid oleic acid, olive oil also supplies vitamin E and certain phytochemicals. Studies indicate that monounsaturated fatty acids may reduce the risk of developing atherosclerosis. Olive oil also supplies polyphenol phytochemicals. If you are watching your

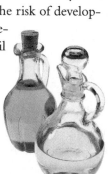

weight, you should keep in mind that while olive oil is a healthy, nutritious alternative to other fat sources, it is, nonetheless, high in calories and should be consumed in moderation.

Maximizing nutrients To preserve flavor, store olive oil in an airtight container in the refrigerator or another cool, dark place, and use as soon as possible. Refrigerated olive oil will solidify, so you have to let it reach room temperature before it can be poured.

olives

Nutrition profile Though a large percentage of the caloric content of olives is fat, it's derived from heart-healthy monounsaturated fats. Olives also contain the antioxidant vitamin E, and polyphenol phytochemicals. It's important to note, however, that most olives are quite high in sodium.

Maximizing nutrients Olives can contribute good flavor to a dish without an overload of sodium if they are chopped or minced. This way you can use a small number of olives but still permeate the dish with their flavor.

onions

Nutrition profile Along with their savory, pungent flavor, onions supply fiber, vitamin C, potassium, and vitamin B_6. Onions, particularly red onions, provide quercetin, an important member of a large group of plant compounds called flavonoids. Onions are also a rich source of a phytochemical called diallyl sulfide.

Maximizing nutrients Chopping or slicing an onion brings its sulfur-containing amino acids into contact with enzymes to form volatile compounds, one of which strikes the tongue, while another irritates the eye, apparently by turning into sulfuric acid. Enzymes released by chopping are also responsible for diminishing the onion's vitamin C content. Cooking, on the other hand, will tame the sulfur compounds and further diminish vitamin C. So for those who admire raw onions, there are some nutritional advantages. However, cooked onions retain their fine fiber content, and as long as they are not boiled in a liquid that does not get consumed, the potassium and vitamin B_6 are retained as well.

oranges

Nutrition profile While most people tend to associate the benefits of oranges and their juice with vitamin C, they may not be aware that oranges are also a good source of folate, potassium, and thiamin. In addition, the whole fruit (as opposed to the juice) has the added benefit of more than 3 g of fiber. Phytochemicals in oranges include citrus flavonoids as well as limonenes.

Maximizing nutrients If making fresh-squeezed orange juice, be sure to refrigerate it in a glass

container: Unlike permeable plastic or waxed paper cartons, glass will prevent oxygen from getting in and diminishing the vitamin C. To get the most limonenes, grate the zest (the colored outer layer of the peel) of the oranges and use it in the dish, too.

oysters

Nutrition profile

Oysters are a good source of protein. And while they contain dietary cholesterol, they are low in saturated fat, which has a more harmful impact on blood cholesterol. Small amounts of heart-healthy omega-3 fatty acids can also be found in oysters. In addition, oysters supply a rich compendium of vitamins and minerals, including thiamin, riboflavin, niacin, vitamin C, vitamin E, and magnesium. Most notable, however, are the oyster's vitamin B_{12}, zinc, selenium, and vitamin D content: A single oyster has, respectively, 300%, 151%, 140%, and 78% of the RDA for these nutrients.

Maximizing nutrients Raw shellfish may harbor various kinds of bacteria and other potentially harmful organisms and should be cooked to avoid food poisoning. For healthful ways to cook oysters, see page 66.

papaya

Nutrition profile Sweet and refreshing, and an impressive source of vitamin C, papaya also supplies fiber, folate, vitamin E, potassium, and the carotenoids beta cryptoxanthin and beta carotene.

Maximizing nutrients Fresh papaya, used in desserts or salsas, will have the most vitamin C. Note, however, that uncooked papaya has a protein-eating enzyme called papain (often used as a meat tenderizer); if raw papaya is left for too long in combination with other ingredients (as in a salad), it will start to break them down and turn them mushy. Cooking papaya (it can be baked like winter squash) will inactivate the papain, and will also make the fruit's carotenoids more bioavailable.

parsnips

Nutrition profile Parsnips provide ample amounts of fiber, especially the soluble fiber pectin, which may lower LDL ("bad") cholesterol levels, thus helping to prevent heart disease. Vitamin C and folate are the most prominent nutrients, but there are also decent amounts of thiamin, vitamin E, iron, and magnesium.

Maximizing nutrients Cooking makes the soluble fiber in the parsnips more bioavailable; heat breaks down the cellulose walls and makes the soluble fiber within more available (this also tenderizes the parsnips as they cook). When cooking parsnips, use a dry-heat method (such as roasting) or a low-moisture method (such as steaming, microwaving, or stir-frying) to retain more of their water-soluble B vitamins.

peaches

Nutrition profile Sweet and juicy, peaches have moderate amounts of fiber, including pectin, which can lower cholesterol. Though the amount of vitamin E in a single peach is only 7% of the RDA, it is an amount worth noting, since it's rare to find this vitamin in a low-fat food.

Maximizing nutrients Cooking peaches makes their soluble fiber more bioavailable, but the vitamin E content will be the same in both cooked and uncooked.

peanuts

Nutrition profile Peanuts are actually legumes, like beans and peas, but their use in cooking more closely resembles that of nuts. Rich in plant protein, peanuts supply vitamin E, folate, niacin, and magnesium, and they also provide a good amount of fiber. Peanuts are low in saturated fat and are a good source of heart-healthy monounsaturated and polyunsaturated fats, as well as cholesterol-lowering plant

sterols. In fact, studies indicate that a diet rich in peanuts (and peanut butter) may help to reduce blood cholesterol. It is important to keep in mind that although peanuts have a favorable fats profile, they are still high in calories and should be eaten in moderation.

Maximizing nutrients Cooking does not adversely affect the nutrients in peanuts, but the proper storage (in the refrigerator or freezer) is important to help prevent their oils from going rancid.

pears

Nutrition profile Juicy and tender, pears offer a good amount of dietary fiber, including the heart-healthy soluble fiber pectin. In part because of their fiber content, pears make a satisfying low-calorie dessert.

Maximizing nutrients A good percentage of the fiber in pears is in the skin or just under it, so unpeeled pears will give you the most fiber. And the bioavailability of the soluble fiber pectin will be somewhat increased when the pears are cooked.

peas, dried

Nutrition profile Low in fat and with a moderate amount of protein, dried peas have an excellent amount of fiber (8 g for ½ cup cooked) and good amounts of the B vitamins folate and thiamin, as well as potassium and iron.

Maximizing nutrients Since dried peas are generally cooked into soups or purees—dishes in which the cooking liquid is not thrown away—even the B vitamins and minerals that leach into the cooking water will be consumed.

peas, fresh

Nutrition profile Peas are low in fat and provide copious amounts of vitamins, minerals, and fiber. Rich in thiamin, riboflavin, niacin, vitamin C, iron, magnesium, and zinc, peas are also a good source of plant protein, though the protein is incomplete because peas lack certain essential amino acids. Just 1 cup of cooked green peas will supply 25% of the RDA for folate and 20% of the RDA for vitamin B_6. Peas also contain the carotenoid lutein. And though fresh peas (in the pod) are not that easy to come by, frozen green peas retain their nutritional value, as well as their flavor.

Maximizing nutrients Heat-sensitive vitamin C and water-soluble B vitamins (folate and B_6) are best preserved if you either quickly steam or microwave peas. Peas can also be cooked in a bit of water along with seasonings and a small amount of unsaturated fat. The seasoned water into which some of the B vitamins have leached then can serve as a a a sauce for the peas.

pecans

Nutrition profile Pecans contain thiamin, zinc, and fiber. They also provide heart-healthy monounsaturated and polyunsaturated fats, which help to lower blood cholesterol, especially when substituted for foods high in saturated fat. Plant sterols are also found in pecans. Still, like other nuts, pecans are high in calories and should be consumed in moderation.

Maximizing nutrients Cooking does not adversely affect the nutrients in pecans, but the proper storage (in the refrigerator or freezer) is important to help prevent their oils from going rancid.

peppers

Nutrition profile Although all bell peppers provide fiber and vitamin B_6, there are some nutritional differences that depend on the color of the pepper. For example, yellow and red bell peppers provide more than twice the amount of vitamin C as green peppers. And red peppers contain 11 times more beta carotene than green. One large bell pepper has only 44 calories. (*See also Chili peppers, page 280.*)

Maximizing nutrients To maximize the bioavailability of the carotenoids, cook peppers with a little monounsaturated fat, such as canola or olive oil. Or, roast peppers and toss in a small amount of olive oil. For vitamin C, eat uncooked peppers, since

this vitamin is easily destroyed by heat.

persimmons

Nutrition profile Persimmons are good sources of vitamin C, beta carotene, and potassium, and are fairly low in calories (60 in 3 ounces). About 90% of persimmons sold in the U.S. are the Hachiya variety, which are astringent when unripe and must be fully ripened and soft before they are edible. Fuyu persimmons, which are edible when they are hard-ripe, have six times more vitamin C—200 mg in 3 ounces, which is more than double the RDA. Carotenoid pigments in persimmons are notable as well; the vivid color of the fruit is due to alpha carotene, beta carotene, and beta cryptoxanthin (which is present in particularly high amounts).

Maximizing nutrients More often than not, persimmons are eaten in their raw state. However, the sturdier Fuyu persimmon can be sautéed in a small amount of oil, thus increasing the availability of the carotenoids. While the peel on the Hachiya persimmon is often highly tannic and bitter, the skin of the Fuyu is tasty and provides a certain amount of fiber.

pine nuts

Nutrition profile Rich in magnesium, monounsaturated fats, and iron, pine nuts (also called pignoli or piñon nuts) are slender, ivory-colored, high-fat nuts that come from several varieties of pine trees. Depending upon where the pine nut is grown, the nutrition content will vary slightly; for example, the European species of pine nuts are richer in protein and lower in fat than the American varieties, but American pine nuts offer more vitamins and minerals.

Maximizing nutrients Cooking does not adversely affect the nutrients in pine nuts, but the proper storage (in the refrigerator or freezer) is important to help prevent their oils from going rancid.

pineapple

Nutrition profile Pineapple is a rich source of vitamin C, thiamin, and the mineral manganese. Both fresh and canned pineapple are widely available, including already cut-up fresh. If you prefer canned, be sure to buy pineapple that is not packed in sugar syrup. The fruit is plenty sweet on its own.

Maximizing nutrients For maximum vitamin C content, eat pineapple uncooked, and cut it up as close to serving time as possible.

pistachios

Nutrition profile Buttery, sweet, and slightly smoky in flavor, the pistachio nut, like most nuts, is also packed with nutritional value. It is a rich source of vitamins B_6 and E, thiamin, iron, magnesium, fiber, and potassium, as well as heart-healthy monounsaturated fatty acids and plant sterols. Its delicate flavored kernel is naturally green and is covered with a fine, thin, pale brown skin that need not be removed before eating.

Maximizing nutrients Cooking does not adversely affect the nutrients in pistachios, but the proper storage (in the refrigerator or freezer) is important to help prevent their oils from going rancid.

plums, fresh

Nutrition profile While they provide a concentration of nutrients in their dried form as prunes, fresh plums are, nonetheless, a decent source of vitamin C and fiber. The plant pigments that make plums purple are called anthocyanins.

Maximizing nutrients For vitamin C retention, plums are best consumed uncooked. But when cooking plums, cook them with their skins on for the most fiber.

plums, dried

Nutrition profile Dried plums (prunes) furnish more than the well-known laxative benefits. Along with providing magnesium, iron, and potassium, dried plums are also a good source of fiber-both soluble and insoluble. And recent research has shed light on the antioxidant potential of dried plums. In fact, in one well-known study they appear at the top of a long list of fruits and vegetables tested for antioxidant status.

Maximizing nutrients Stewing dried plums makes their soluble fiber more bioavailable.

pomegranates

Nutrition profile The juicy, sweet seeds of a pomegranate provide vitamin B_6, vitamin C, and potassium. Pomegranates have a wealth of phytochemicals, including ellagic acid, catechins, and anthocyanins, the pigments that lend pomegranates their crimson color.

pork

Nutrition profile Pork supplies significant amounts of thiamin, riboflavin, niacin, and selenium as well as good amounts of vitamin B_6, vitamin B_{12}, iron, potassium, zinc, and high-quality protein. As with beef, the guidelines for including pork in your diet are to choose lean cuts (such as tenderloin and center loin or extra-lean ham), to eat small portions (3 ounces cooked), and to trim all visible fat before cooking. However, unlike beef, you can't rely on a grading system for pork to give you a clue to the fat content of the cut.

Maximizing nutrients For healthful ways to cook pork, see page 82.

potatoes

Nutrition profile Potatoes are a good source of vitamin C, thiamin, iron, niacin, and fiber, and they also supply ample amounts of potassium. In addition, one large baked potato gives you almost 50% of the RDA for vitamin B_6.

Maximizing nutrients Try to eat potatoes with the skin, where most of the iron and fiber are found. And whenever possible, regardless of the cooking method, cook whole unpeeled potatoes to preserve most of the water-soluble B vitamins; you can peel them after they're cooked. If a recipe calls for cooking cut-up potatoes, you can minimize the loss of B vitamins by steaming the potatoes (although most recipes would call for boiling them).

pumpkin

Nutrition profile Low in fat and nutritious, pumpkins offer more than their mild, sweet flavor, they also provide a rich bounty of beta carotene as well as fiber, potassium, riboflavin, and vitamins C and E. Other carotenoids such as alpha carotene and lutein are also found in pumpkin. Canned pumpkin puree, by far the most common form of pumpkin in the American diet, is more nutritious than fresh: ½ cup has more beta carotene than a standard supplement (15,000 IU), plus a good amount of fiber, iron, and other minerals, but just 40 calories.

Maximizing nutrients Cooking or eating pumpkin with a small amount of unsaturated oil will improve the body's ability to absorb the fat-soluble carotenoids and vitamin E.

pumpkin seed oil

Nutrition profile Pumpkin seed oil is rich in oleic acid and linoleic acid, both unsaturated fats that may prevent hardening of the arteries and reduce LDL cholesterol levels in the blood. The oil also contains plant sterols.

Maximizing nutrients To prevent pumpkin seed oil from going rancid, make sure to keep it refrigerated and away from direct sunlight or heat. It is also best and most flavorful if added toward the end of cooking, since direct heat (*e.g.*, in a skillet) breaks it down and dissipates its fragrance.

pumpkin seeds

Nutrition profile A good source of magnesium, zinc, vitamin E, and iron, pumpkin seeds serve as an ideal snack as well as a tasty addition to a variety of recipes. One ounce of pumpkin seeds will give you 36% of the RDA for magnesium, and 21% of the RDA for vitamin E. In addition, these flavorful morsels provide both essential and unsaturated fatty acids, as well as plant sterols.

Maximizing nutrients Cooking does not adversely affect the nutrients in pumpkin seeds, but the proper storage (in the refrigerator or freezer) is important to help prevent their oils from going rancid.

quince

Nutrition profile Quince provides substantial amounts of fiber, including cholesterol-lowering soluble fiber pectin, and vitamin C.

Maximizing nutrients Quince must be cooked to be edible, but its substantial soluble fiber content will be made more bioavailable in the process.

quinoa

Nutrition profile An ancient grain, quinoa (pronounced KEEN-wah) is not a true grain, but it looks like one and has similar uses. A highly nutritious food, quinoa supplies riboflavin, vitamin E, iron, magnesium, potassium, zinc, and fiber. But one nutrient that distinguishes quinoa from most other plant foods is its high level of lysine, an amino acid necessary for the synthesis of protein, making it one of the best sources of plant protein.

Maximizing nutrients Cook quinoa in a minimum of water (as you would cook rice) to conserve nutrients that leach into the cooking water. Eating quinoa with a food high in vitamin C will improve the body's ability to absorb its nonheme iron.

radicchio

Nutrition profile Deep burgundy red with white ribs, radicchio resembles a small head of cabbage. Two cups of this member of the chicory family will yield only 18 calories and 12% of the RDA for both vitamin E and folate.

radishes

Nutrition profile These sharp-flavored root vegetables are low in calories and a good source of vitamin C (29% of the RDA in 1 cup of red radish slices). And, like their cruciferous relatives, radishes possess phytochemicals.

Maximizing nutrients Radishes are most commonly eaten uncooked, which will provide the maximum amount of vitamin C.

raisins

Nutrition profile These sweet dried grapes are a concentrated source of the nutrients (as well as calories and sugar) found in the whole fruit. They are rich in iron, potassium, and soluble and insoluble fiber. And raisins made from red and purple grapes that are cured indoors (*i.e.,* not in the sun) have small amounts of resveratrol, a phytochemical found in the skins.

Maximizing nutrients If you cook raisins in a liquid high in vitamin C (such as orange juice), even though some of the liquid's vitamin C will be diminished, it will still help make the nonheme iron present in raisins more bioavailable.

raspberries

Nutrition profile Fragrant, delicate, and sweet, raspberries are low in calories and offer an impressive amount of vitamin C (1 cup provides 34% of the RDA) and a good amount of dietary fiber, much of it coming from the seeds. In addition, raspberries get their color from phytochemicals called anthocyanins.

Maximizing nutrients Try to eat raspberries fresh, because cooking can destroy some of their vitamin C. If making a raspberry sauce, do not strain out the seeds in order to get the benefit of their fiber.

rhubarb

Nutrition profile The thick, celerylike stalks of rhubarb supply a hefty amount of fiber as well as vitamin C, potassium, and manganese. And while rhubarb has some calcium, it also has high levels of substances called oxalates, which interfere with the body's absorption of the plant's calcium content. Don't eat rhubarb leaves since they are toxic.

Maximizing nutrients Rhubarb is most commonly cooked with sugar to sweeten it, a process that increases the calories and greatly diminishes its vitamin C content. On the plus side, cooking makes its soluble fiber more bioavailable. One trick to keeping calories down in sweet rhubarb dishes is to cook them with sweet fruits (such as apples), decreasing the amount of sugar required.

rice

Nutrition profile Highly nutritious and low in fat, rice is a valuable source of complex carbohydrates, vitamins, minerals, and fiber—no wonder rice is a staple food for a large segment of the world's population. When white rice is refined, it is milled and polished, a process that removes the bran and germ as well as valuable nutrients. Most white rice in the U.S., however, is enriched with thiamin, niacin, folate, and iron. Enriched white rice is a good source of these nutrients, as well as fiber and selenium.

Brown rice, which has only the outer hull removed, retains—along with its bran layer—thiamin, niacin, and vitamin B_6. Because the bran is not milled away, brown rice has five times more fiber than white rice, supplying 3.5 g of fiber per 1-cup serving. Furthermore because brown rice retains the bran and the germ, it also provides phytochemicals, including oryzanol, which is found in the rice's outer layer.

Maximizing nutrients When cooking rice, do not rinse it before (or after), because that washes away essential nutrients (possible exception: rice purchased in bulk, which may need cleaning). Also avoid cooking rice with excess water to retain its B vitamins.

rutabagas

Nutrition profile Rutabagas (yellow-fleshed turnips) supply good amounts of both insoluble and cholesterol-lowering soluble fiber. These sweet and slightly pungent root vegetables also contain beta carotene, B vitamins, and a sizable amount of potassium and vitamin C.

Maximizing nutrients Although cooking rutabagas diminishes their vitamin C, they still have a respectable amount: 1 cup of cooked rutabaga cubes provides over 35% of the RDA. Rutabagas are best cooked in low-moisture methods, such as steaming or microwaving.

rye

Nutrition profile Along with its distinctive, hearty taste, rye supplies fiber, protein, magnesium, thiamin, niacin, iron, zinc and ample amounts of the antioxidant mineral selenium. Whole rye also contains phytochemicals called saponins.

salmon

Nutrition profile Salmon is one of the top sources of omega-3 fatty acids, which may make the heart less susceptible to dangerous, sometimes fatal, rhythm abnormalities. Salmon also supplies protein, thiamin, niacin, vitamin B_6, vitamin D, potassium, selenium, and an impressive amount of vitamin B12. Canned salmon containing the soft, edible bones will also provide a decent amount of calcium. Canned salmon is usually packed in its own oil, which also supplies omega-3s. And while salmon contains cholesterol, it is low in saturated fat, which is more of a health risk than dietary cholesterol.

Maximizing nutrients Salmon is best cooked with dry-heat methods such as broiling, roasting, or grilling.

sardines

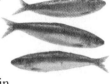

Nutrition profile Sardines provide high-quality protein minus the artery-clogging saturated fat present in other high-protein foods. In addition, sardines are a source of bone-strengthening vitamin D, and a 3-ounce serving of canned sardines with bones contains over 25% of a day's requirement for calcium. In addition, sardines provide omega-3s, polyunsaturated fats that may help lower the risk of heart disease.

Maximizing nutrients Fresh sardines can be baked, grilled, or pan-fried. Remove canned sardines from the oil they may have been packed in and consume the sardines bones and all.

scallions

Nutrition profile Scallions have a distinct nutritional advantage over other members of the onion family: Their green tops, which can be enjoyed along with the white part, provide beta carotene, while the bulb provides a respectable amount of vitamin C. And because they are related to onions, scallions contain a number of phytochemicals, including diallyl sulfide.

Maximizing nutrients Regardless of what the recipe may say, use as much as possible of the dark green tops to maximize the amount of beta carotene you'll be getting. Uncooked scallions will have the most vitamin C, but cooking scallions (especially with a small amount of unsaturated oil) will improve the bioavailability of the beta carotene.

scallops

Nutrition profile Scallops, in spite of their very rich texture and flavor, are quite low in calories—only 120 calories for 6 large sea scallops. Unlike most other shellfish, scallops are extremely low in cholesterol, and have modest amounts of heart-healthy omega-3 fatty acids. Scallops are a good low-fat source of protein and are rich in vitamin B_{12}, vitamin E, potassium, and magnesium.

Maximizing nutrients The vitamins and minerals in scallops are not affected by heat, but their texture is. Cook them briefly to keep them from getting tough.

sesame seeds

Nutrition profile Sesame seeds have 55 calories and 5 g of fat per tablespoon. They supply some vitamin E, iron, and zinc, and are an essential part of many

S

cuisines. Sesame seeds come unhulled (with the bran and thus more nutrients) or hulled. And along with healthful polyunsaturated and monounsaturated fats, sesame seeds contain phytochemicals.

Maximizing nutrients Cooking does not adversely affect the nutrients in sesame seeds, but the proper storage (in the refrigerator or freezer) is important to help prevent their oils from going rancid.

shallots

Nutrition profile Shallots resemble both onions and garlic (and have a flavor that falls somewhere between the two). They are a good source of vitamin B_6, though you would have to eat about ¼ cup cooked (not impossible) to get more than 10% of the RDA for this vitamin. Shallots also contain phytochemicals, specifically, sulfur compounds, that are present in onions and other members of the *Allium* family.

shiitake mushrooms

Nutrition profile Very low in calories, full of meaty texture and flavor, shiitake mushrooms are a good addition to a meatless and/or heart-healthy diet. Like many other mushrooms, shi-

itakes are a good source of B vitamins (riboflavin, niacin, and B_6). They also have excellent amounts of the antioxidant mineral selenium: 65% of the RDA in 1 cup. These mushrooms also contain a phytochemical called lentinan.

Maximizing nutrients For dried shiitakes, when you soak them to reconstitute them, use the soaking water in the recipe. This not only adds flavor to the dish, but also uses whatever B vitamins might have leached into the soaking water.

shrimp

Nutrition profile Shrimp are low in both calories (only 35 calories for about 6 medium shrimp) and saturated fat. Although shrimp have about twice as much cholesterol as meat, their fat is largely polyunsaturated, and includes heart-healthy omega-3 fatty acids. Shrimp have very good amounts of vitamin B_{12} and the antioxidant mineral selenium; they also supply protein, niacin, vitamin D, iron, and zinc.

Maximizing nutrients The nutrients in shrimp are not adversely affected by heat, but the texture is. Brief cooking keeps the shrimp from getting tough.

soybeans

Nutrition profile Soybeans are a rich source of B vitamins (thiamin, riboflavin, B_6, and folate), iron, potassium, magnesium, and cholesterol-lowering plant sterols. And 1 cup of cooked soybeans will give you 22% of the RDA for vitamin E.

Unlike other legumes, soybeans have all the essential amino acids required for the building and maintenance of human body tissues. It is this high-quality protein that distinguishes them from other legumes. Studies show that when substituted for animal protein in the diet, soy protein helps to reduce LDL cholesterol and triglycerides without having an adverse effect on the beneficial HDL cholesterol.

Along with their impressive nutritional make-up, soybeans contain isoflavones, phytochemicals that have been the subject of intense study.

Maximizing nutrients Mature (dried) soybeans take quite a long time to cook and may lose some of their water-soluble vitamins and minerals to the cooking water, but the protein and fat-soluble vitamin E will be fine. Fresh, green soybeans (also called edamame) have many of the same benefits as the mature beans and can be cooked very quickly with a minimum of liquid—in a steamer or microwave—thus preserving more of their water-soluble nutrients. And eating soybeans with foods high in vitamin C will improve the body's ability to absorb their nonheme iron.

soyfoods

Nutrition profile Soyfoods are derived from soybeans, well known for their superior nutritional value and health benefits (*see Soybeans, opposite page*). Soyfoods—which include tofu (*see page 301*), TSP (*see page 301*), miso, soy protein powder (or soy flour), tempeh, and soymilk— share the health benefits of the soybean to a greater or lesser extent depending on the particular product.

For some time it has been known that soy protein, when substituted for animal protein in the diet, lowers total and LDL ("bad") cholesterol and triglycerides without lowering HDL ("good") cholesterol, though no one knows why. The FDA has now authorized a nutrition label claiming that at least 25 g of soy protein a day, as part of a low-fat diet, can lower blood cholesterol levels in people who have high cholesterol. Soyfoods containing at least 6.25 g of soy protein per serving are allowed to bear the FDA-approved health claim label.

Despite this, researchers still disagree about whether it's the protein or some other substance in soy that provides these heart-healthy benefits. It is possible that it's the soy isoflavones (see below), perhaps acting as antioxidants, that are responsible. In addition, scientists are also look-

ing at other cardioprotective components of soy, such as fiber.

Soyfoods contain phytochemicals called isoflavones, which may help relieve the hot flashes associated with menopause and possibly reduce the risk of certain hormone-related types of cancer. But the actual isoflavone content of soyfoods varies with the product: For example, 1 cup of soymilk provides about 24 mg isoflavones, but 1 cup of cooked soybeans will give you almost four times that amount (95 mg).

Maximizing nutrients To preserve phytochemical content, minimize cooking time for tofu and miso by adding them late in the cooking process.

spaghetti squash

Nutrition profile Spaghetti squash is a winter squash whose name alludes to its long yellow spaghetti-like strands that can be pulled out with a fork after it's cooked. Not only do the strands resemble spaghetti, but they can also serve as a low-calorie pasta substitute. In addition to its low calorie count—an 8-ounce serving contains only about 75 calories—spaghetti squash provides fiber, vitamin B$_6$, and some beta carotene.

Maximizing nutrients Baking or

microwaving spaghetti squash is the best way to preserve the vitamin B$_6$.

spinach

Nutrition profile Highly nutritious, spinach has plentiful amounts of folate, magnesium, thiamin, riboflavin, vitamins B$_6$, C, and E, zinc, and the carotenoids beta carotene and lutein. It's important to note that while spinach does provide iron—and also calcium—these minerals cannot be completely used by the body because the vegetable also contains compounds called oxalates, which interfere with the absorption of these minerals.

Maximizing nutrients While raw spinach is a healthy addition to salads, to reap the full benefits from this leafy green, eat it cooked at least some of the time. Cooking helps to convert the lutein and beta carotene in spinach into more bioavailable forms. In addition, cooking or eating spinach with a small amount of healthful, unsaturated fat such as olive oil will help the body absorb the carotenoids more efficiently.

strawberries

Nutrition profile Strawberries provide dietary fiber and more vitamin C than any other berry (1 cup supplies 96%

of the RDA for this antioxidant vitamin). Strawberries also contain phytochemicals, such as anthocyanins and ellagic acid.

Maximizing nutrients It's best to eat strawberries fresh, because cooking can destroy some of their vitamin C.

summer squash

Nutrition profile Summer squash is actually a category of squash with soft edible skin and tender, light-colored flesh. Included in this category are zucchini (*see page 303*) and yellow squash. Yellow-skinned summer squash—which comes in both straight and crook-necked varieties—are what most people mean when they say summer squash. Yellow summer squash is extremely low in calories (about 19 per cup of raw sliced squash) and has decent amounts of vitamin C (about 13% of the RDA in a cup), fiber, potassium, and magnesium.

Maximizing nutrients Summer squash can be eaten both raw and cooked. Raw squash (as in a vegetable slaw) will be higher in vitamin C, which is partially destroyed by heat. When cooking squash, be careful not to use too much fat, because the spongy flesh of the squash soaks up fat easily.

S

sunflower seeds

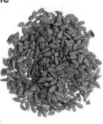

Nutrition profile Sunflower seeds furnish thiamin, vitamin B_6, folate, iron, magnesium, selenium, zinc, protein, fiber, and an exceptional amount of the antioxidant vitamin E (1 ounce will give you 95% of the RDA). The seeds also contain an essential fatty acid that may help lower the risk of stroke and heart disease, as well as certain phytochemicals such as lignans and phenolic acids. While nutrient-dense sunflower seeds offer a good array of vitamins and minerals, they are rather high in calories; if you are watching your weight, try to include them in your diet in moderation.

Maximizing nutrients Cooking can diminish the folate in sunflower seeds, but most of the nutrients in these seeds are fairly heat stable. The proper storage (in the refrigerator or freezer) is also important to help prevent their oils from going rancid.

sweet potatoes

Nutrition profile Among the most nutritious of vegetables, sweet potatoes are low in calories (about 143 calories per medium-sized sweet potato) and high in nutrients such as vitamin B_6,

vitamin C, iron, and potassium. Furthermore, one sweet potato provides over 25% of the RDA for vitamin E, which is highly unusual since most sources of this antioxidant vitamin tend to also be high in fat. Certain sweet potatoes with deep orange flesh contain excellent amounts of beta carotene. In fact, one sweet potato supplies just over 100% of the recommended intake for beta carotene (the darker the flesh of a sweet potato, the more beta carotene). These delicious vegetables also contain other carotenoids such as lutein and zeaxanthin.

Maximizing nutrients Cook whole sweet potatoes with a dry-heat or minimum-liquid method, such as roasting, baking, microwaving, or steaming. And whenever possible, regardless of the cooking method, cook whole unpeeled potatoes to preserve most of the water-soluble B vitamins; you can peel them after they're cooked—though eating the sweet potatoes with the skin provides an extra measure of fiber. If a recipe calls for cooking cut-up sweet potatoes, you can minimize the loss of B vitamins by steaming them (although most recipes would call for boiling them).

swiss chard

Nutrition profile One cup of cooked Swiss chard will yield more than 30% of the RDA for magnesium, beta carotene, and vitamin C. And for a low-fat food, you will be getting an unusually high amount of vitamin E—1 cup of cooked chard gives you 22% of the RDA for this antioxidant vitamin. Moreover, Swiss chard is extremely rich in potassium and fiber, and also supplies a tremendous amount of vitamin K, which is needed for bone formation. Though it contains iron, Swiss chard also contains oxalates, compounds that will interfere with the mineral's absorption by the body.

Maximizing nutrients Most of Swiss chard's nutrients will be made more available to the body through cooking, except for the vitamin C, which is partially destroyed by heat. To make the fat-soluble beta carotene bioavailable, cook the chard with a small amount of fat, such as healthful monounsaturated olive oil.

tangerines

Nutrition profile Highly nutritious, tangerines supply vitamin C (an average-sized tangerine supplies about 26 mg, or 29% of the RDA), thiamin, and some heart-healthy soluble pectin fiber. Tangerines also provide the carotenoids beta cryptoxanthin, lutein, zeaxanthin, and beta carotene. In addition, citrus flavonoids called tangeretin, nobiletin, and hesperidin are found in tangerines.

tofu

Nutrition profile Tofu is highly nutritious and, when substituted for foods high in saturated fat, is a heart-healthy ingredient that offers a wide range of nutrients. In addition to soy protein and phytochemicals called isoflavones, tofu has magnesium, selenium, and zinc. And the type of tofu made with a calcium salt (check the label to be sure) can also contribute to your calcium needs.

Maximizing nutrients Firm and extra-firm tofu take well to broiling, grilling, baking, sautéing, and stir-frying. Softer types can replace all or some of the cream cheese in cheesecake, can be added to puddings, or pureed to make salad dressings. Cooking does not adversely affect the nutrient content of tofu.

tomatillos

Nutrition profile At only a little bit more than 42 calories, one cup of chopped or diced tomatillos will give you 15% of the RDA for niacin, 17% for vitamin C, and 12% for potassium.

Maximizing nutrients Tomatillos can be eaten raw or cooked. Raw tomatillos will have the most vitamin C. But you can cook whole, unpeeled tomatillos very briefly in boiling water or in a steamer to soften them

slightly. This quick cooking will minimize the loss of vitamin C.

tomatoes

Nutrition profile Ever-popular, tomatoes supply fiber, thiamin, vitamin B_6, potassium, and lots of vitamin C: One medium tomato will give you 66% of the RDA for vitamin C. Tomatoes—especially in cooked, condensed forms such as tomato paste, juice, sauce, ketchup, and puree—are an important source of the carotenoid, lycopene. They also contain a phytochemical called quercetin.

Maximizing nutrients Heat and oil enhance absorption of lycopene and beta carotene, though some vitamin C is lost. So, for the most vitamin C, eat tomatoes uncooked.

TSP (TVP)

Nutrition profile The initials TSP stand for Textured Soy Protein, a substance that is usually made from defatted soy flour. Highly nutritious, a 1-ounce serving will give you a hefty amount of fiber (5 g) and protein (15 g), as well as 14% of the RDA for thiamin, 21% for folate, 16% for iron, 21% for magnesium, 23% for potassium, and 14% for zinc. TSP is used to add a chewy, meatlike texture to a wide variety of foods. Though this vegetable protein is technically called TSP, many supermarkets and health-food stores market it under the proprietary brand name "TVP." TSP is a useful ingredient because it absorbs flavors well and is available in powder form, chunks, slices, and dried granules.

tuna

Nutrition profile One of the more popular fish, tuna is a good source of protein, has little fat, and is rich in healthful omega-3 fatty acids—which help reduce blood clotting and may lower the risk of coronary artery disease and fatal heart attacks. Tuna also has plentiful amounts of thiamin, niacin, vitamin B_6, vitamin B_{12}, and selenium. The canned form (particularly albacore) is also a rich source of nutrients, including omega-3s (though these beneficial fats are not listed on the label).

Maximizing nutrients Cook tuna with dry-heat or low-fat methods, such as broiling, grilling, or stir-frying.

turkey

Nutrition profile Turkey is an excellent source of protein, riboflavin, niacin, vitamin B_6, vitamin B_{12}, selenium, iron, and zinc. While most of the fat in turkey is found in the skin, turkey meat is so low in fat that eating 3 ounces of roasted breast meat with skin would furnish only 130 calories and less than 1 g fat. The dark meat is higher in fat than the light meat, but it is still relatively lean if eaten without the skin.

Maximizing nutrients For healthful ways to cook turkey, see page 122.

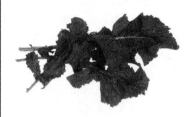

turnip greens

Nutrition profile Turnip greens are nutritious, with a 1-cup serving of cooked greens offering 43% of the recommended daily intake for beta carotene, 44% of the RDA for vitamin C, and 42% of the RDA for folate. In addition, these sharp-tasting greens also have isothiocyanates, indoles, and sulforaphane, phytochemicals found in cruciferous vegetables.

Maximizing nutrients To preserve folate content, cook turnip greens in very little liquid (or incorporate the cooking liquid into the dish) and use a small amount of unsaturated oil (such as olive oil or canola oil) to enhance the bioavailability of the beta carotene.

turnips

Nutrition profile These sweet, crisp vegetables supply good amounts of fiber and they also contain a surprisingly high concentration of vitamin C: 1 cup of cooked turnip cubes provides about 20% of the RDA.

Maximizing nutrients Cooking

will diminish vitamin C, but it increases the availability of the soluble fiber.

walnuts

Nutrition profile Not only are walnuts a good source of vitamin B_6 and magnesium, but they (and their oil) contain alpha-linolenic acid (ALA), a heart-healthy omega-3 fatty acid that research suggests may help prevent heart attacks. And the monounsaturated fats and polyunsaturated fats in walnuts can also lower blood cholesterol, especially when substituted for saturated fat in the diet. Walnuts also contain plant sterols. Go easy on walnuts, though, because like all nuts, they are calorie-dense (7 walnut halves have almost 100 calories).

Maximizing nutrients Cooking does not adversely affect the nutrients in walnuts, but the proper storage (in the refrigerator or freezer) is important to help prevent their oils from going rancid.

watercress

Nutrition profile This peppery member of the mustard family provides fiber, potassium, beta carotene, and, most notably, vitamin C: Just 2 cups of uncooked watercress supplies an impressive one-third of the

RDA for this indispensable vitamin. Watercress and its cruciferous cousins are known to be excellent sources of a family of phytochemicals called isothiocyanates. And scientists are studying a phytochemical in watercress called phenylethyl isothiocyanate (PEITC).

Maximizing nutrients Watercress is most commonly eaten uncooked, which will provide the most vitamin C. But this green is also good cooked, which will improve the availability of its carotenoids, especially if it's cooked (or served) with a small amount of unsaturated oil.

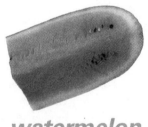

watermelon

Nutrition profile Low in calories, and rich in sweet, refreshing flavor, this all-American summertime favorite offers vitamin B_6, vitamin C, potassium, and lycopene, a carotenoid that gives red color to certain foods.

wheat

Nutrition profile The nutritional value of wheat is determined by how it is processed. For example, removing the germ and bran from wheat results in refined white flour, which lacks many nutrients (though iron and B vitamins are replaced when white flour is enriched). And conversely, because whole wheat retains its natural bran and germ, it retains a full range of nutrients (see below), as well as phytochemicals called saponins and lignans.

Wheat germ, the wheat kernel's embryo, contains a fair amount of highly polyunsaturated fat. It also supplies about 30% of the RDA for thiamin, vitamin E, and zinc; 20% of the RDA for folate; and 10% for iron and riboflavin. Defatted wheat germ is available, but it's lower in vitamin E.

Wheat bran is the kernel's outer shell and contains a whopping 12 g of fiber per ounce. One ounce contains 40% of the RDA for both niacin and magnesium, plus 20 to 40% of the RDA for iron. It has 60 calories and 5 g of protein, but just 1 g of fat.

Maximizing nutrients When soaking cracked wheat, such as bulgur, use a minimum of water so the water-soluble B vitamins are not lost. This is a little less important when cooking whole wheatberries, because the bran layer protects the nutrients on the inside from leaching too much into the cooking water.

wild rice

Nutrition profile Delicate and chewy, wild rice isn't really rice at all, but the seed of an aquatic grass. Still, most people tend to regard wild rice as an exotic form of real rice. Wild rice has more protein than regular rice, and it also provides some zinc.

yogurt

Nutrition profile Along with its satisfying creamy texture and subtly tart flavor, yogurt also offers an impressive nutritional profile. Yogurt supplies calcium, protein, B vitamins (especially B_{12}), and minerals. Yogurt can definitely play a role in a healthy diet, if you stick to the nonfat or low-fat kind.

Maximizing nutrients Yogurt can be used as a low-fat alternative to sour cream in many recipes.

zucchini

Nutrition profile Zucchini is low in calories (only 25 calories per cup cooked) and provides a good amount of vitamin C, potassium, fiber, and carotenoids such as beta carotene. It is also a leading source of lutein and zeaxanthin, carotenoid pigments.

Maximizing nutrients Zucchini can be eaten both raw and cooked. Raw squash will be higher in vitamin C, which is partially destroyed by heat. If you prefer cooked zucchini, try steaming or microwaving it, or sautéing it in a small amount of oil, which will help maximize the absorption of its carotenoids.

Z

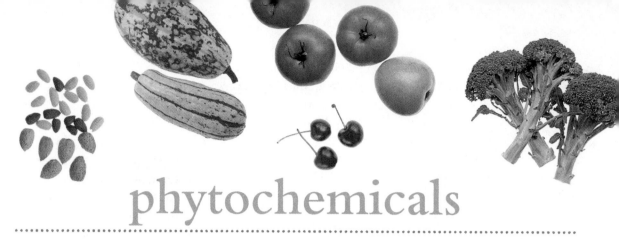

phytochemicals

An amazing 4,000 phytochemicals (which means "plant chemicals") have been identified so far, and many more remain to be discovered. Only about 150 phytochemicals have been intensively studied, and what follows is a thumbnail description of some of the more prominent of them.

alpha-linolenic acid An essential fat similar to omega-3 fatty acids, alpha-linolenic acid (ALA) must be acquired through the diet because the body does not manufacture it. Studies suggest that ALA can substantially cut the risk of heart attacks and may possibly have anti-inflammatory actions as well. Canola oil, ground flaxseed, soybean oil, purslane, and walnuts are notable sources of ALA.

anthocyanins Members of the FLAVONOID phytochemical family, anthocyanins are pigments responsible for the red and blue colors of fruits and vegetables, including apples, berries, cherries, plums, pomegranates, and red cabbage. Preliminary laboratory research suggests that anthocyanins have potent ANTIOXIDANT properties.

antioxidants Antioxidants are a large group of substances—including certain vitamins, minerals, and phytochemicals—that are found in abundance in fruits, vegetables, and whole grains. What defines an antioxidant is its ability to help defend plants and our bodies against highly damaging forms of oxygen called free radicals. Generated in the environment as well as in the body, free radicals accelerate aging and contribute to disease. Antioxidants seek out and quench these unhealthy free radicals.

beta carotene The best known member of the CAROTENOID family, beta carotene is an orange pigment that is converted by the body into vitamin A. Beta carotene also acts as an ANTIOXIDANT, mopping up free radicals that may promote cancer and cataracts. Apricots, broccoli, butternut squash, cantaloupe, carrots, peppers, pumpkin, spinach, and sweet potatoes are rich sources of beta carotene.

beta cryptoxanthin A member of the CAROTENOID family, this pigment is plentiful in orange-colored fruits, including peaches, oranges, tangerines, nectarines, papayas, and persimmons. In addition to being an ANTIOXIDANT, beta cryptoxanthin has shown promise in blocking tumor cell growth and is under investigation for its potential to help suppress the growth of malignant cervical cells.

betacyanin This deep red to red violet plant pigment is found in a few plant foods such as beets, red Swiss chard, and amaranth leaves, and is being studied for its anticancer potential.

beta glucan Beta glucan (a complex glucose polymer) is the soluble portion of dietary fiber. Beta glucan plays a special role in lowering total and LDL ("bad") blood cholesterol by blocking the absorption and production of cholesterol in the body. Oats and barley are the best sources of beta glucan.

capsaicin Found in the soft seed-bearing ribs inside chili peppers, this flavonoid phytochemical gives the peppers their characteristic fiery taste—the hotter the pepper, the higher the concentration of capsaicin. The anticancer and cardio-protective properties of capsaicin are under review, in addition to its potential to neutralize free radical damage. In topical ointments, capsaicin is used to alleviate the discomfort of arthritis and shingles.

carotenoids Dozens of these yellow-orange pigments in fruits and vegetables are converted into vitamin A by our bodies. Carotenoids are robust ANTIOXIDANTS and may possibly guard against cancer, heart disease, and age-related vision problems. BETA CAROTENE, alpha carotene, BETA CRYPTOXAN-THIN, LUTEIN, LYCOPENE, and ZEAXANTHIN are notable carotenoids. Leading carotenoid sources are carrots, kale, peppers, pumpkin, tangerines, sweet potatoes, butternut squash, and tomatoes. Processing and cooking (with a bit of oil) enhance the absorption of carotenoids.

catechins Noted for their potent ANTIOXIDANT properties, catechins are a group of POLYPHENOL phytochemicals. The four major types of catechins are epicatechin (EC), epigallocatechin gallate (EGCG), epigallocatechin (EGC), and gallocatechin (GC). Promising research suggests that catechins may help to protect against cancer and impede harmful plaque buildup in arteries. High amounts of catechins are found in apples, dark chocolate, grapes, pomegranates, raspberries, red wine, and tea. EGCG is a particularly potent type of catechin in tea.

chlorogenic acid Found in many fruits and vegetables, this phytochemical is believed to act as an ANTIOXIDANT. Chlorogenic acid may possibly exert anticancer actions as well; it is under investigation for its potential to block the conversion of nitrates into cancer-causing nitrosamines. Berries, cherries, kiwifruit, and tomatoes contain chlorogenic acid.

citrus flavonoids Found in citrus fruit, this collection of disease-fighting phytochemicals includes HESPERIDIN, NARINGIN, NOBILETIN, and TANGERETIN. Citrus flavonoids may neutralize free radicals and inhibit blood clotting, according to experimental research.

daidzein Along with GENISTEIN, daidzein is one of the major ISOFLAVONES found in soyfoods. Although research is in the early stages, some evidence suggests daidzein may exert mild estrogenic

effects as well as offer cardiovascular and anti-cancer benefits.

diallyl sulfide Abundant in *Allium* vegetables such as leeks, onions, and garlic, this robust compound may possibly lower the risk of certain forms of cancer, including colon and stomach cancer. Preliminary findings suggest that diallyl sulfide helps to stimulate cancer-fighting enzymes in our bodies that detoxify carcinogens.

dithiolthiones These compounds may help to fight cancer by mobilizing protective enzymes in the liver, according to preliminary evidence. Dithiolthiones are particularly plentiful in broccoli.

EGCG The most potent of the CATECHIN phytochemicals, EGCG is a particularly powerful ANTIOXIDANT and may have even more antioxidant power than vitamin E, according to laboratory findings. Both substances quench disease-causing free radicals. Green tea is an especially rich source of EGCG.

ellagic acid An ANTIOXIDANT phytochemical, ellagic acid disarms cell-damaging free radicals. Studies in laboratory animals suggest that ellagic acid may exert additional anticancer actions as well. Appreciable amounts of ellagic acid are found in berries, grapes, nuts, and pomegranates.

flavonoids A large class of phytochemicals, flavonoids include ANTHOCYANINS, QUERCETIN, ISOFLAVONES, and a group of compounds often referred to as CITRUS FLAVONOIDS. Flavonoids neutralize disease-causing free radicals and may also help to suppress the growth of tumor cells and protect against heart disease. Fruits, vegetables, legumes, whole grains, tea, and wine contain various types of flavonoids.

genistein Like DAIDZEIN, genistein is a PHYTOESTROGEN with mild estrogenic properties. According to a recent review, genistein may help to protect against hormone-related cancers, such as breast cancer. Genistein is also thought to be an ANTIOXIDANT. Soyfoods contain variable amounts of genistein; whole soybeans, soy flour, textured soy protein, soy milk, tempeh, tofu and soy nuts are the best sources.

glucosinolates Upon ingestion, these powerful compounds are converted into INDOLES, ISOTHIOCYANTES, and SULFORAPHANE. According to laboratory studies, glucosinolates exert numerous anticancer actions; they appear to detoxify carcinogens, impede cancer cell replication, and raise levels of cancer-fighting enzymes in the body. Brussels sprouts, kale, watercress, and other cruciferous vegetables contain substantial quantities of glucosinolates.

hesperidin This CITRUS FLAVONOID works synergistically with vitamin C to exert antioxidant abilities.

indole-3-carbinol A member of the INDOLE family, indole-3-carbinol is believed to interrupt the growth of tumor cells and be particularly protective against hormone-related cancers, including breast and prostate cancer. Broccoli is a rich reservoir of indole-3-carbinol.

indoles Members of the GLUCOSINOLATE family, indoles are under review for their potential to reduce the risk of hormone-related cancers, including breast and prostate cancer. Indoles appear to elevate levels of anticancer enzymes, block some of the actions of estrogen, and suppress the harmful effects of carcinogens. Cruciferous vegetables, such as cabbage, kohlrabi, and turnip greens, contain indoles.

isoflavones A widely studied class of PHYTOESTROGENS, isoflavones have mild estrogenic properties. Isoflavones are under investigation for their ANTIOXIDANT and anticancer actions, as well as their potential benefits for bones, blood vessels, the brain, and the heart. Soyfoods are rich in isoflavones; particularly high amounts are found in dried soybeans, soybean sprouts, soynuts, tempeh, and soy flour.

isothiocyanates Similar to INDOLES, isothiocyanates are cancer-fighting compounds in broccoli, kale, mustard greens, and other cruciferous vegetables. Research findings suggest that isothiocyanates may possibly halt tumor growth, mobilize protective enzymes in the body, and detoxify carcinogens. A certain type of isothiocyanate in watercress (called PEITC) has shown promise in neutralizing carcinogens associated with lung cancer. One intensely studied and particularly potent isothiocyanate is SULFORAPHANE.

lignans In addition to being a type of fiber, lignans are converted in the intestines into estrogen-like substances called enterodiol and enterolactone, which may have anti-tumor properties. Lignans are also thought to defend cells against free radical damage. Whole grains contain lignans, and flaxseed is a concentrated source. Although lignans are destroyed in the process of making flaxseed oil, some processors add lignans back into the oil (check the label).

limonenes Citrus peels are high in limonene phytochemicals, which seep into the juice of citrus fruit. Preliminary findings suggest that limonenes may work against carcinogens and tumors, possibly lowering the risk of certain forms of cancer. Lemon and lime skins are especially rich in limonenes, and seasonings such as caraway, coriander, and thyme, contain limonenes.

lutein This antioxidant carotenoid teams up with ZEAXANTHIN to form the yellow pigment of the eye's retina. Lutein shields the retina from harmful ultraviolet rays and may help to ward off age-related vision problems, including cataracts and macular degeneration. Corn is a rich source of lutein; other good sources are celery, egg yolks, kiwifruit, peas, pumpkin, red grapes, spinach, yellow squash, and zucchini.

lycopene An important relative of BETA CAROTENE, this plant pigment makes tomatoes red. Preliminary research suggests that diets rich in lycopene may lower the risk of cancer of the prostate, bladder, breast, cervix, digestive tract, and lung. Lycopene may protect against coronary artery disease as well. Tomato sauces and other processed tomato products are the best sources of lycopene. Raw tomatoes, pink grapefruit, watermelon, and guava also contain appreciable amounts. Processing and cooking with a small amount of fat or oil make lycopene and other carotenoids easier to absorb.

naringin This CITRUS FLAVONOID gives grapefruit its characteristic bitter flavor. Naringin is believed to enhance our perception of taste by stimulating the taste buds.

nobiletin A CITRUS FLAVONOID found primarily in tangerines, nobiletin is being studied for its potential to block the excessive cell growth associated with cancer. In addition, nobiletin appears to have anti-clotting activities that keep blood cells from clumping together.

oleuropein Found in olive oil, this phytochemical appears to scout out and destroy free radicals. In addition, preliminary findings suggest oleuropein may have anticancer and heart-healthy attributes as well.

oryzanol Also called gamma oryzanol, this phytochemical is under investigation for its cardiovascular benefits. Oryzanol is found in grains, particularly in the outer layer of brown rice, and is also derived from rice bran oil.

PEITC Found in concentrated amounts in watercress, PEITC is a type of ISOTHIOCYANATE that may have anticancer potential.

phenolic compounds This broad class of phytochemicals appears to halt free radical damage to cells and may have additional cancer-fighting properties. CHLOROGENIC ACID and ELLAGIC ACID are both types of phenolic compounds.

phytoestrogens These plant compounds are converted into estrogen-like substances in the digestive tract. ISOFLAVONES, LIGNANS, and coumestans are the three major forms of phytoestrogens Research is underway to explore their potential favorable effects on bone, blood cholesterol, the brain, blood vessels, and the heart. Soy is particularly high in phytoestrogens; certain herbs, seeds, and whole grains also contain phytoestrogens.

plant sterols These naturally occurring plant compounds are chemically similar to cholesterol. Some plant sterols are not absorbed by the digestive tract and block the absorption of cholesterol into the bloodstream. SAPONINS are a type of plant sterol.

polyphenols A class of phytochemicals that includes FLAVONOIDS, PHENOLIC COMPOUNDS, and CAPSAICIN.

procyanidins In addition to being potent ANTIOXIDANTS, these FLAVONOID phytochemicals may inhibit bacteria from sticking to the urinary tract and starting an infection. Procyanidins are found in blueberries and are particularly abundant in cranberries.

quercetin A FLAVONOID, quercetin is under review for its ANTIOXIDANT potential, and its ability to act as an antihistamine, and to suppress the growth of cancer cells. Quercetin may also guard against heart disease by reducing the oxidation of LDL ("bad") cholesterol. Apples, berries, cherries, red onions, red and purple grapes, tea, and tomatoes are leading sources of quercetin.

resveratrol Resveratrol is a FLAVONOID phytochemical. According to initial laboratory findings, resveratrol may possibly neutralize free radicals, suppress tumor growth, and contribute to normal levels of cholesterol. Significant amounts of resveratrol are present in peanuts, peanut butter, red and purple grapes, and red wine.

saponins These PLANT STEROLS are present in legumes, nuts, oats, and whole grains. By binding to cholesterol and toxins in the intestines, saponins are thought to lower blood cholesterol and prevent DNA damage from carcinogens.

sulforaphane This robust phytochemical in cruciferous vegetables is under intense investigation for its potential to reduce cancer risk. Sulforaphane appears to detoxify carcinogens as well as stimulate the body's own cancer-protective enzymes. Broccoli and especially broccoli sprouts are believed to be the best sources of sulforaphane.

tannins Also known as PROCYANIDINS.

tangeretin Found primarily in tangerines, this CITRUS FLAVONOID may possess potential anticancer and immune-enhancing properties.

zeaxanthin Like LUTEIN, zeaxanthin is a CAROTENOID in the retina that may promote healthy vision and possibly protect against cataracts and macular degeneration, a leading cause of blindness in older people. Foods highest in zeaxanthin are corn, egg yolks, honeydew melon, mango, orange bell peppers, and oranges.

RECOMMENDED INTAKES FOR VITAMINS & MINERALS

The chart on this page features two sets of figures recently issued by the Food and Nutrition Board of the National Academy of Sciences to help people improve the nutritional quality of their diets.

Recommended Dietary Allowances (RDAs) are optimum levels of nutrients sufficient to prevent deficiency diseases and also promote good health in most of the population. When too little data exists for a particular nutrient to set an RDA, the Food and Nutrition Board has set an Adequate Intake (AI).

Upper Levels (ULs), also called Tolerable Upper Intake Levels, are the highest amount of a vitamin or mineral that can be taken without any risk of an adverse effect to healthy individuals. For most nutrients, exceeding the ULs is possible only by taking dietary supplements or fortified foods. Some nutrients do not have a UL because no data exist to set a specific figure.

The figures listed are for adults only. Recommended intakes for pregnant and lactating women can differ and are not included here.

Vitamins	Recommended Dietary Allowance (RDA)**	Upper Level (UL)**
Biotin	30 mcg*	None established
Folate (Folic acid)	400 mcg	1,000 mcg (from supplements and fortified foods)
Niacin	Women: 14 mg Men: 16 mg	35 mg (from supplements and fortified foods)
Pantothenic acid	5 mg*	None established
Riboflavin	Women: 1.1 mg Men: 1.3 mg	None established
Thiamin	Women: 1.1 mg Men: 1.2 mg	None established
Vitamin A	Women: 700 mcg Men: 900 mcg	10,000 IU (3,000 mcg)
Vitamin B$_6$	Women to age 50: 1.3 mg Women over 50: 1.5 mg Men to age 50: 1.3 mg Men over 50: 1.7 mg	100 mg
Vitamin B$_{12}$	2.4 mcg	None established
Vitamin C	Women: 75 mg Men: 90 mg	2,000 mg
Vitamin D	To age 50: 200 IU Ages 51-70: 400 IU Over 70: 600 IU	2,000 IU
Vitamin E	15 mg	1,000 mg (1,000 IU synthetic, 1,500 IU natural)
Vitamin K	Women: 90 mcg* Men: 120 mcg*	None established
Minerals		
Calcium	To age 50: 1,000 mg* Over 50: 1,200 mg*	2,500 mg

*Adequate Intake (AI) **RDA and UL values are for adults only

Minerals	RDA**	UL**
Chromium	Women to age 50: 25 mcg* Women over 50: 20 mcg* Men to age 50: 35 mcg* Men over 50: 30 mcg*	None established
Copper	900 mcg	10 mg
Iodine	150 mcg	1.1 mg
Iron	Women to age 50: 18 mg Women over 50: 8 mg Men: 8 mg	45 mg
Magnesium	Women to age 30: 310 mg Women over 30: 320 mg Men to age 30: 400 mg Men over 30: 420 mg	350 mg
Manganese	Women: 1.8 mg* Men: 2.3 mg*	11 mg
Molybdenum	45 mcg	2 mg
Phosphorus	700 mg	Up to age 70: 4,000 mg After age 70: 3,000 mg
Selenium	55 mcg	400 mcg
Zinc	Women: 8 mg Men: 11 mg	40 mg

Other Recommended Intakes

For a few nutrients, existing evidence isn't sufficient to establish a requirement. The intakes listed below are based on guidelines established by various health organizations and experts, including the Food and Nutrition Board.

Carotenoids

There is no established daily intake for carotenoids. Some carotenoids are converted by the body into vitamin A; you can meet the RDA for vitamin A by consuming 11 milligrams of beta carotene a day. No specific group of carotenoids can be singled out for providing disease prevention benefits. The Food and Nutrition Board advises eating more carotenoid-rich fruits and vegetables. Don't take beta carotene supplements. Smokers in particular should avoid high doses of beta carotene, which are associated with an increased risk of lung cancer.

Potassium

Nutritionists generally recommend that adults consume 3,000 milligrams of potassium per day.

Sodium

Try to limit daily intake to 2,400 milligrams.

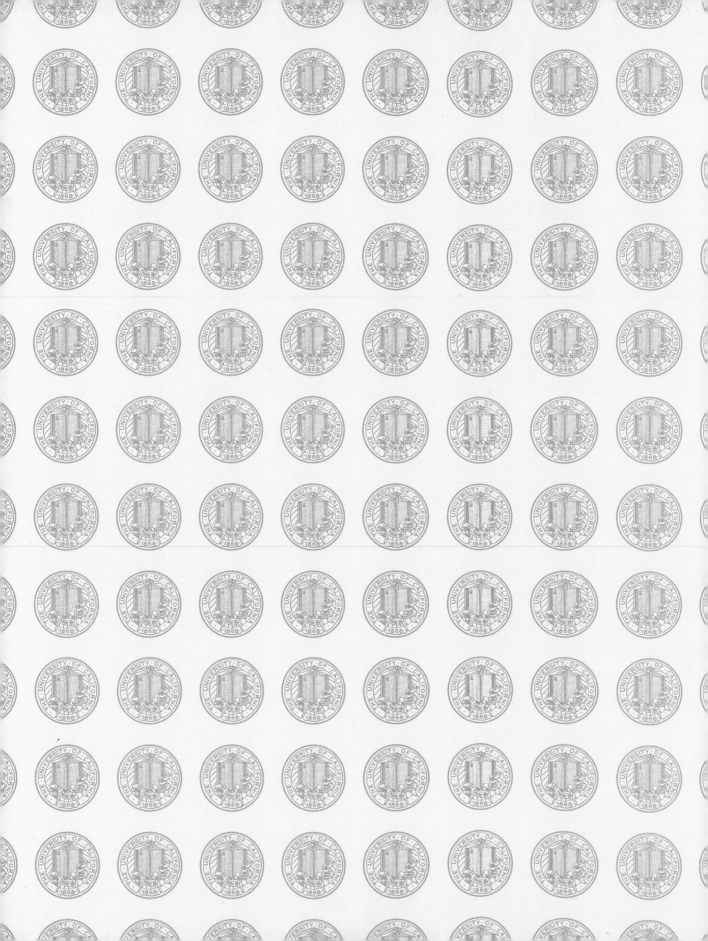